Tinnitus Retraining Therapy
Implementing the Neurophysiological Model

Tinnitus and oversensitivity to sound are common, and hitherto incurable, distressing conditions that affect about 17% of the population. Pawel Jastreboff's identification of the mechanisms by which tinnitus and decreased sound tolerance occur has led to a new and effective treatment called Tinnitus retraining therapy (TRT). Audiologists, ENT specialists, psychologists and counsellors around the world currently practice this technique, with success rates of around 80%.

TRT, the treatment developed by the authors from the model, has already proved to be the most effective and most widely practiced tinnitus treatment worldwide. This book presents a definitive description and justification for the Jastreboff neurophysiological model of tinnitus, outlining the essentials of TRT, reviewing the research literature supporting its claims and providing an expert critique of other current therapeutic practices.

Pawel Jastreboff is Professor and Director of the Tinnitus and Hyperacusis Center in the Department of Otolaryngology at Emory School of Medicine, Atlanta, USA. He is the author of the neurophysiological model of tinnitus and developer of tinnitus retraining therapy.

Jonathan Hazell is Honorary Consultant Surgeon at the University College London Hospitals and Director of the Tinnitus and Hyperacusis Centre in London. He was the first to apply Pawel Jastreboff's neurophysiological model of tinnitus to clinical practice.

T0213314

Tinnitus Retraining Therapy

Implementing the Neurophysiological Model

Pawel J. Jastreboff, Ph.D., Sc.D.

Professor and Director, Emory University School of Medicine, Tinnitus & Hyperacusis Center, Atlanta, USA

and

Jonathan W. P. Hazell, FRCS

Director Tinnitus and Hyperacusis Centre, and Honorary Consultant Surgeon, University College London Hospitals, London, UK

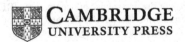
CAMBRIDGE
UNIVERSITY PRESS

CAMBRIDGE UNIVERSITY PRESS
Cambridge, New York, Melbourne, Madrid, Cape Town, Singapore, São Paulo, Delhi

Cambridge University Press
The Edinburgh Building, Cambridge CB2 8RU, UK

Published in the United States of America by Cambridge University Press, New York

www.cambridge.org
Information on this title: www.cambridge.org/9780521592567

First published 2004
Third printing 2007
This digitally printed version 2008

A catalogue record for this publication is available from the British Library

Library of Congress Cataloguing in Publication data
Jastreboff, Pawel J.
Tinnitus retraining therapy: implementing the neurophysiological model /
Pawel J. Jastreboff & Jonathan W. P. Hazell.
    p.   cm.
Includes bibliographical references and index.
ISBN 0 521 59256 9
1. Tinnitus – Patients – Rehabilitation.   2. Tinnitus – Treatment.   I. Hazell, Jonathan W. P.
II. Title.
RF293.8.J37   2004   617.8 – dc22   2003069730

ISBN 978-0-521-59256-7 hardback
ISBN 978-0-521-08837-4 paperback

To our wives Margaret and Rena, whose continuous encouragement, criticism and contributions have made this book a reality.

Contents

Preface

A number of books written in the past on the subject of tinnitus were aimed at readers who had an advanced knowledge of physiology of the auditory system. They were often difficult to understand, even for professionals from other medical fields, and frequently for audiologists as well. They were much too complex for the average patient, who searched the professional literature to find answers and possible solutions to their problems. Most of these books had chapters written by different authors, who each present their own approach to tinnitus. We believe that there is a need for a book focused at presenting a specific tinnitus treatment in a coherent and yet critical way.

Accordingly, this book does not cover all the different theories and managements of tinnitus, but it does present a singular and novel approach, tinnitus retraining therapy (TRT), against a background of other treatments without attempting to describe them in detail. Chapter 1 provides the reader with definitions of tinnitus and decreased sound tolerance. Chapter 2 describes the neurophysiological model of tinnitus, which forms the theoretical basis for TRT, and Ch. 3 presents TRT and specific aspects of the TRT protocol. Chapter 4 discusses the outcome of TRT in clinical practice. Chapter 5 introduces possibilities for tinnitus prevention and Ch. 6 presents a critical overview of the approaches presently used to treat tinnitus, pointing out their strengths and limitations. Finally, Ch. 7 summarizes the book and presents our conclusions.

At the end of the 1980s, P. J. Jastreboff introduced the neurophysiological model of tinnitus (first published in 1990 (Jastreboff, 1990)), and a basic version of its clinical implementation, presently known as TRT. The model and its clinical implementation were based on scientific studies on the development of an animal model of tinnitus (Jastreboff et al., 1988), experiments on the mechanisms of tinnitus (Jastreboff & Sasaki, 1986, 1994), as well as detailed study of the literature. The ideas were first presented to Jonathan Hazell and Jacqui Sheldrake in 1988, who made TRT the focal point of their joint clinical work with tinnitus patients, and they were first to implement it in clinical practice. Immediately, it became evident that patients were improving much more rapidly than with a program of "partial masking" and coping strategies, that had been employed previously. TRT has been further refined by the authors during the following years, both in the USA and the UK, and undergoes continuous modifications aimed at shortening the time needed for treatment and enhancing its effectiveness.

The neurophysiological model of tinnitus, on the one hand, has been rigorously tested by its constant exposure to professionals and patients, and to our knowledge the model has never been challenged. TRT, on the other hand, like many other new treatments, has been vigorously attacked and questioned. The important message is that the model appears very robust, while TRT, like other treatments, is continuously evolving and improving with time. Many professionals around the world now use TRT, finding the best way of implementing it in different medical systems and cultures to provide best help to tinnitus and hyperacusis sufferers.

We have attempted to present the neurophysiological model in a clear way, but the principles on which it is based and its mechanisms are complex and their understanding requires knowledge from various areas of neuroscience. As a good understanding of the model is crucial for optimal implementation of TRT and achieving control of tinnitus, a special effort has been made to provide explanation for various concepts of neuroscience, mechanisms and processes involved in the model. Furthermore, we have illustrated these concepts with diagrams and parables from everyday life to facilitate their comprehension. Nevertheless, the readers may need to supplement this text with additional readings, suggested in the references, depending on their level of knowledge of neuroscience and audiology.

There are few, if any, health sciences or medical methods that can be learned from a book alone. TRT is no exception, and we know from our own teaching of the subject during TRT courses that the proper use of TRT only comes from a combination of a full understanding of the theory followed by significant practical experience of its use with patients. Reading this book will not enable you to practice TRT. Rather we hope that it will enthuse professionals to learn more about TRT and encourage patients to seek TRT as a primary treatment for their tinnitus and hyperacusis.

Throughout the book, we attempt to write each chapter so that it can be read independently from the others. At the beginning of each chapter, there is a short summary of information contained in the chapter, together with a list of main conclusions. Through the text, extra comments and descriptions of more complex issues are presented in footnotes. To ease comprehension and facilitate browsing through the book, highlights of the text are presented on the margins with a shaded background. Finally, the Glossary provides the definition of terms used in the text and a list of abbreviations.

Acknowledgments

We are indebted to John Graham FRCS for critical appraisal of an earlier draft of the manuscript. The work has been partially supported by grants from the National Institutes of Health, National Institute for Deafness and other Communicative Disorders (grants R01 DC 00445 and DC 00299) (PJJ), and by the Royal National Institute for Deaf People (grant 621-089) (JWPH). Initial versions of some figures were published in *Proceedings of the Fifth International Tinnitus Seminar* (Jastreboff, 1996a,b), in Jastreboff, Gray & Gold (1996), and in Jastreboff (1998).

Acknowledgements

Introduction

Tinnitus is a symptom recognized for thousands of years. However, most definitions presently in use are neither sufficiently specific nor physiological in basis. Many definitions include objective sounds originating in the head and neck areas (*somatosounds*) and auditory hallucinations. This has frequently misdirected research clinical approaches. A definition of tinnitus as an auditory phantom perception was proposed in the early 1990s (Jastreboff, 1990, 1995); it is discussed here and used throughout this book. Decreased sound tolerance and its components hyperacusis and misophonia are defined and discussed. They frequently accompany tinnitus, similarly to hearing loss, but they do not have significant recognition in the literature.

1.1 Definitions of tinnitus

1.1.1 Commonly used definitions of tinnitus

Tinnitus is defined by the American National Standards Institute (ANSI, 1969) as "the sensation of sound without external stimulation." Another common description was proposed in the Committee on Hearing, Bioacoustics and Biomechanics (CHABA) report *Tinnitus Facts, Theories, and Treatments*, which defines tinnitus as "the conscious experience of sound that originates in the head" (McFadden, 1982). Both definitions include the auditory hallucinations of schizophrenia, a variety of somatosounds such as palatal myoclonus, abnormal opening or patency of the eustachian tube, temporomandibular joint disease, spontaneous otoacoustic emissions and sounds (bruits) of vascular origin (see Ch. 6; Champlin, Muller & Mitchell, 1990; Harris, Brismar & Cronqvist, 1979; Hazell, 1990b; Hentzer, 1968; Jastreboff, Gray & Mattox, 1998; McFadden, 1982) as well as sensation resulting from a malfunction of the cochlea or auditory nerve (Jastreboff, 1990; Moller, 1984). Obviously, this broad definition invites a discussion of many different phenomena unrelated to tinnitus problems. Traditional definition of tinnitus as any sound generated within the head, without regard for underlying mechanism(s) or possible origin, invites discussion of phenomena unrelated to tinnitus problems and promotes categorization of tinnitus by symptoms alone.

Traditional definition of tinnitus as any sound generated within the head, without regard for the underlying mechanism(s) or possible origin, invites discussion of phenomena unrelated to tinnitus problems and promotes categorization of tinnitus by symptoms alone.

In the past tinnitus has been classified by various divisions, such as subjective/objective and peripheral/central tinnitus (McFadden, 1982). However, these categories were not clearly defined, and they involved significant overlap. Let us look at the most common division into *subjective* and *objective* tinnitus. Objective tinnitus (or some component of it) could be heard by an observer, and subjective tinnitus was heard by the sufferer alone. With better knowledge of the auditory system and better measurement techniques, some cases of tinnitus previously considered to be subjective can now be measured in an objective manner and heard after appropriate processing and amplification, for example patients with spontaneous otoacoustic emissions. These cases therefore become objective or at least have an objective component.

Another problem is that, while so-called objective tinnitus may be strongly associated with an audible generator, nevertheless, the perception resulting from such a source may be quite different, and in some cases not even detected by the owner. Certain spontaneous otoacoustic emissions can be detected by an external observer but are not perceived by the person generating them. It is impossible to predict if a given spontaneous otoacoustic emission is perceived or not, and a complex psychoacoustical approach is needed to associate spontaneous otoacoustic emission with perception of a sound (Penner, 1992; Penner & Burns, 1987). Classification into objective/subjective tinnitus is completely dependent on the sensitivity of the methods used to detect the somatosounds.

The definition proposed in the CHABA report results in a paradox. If it is understood as referring to sound originating in the head, then the majority of tinnitus cases would be excluded since there is no sound that can be detected. If the definition is understood as referring to the perception originating in the head, then all external and internal sounds would be included since all perception occurs in the head. While this definition attempts to restrict the origin of the sound to the head of the owner, it includes both real sounds, which can be detected by an external observer (somatosounds), and hallucinations related to schizophrenia, in addition to tinnitus. The sound perception generated by cochlear implants would also need to be included.

Other definitions were equally broad and not very precise. For example, the definition proposed during the CIBA symposium on tinnitus in 1981 stated, "The sensation of sound not brought about by simultaneously applied mechano-acoustic or electrical signals" (anon., 1981a) and, therefore, includes somatosounds generated anywhere in the whole body.

Another definition "Tinnitus is an aberrant perception of sound reported by a patient that is unrelated to an external source of stimulation" (Shulman, 1988) is similar to the previous one, with the additional assumption that tinnitus perception is abnormal. This is contradicted by the fact that tinnitus can be induced in 94% of the population by a few minutes of sound deprivation (Heller & Bergman, 1953).

Berrios *et al.*, have chosen a different approach and defined tinnitus as a formless hallucination (Berrios, 1991; Berrios & Rose, 1992). They pointed out that tinnitus belongs to the physiological/medical otological field rather than the psychological/psychiatric area. During the twentieth century, the subject has been passed from psychiatry to otolaryngology (where it was known as *tinnitus aurium* – tinnitus of the ear) and back several times. However, none of the models of tinnitus developed by surgeons, or psychiatrists, was successful in helping the patient. One difficulty in achieving agreement regarding the mechanisms of tinnitus and its definition might be the bias towards the hallucinatory type of phantom perception, more frequently encountered by psychiatrists, as opposed to the simpler (tonal or noise-like) perceptions seen by otolaryngologists. The labeling of tinnitus as either tinnitus aurium or hallucination had a powerful impact on thinking about mechanisms of tinnitus and was responsible in large part for the past approaches to treatment.

As a consequence of traditional definitions of tinnitus as any sound generated within the head, classifications were based on lists of mutually exclusive types of tinnitus with clear separation of their boundaries, for example eustachian tube tinnitus, palatal tinnitus, stapedial tinnitus, 8 kHz hearing loss tinnitus, Ménière's tinnitus, VIII nerve tinnitus, vestibular schwannoma tinnitus, cochlear nuclei tinnitus, vascular compression tinnitus, caffeine tinnitus, presbycusis tinnitus, etc. This approach creates complex, multilevel definitions that frequently require redefining as we increase our knowledge of the functioning of the auditory system and the brain.

1.1.2 Tinnitus as a phantom perception

The proposed new definition of tinnitus used here restricts the use of the word tinnitus to one unique phenomenon: a phantom auditory perception (Jastreboff, 1990, 1995). The definition is "The perception of sound that results exclusively from activity within the nervous system without any corresponding mechanical, vibratory activity within the cochlea, and not related to external stimulation of any kind" (Jastreboff, 1995). If there is a vibratory component in the cochlea, which can be related to the perception of sound, it is categorized as a *somatosound* (Jastreboff & Jastreboff, 2003a).

> Tinnitus is the perception of sound that results exclusively from activity within the nervous system without any corresponding mechanical, vibratory activity within the cochlea, and not related to external stimulation of any kind.

From a historical perspective it is quite interesting that the above definition of tinnitus is the exact opposite of the first scientific attempt proposed in 1683 by Duverney to define tinnitus as "True," perceived by external observer, and "False," heard only by the subject (Stephens, 1984).

1.1.3   Justification of proposed definition

The proposed definition is based on several lines of evidence. One comes from the dissimilarity of tinnitus perception from the perception of external sounds. The results of psychoacoustical evaluation (audiometric testing) of tinnitus patients show that they perceive tinnitus as a sound completely different from anything previously experienced in their external environment. Hazell used a music synthesizer in an attempt to match tinnitus perception in 200 patients (Hazell, 1981). Although near matches were achieved, it was never possible to imitate the tinnitus sound the patient heard exactly. This finding was later confirmed by a careful research study (Penner, 1993). Subjects in this study were attempting to resynthesize their tinnitus and complex external sounds using combinations of pure tones with varying frequency, amplitude and phase. This study fully confirmed Hazell's finding of the inability to match tinnitus perfectly with any combination of external tones. Notably, using the same technique, Penner achieved perfect matching of complex external sound by a combination of pure tones. These results indicate that tinnitus patients perceive tinnitus as a sound completely different from anything previously experienced in their external environment.

> Tinnitus patients perceive tinnitus as a sound completely different from anything previously experienced in their external environment.

If tinnitus has a vibratory correlate in the cochlea then suppression of its perception should follow the rules of acoustical masking. The psychoacoustical masking of sound is defined as "the amount by which the threshold of audibility for one sound is raised by the presence of another (masking) sound" (Moore, 1995). Masking is commonly understood as the total disappearance of perception of a sound owing to the presence of a masking sound. Pure tones of varying frequency and intensity are used to characterize the properties of masking. Two tones (one that is masked, and the other acting as masker) have to be within a certain frequency range, which is referred to as a critical band, for masking to occur. The critical band is defined as a narrow band of frequencies surrounding the masked tone contributing to the masking of the tone (Moore, 1995). Predominant opinion is that the masking results from mechanical interaction of the vibration of two adjacent parts of the basilar membrane in the cochlea. Two tones that are separated by more than the critical band width cannot mask each other, however loud the masker. When the masking tone is within the range of the critical band, the frequency distance of one tone from the other determines the extent of the increase in a threshold of detection of the masked tone in the presence of the second (masker), with stronger masking occurring when the tones are closer. As a result, there is a V-shaped masking curve of intensity of the first tone required to "cover" the second when the intensity and frequency of the masked tone are kept constant (Moore, 1995; Zwicker & Schorn, 1978). This rule applies to all external sounds and to sounds made by the body (somatosounds).

Contrary to the masking of external sounds, it is possible to abolish the perception of tinnitus sounds by pure tones of a similar intensity regardless of their frequency.

Contrary to the masking of external sounds, it is possible to abolish the perception of tinnitus sounds by pure tones of a similar intensity regardless of their frequency (Feldmann, 1971). This proves that "masking" of tinnitus does not involve a mechanical interaction of basilar membrane movements, does not depend on the critical band principle and, therefore, has to occur at a higher level within the auditory pathways. Consequently, the elimination of the perception of tinnitus by another sound should be labeled suppression rather than "masking," as is commonly used. Unfortunately, Feldmann's fundamental discovery has been widely disregarded, resulting in focusing attention on masking rather than suppression and in producing tinnitus instruments tuned to the dominant perceived pitch of tinnitus.

The elimination of the perception of tinnitus by another sound should be labeled suppression and not "masking," as is commonly used.

In the case of masking an external tone, a much higher intensity of masker is always needed when the masker is applied to the opposite ear than when both sounds are applied to the same ear. This is usually not the case with tinnitus suppression by a contralateral sound, which can be equally, or even more, effective in suppressing tinnitus as sound applied to the ear where the tinnitus is localized (Feldmann, 1971). The independence of tinnitus suppression from the frequency of the external tone was noticed in 1969 (Feldmann, 1969a), but the term minimal masking level was used inappropriately to describe the minimal level of external sound required to make the tinnitus inaudible. As this effect on tinnitus is one of acoustic suppression the terms "suppression" and "minimal suppression level" should be used instead.[1]

Sound applied to the opposite ear contralaterally (can be equally, or even more), effective in suppressing tinnitus as sound applied to the ear where the tinnitus is localized.

Cyclical fluctuation of loudness of perceived sound occurs when two pure tones that are very close in frequency are presented together. This phenomenon is called *beating of tones*, and the cyclical rate of the loudness change equals the difference of the two frequencies. This phenomenon has not been achieved during attempts to produce beating with tonal tinnitus (perceived as being similar to a pure tone) and an externally applied pure tone.

Tinnitus beats with external tones do not occur.

The phenomenon of disappearance of tinnitus perception after exposure to loud sound was first described by Feldmann (1971a). This effect can last for seconds, minutes or, very rarely, hours or days and was called *residual inhibition*. It cannot be explained by any changes in cochlear function and has not been reported for external tones. It can, however, be easily explained by the rebound phenomenon.[2]

Residual inhibition is observed in some patients after tinnitus suppression.

All these properties of tinnitus strongly indicate that the interaction of tinnitus and external sounds does not occur at the level of the cochlea. Let us consider a situation where tinnitus is related to malfunction of a small area of the cochlear basilar membrane. In this case, the subject would perceive "tonal" tinnitus, as only a small group of auditory nerve fibers tuned to close-by frequencies would be stimulated. By using an external tone with frequency corresponding to the pitch of tinnitus, it should be possible to suppress the tinnitus much more easily than with tones of different frequency. Therefore, the observation that tinnitus suppression does not depend on the frequency of the external sound argues against the cochlea playing a dominant role. The absence of a beating phenomenon also argues against any kind of a mechanical tinnitus-related vibration occurring in the cochlea. In the rare condition when perception of sound results from spontaneous otoacoustic

---

[1] Psychoacoustically masking within the cochlea reflects the mechanical interaction of two traveling waves on the basilar membrane induced by two sounds in the cochlea. The interaction of these two waves depends upon the frequency relationship between the signal and the masking sound, and also on the frequency difference between the two. The frequency range within which the signal is affected by the masker is known as the critical band.

[2] The rebound phenomenon is well recognized in neurophysiology. If the activity of a neuron, as the result of sound stimulation, is increased, cessation of the signal frequently results in activity decreasing below the previous level of spontaneous activity occurring before stimulation. If stimulation was causing inhibition of neuronal activity, then switching off the sound results in an enhancement of spontaneous activity for some time. After a while, the neuronal activity returns to the pre-stimulus level.

emissions, frequency-specific suppression of perceived somatosound is observed (Penner, 1992; Penner & Burns, 1987).

1.2 Categories of phantom auditory perception

The definition of tinnitus that we use states that tinnitus is equivalent to a phantom auditory sensation (Jastreboff, 1990). There are a number of quite different auditory experiences that are included in this definition of tinnitus.

Tinnitus is equivalent to a phantom auditory sensation.

Tinnitus can be perceived as a formless sound, either tonal or complex in nature, that resembles (although it is never identical with) environmental sounds, for example hissing, ringing, buzzing, cicadas, escaping steam, fluorescent light, running engine, static, humming, etc. These descriptions of tinnitus are by far the most common reported. It is believed that this kind of perception occurs as a result of abnormal neuronal activity at a subcortical level of the auditory pathway. The cortex plays a predominantly passive role.

Perception of a formless sound (e.g., hissing, ringing, buzzing, cicadas, escaping steam, fluorescent light, running engine, static, humming, etc.) is by far the most common experience of tinnitus.

Auditory imagery is the phantom perception of well-known musical tunes or of voices without any understandable speech (Berrios, 1991; Berrios & Rose, 1992; Goodwin, 1980). This perception is much less frequent; nevertheless, it is well documented and occurs primarily in older people with hearing loss. It is presumably a central type of tinnitus involving reverberatory activity within neural loops at a high level in the auditory cortex.

Auditory imagery is the phantom perception of musical tunes or of voices without any understandable speech. It is presumably a central type of tinnitus involving reverberatory activity within neural loops at a high level in the auditory cortex.

The definition of tinnitus as a phantom auditory perception does not exclude phantom perception of understandable speech, frequently commanding the subject to perform specific tasks. This type of perception is a hallmark of schizophrenia (Cloninger et al., 1985; Heilbrun et al., 1986), and presumably results from stimulation of cortical speech centers caused by significant malfunctioning of the brain. In clinical practice, there is a tendency to separate schizophrenic from tinnitus patients because of the different approaches to treatment. Nevertheless, there are a number of reasons to include understandable speech as a form of tinnitus.

The definition of tinnitus as a phantom auditory perception does not exclude phantom perception of understandable speech, which is a hallmark of schizophrenia.

There is no clear distinction between "central" and "cortical hallucinatory" tinnitus in the classical definition, except in the complexity of perceived sound. According to the proposed definition of tinnitus, "hearing voices" indicates that abnormal cortical activity causes excitation of the cortical area involved in speech perception. There is no real difference whether speech areas of the brain are excited by electrical stimulation of the cortex or whether this is an abnormal pattern of spontaneous cortical activity affecting cortical speech areas, as happens in schizophrenia. It has been shown that complex auditory (Berrios, 1991; Hammeke, McQuillen & Cohen, 1983; Klostermann, Vieregge & Kömpf, 1992) or visual (Schultz & Melzack, 1991) hallucinations also occur without any psychiatric disorder.

Some schizophrenics experience tinnitus, perceived as a formless sound. In a group of six patients, the auditory hallucinations were unchanged despite amelioration of tonal tinnitus as a result of therapy (J. W. P. Hazell, personal communication).

1.3   Other phantom perceptions

Tinnitus is not unique in being a phantom perception. The concept of phantom perception involves both the philosophy of perception as well as everyday clinical problems. The best recognized other perceptions are phantom limb and phantom pain: the feeling of a limb "being there" or being painful after amputation (Melzack, 1989, 1990, 1992; Wyant 1979).

There are a number of other phantom perceptions, e.g., phantom limb, pain, taste and smell.

Setting aside philosophical aspects of the problem, the main question is whether phantom sensation, as perceived by a patient, differs from their perception of the external world. Melzak, in a series of elegant papers (1989, 1990, 1992), presented convincing data supporting the theory that: "*The experience of a phantom limb has the quality of reality because it is produced by the same brain processes that underline the experience of the body when intact; neural networks in the brain generate all the qualities of experience that are felt to originate in the body, so that inputs from the body may trigger or modulate the output of the networks, but are not essential for any of the qualities of experience.*" He further argued that similar mechanisms are involved in phantom seeing and phantom hearing, including tinnitus (Melzack, 1992; Schultz & Melzack, 1991). Other phantom perceptions include taste and smell (Bartoshuk *et al.*, 1994; Jastreboff, 1990; Kveton & Bartoshuk, 1994; Snow *et al.*, 1991).

Similar mechanisms to tinnitus are involved in phantom seeing.

1.4   Tinnitus-related neuronal activity

The observation that tinnitus suppression does not depend on the frequency of the external sound argues against the cochlea playing a dominant role.

Another possibility is that perception of tinnitus results from neuronal activity within the auditory pathways that is similar to the activity produced by external sounds. If this were so, we should still observe frequency-specific masking, which is not the case. In addition, ipsilateral suppression (masking) should be more effective than contralateral. This makes it unlikely that the perception of tinnitus arises from neuronal activity similar to that evoked by external sounds.

Neuronal activity responsible for tinnitus perception cannot be induced by any combination of external sounds.

The logical conclusion is that the neuronal activity responsible for tinnitus perception cannot be induced by any combination of external sounds (Jastreboff, 1990, 1995). Animal research, where tinnitus-related neuronal activity from the auditory pathway has been recorded, supports this concept and shows that this activity consists of bursts of very high frequency discharges, which are typically associated with epilepsy (Chen & Jastreboff, 1995). This finding has great relevance to some of the puzzles of tinnitus that will be discussed in subsequent chapters.

Perception of tinnitus has been related to abnormal synchronization of auditory nerve activity (Moller, 1984), imbalanced activity of type I and type II afferent fibers in the auditory nerve (Tonndorf, 1987), discordant damage to outer hair cells (OHC) and inner hair cells (IHC) systems (Jastreboff, 1990, 1995) or central abnormalities (Hammeke *et al.*, 1983; Jastreboff, 1990; Moller, 1992). The final result is the same: perception of a sound without any corresponding mechanical vibrations in the cochlea.

1.5   Processing of sounds within the brain

The perception of all external sounds involves a number of brain centers outside the auditory pathways. To evaluate a sound, it is necessary to compare its pattern with other patterns stored in auditory memory. Depending on its significance and past association, perception of the sound will induce various reactions and emotions. In this respect, perception of tinnitus obeys the same general rules and mechanisms as perception of external sounds. The neurophysiological model of tinnitus, discussed later in the book, stresses this aspect very strongly. Many centers within the brain are involved in tinnitus emergence, persistence and its consequent severity.

Depending on significance and past association, perception of a sound will induce various reactions and emotions. Many centers within the brain are involved in tinnitus emergence, persistence and its consequent severity.

The processing of any type of information (including tinnitus-related activity) within the nervous system occurs at several levels and involves pattern recognition, memory and interconnection with other systems, particularly the limbic and autonomic nervous systems. As a result, this model directs our attention away from the concept of tinnitus "belonging" to a place or anatomical site and suggests that it is associated within many centers throughout the nervous system. This activity is changeable, volatile and subject to plasticity (*reprogramming*), which is reflected in patients' behavior in creating new associations, reflex responses and memories. It is this plasticity of the nervous system, properly directed and utilized, that makes it possible to provide patients with relief from their tinnitus.

1.6   Tinnitus duration and epidemiology

The proposed definition disregards tinnitus duration. The episodes of tinnitus can be very short (as in temporary tinnitus following noise exposure or very high dose of aspirin) or it may be continuous. The frequently used criterion of five minutes duration of perception of sound to be classified as tinnitus (MRC-IHR, 1981b) is arbitrary and does not have any clear theoretical or clinical basis or relevance. The time factor is irrelevant for mechanisms of tinnitus generation, regardless of what theory of tinnitus is proposed. From the patient's point of view, however, where the annoyance of tinnitus is certainly related to its duration, this is only one of many parameters determining distress.

The time duration of tinnitus is only one of many parameters determining distress.

Epidemiological studies have shown that temporary tinnitus is a very common symptom experienced by people of all ages (Coles, 1996). There are many factors recognized as most frequently associated with tinnitus: noise exposure, head trauma, some otologic problems, medical conditions and exposure to ototoxic substances. Eventually, while only 0.5–2% of people are significantly affected by tinnitus, various studies estimate that 6–30% of people experience continuous tinnitus (Coles, 1987, 1996; Davis, 1996; Davis & El Refaie, 2000; George & Kemp, 1991). The degree of distress, annoyance, emotional discomfort, sleep problems and interference with day-to-day activities are factors that differentiate people who simply experience tinnitus from those who need help and clinical attention (i.e., have clinically significant tinnitus).

1.7 Comments on somatosounds

The term somatosound refers to the perception of mechanically generated internal body sounds.

The term *somatosound* refers to the perception of internal body sounds (Jastreboff, 1995; Jastreboff *et al.*, 1998). Our proposed definition of tinnitus specifically excludes somatosounds, although they have commonly been considered as tinnitus and included in the same diagnostic category. Somatosounds originate from many different sources, such as turbulent blood flow in the carotid artery, the sound of contracting muscles within the mouth and head area, or the perception of spontaneous otoacoustic emission generated by OHC within the inner ear (Jastreboff *et al.*, 1998).

Including somatosounds within the definition of tinnitus is misleading as they are real sounds mediated through the normal transmission process in the cochlea and can be traced to an acoustic generator.

We believe that including somatosounds within the definition of tinnitus is misleading for two reasons. First, somatosounds, since they are real sounds mediated through the normal transmission process in the cochlea, can be masked in a frequency-specific manner, just as external tones can be, and with masking characteristics differing from those of tinnitus. Although habituation techniques, to be described below, can be applied to somatosounds as well as tinnitus, it may be worthwhile considering the use of frequency-specific masking of these sounds in some cases. Second, somatosounds can be traced to an acoustic generator in a specific location and may be amenable to medical or surgical treatment, for example disobliteration of carotid artery stenosis. In the case of spontaneous otoacoustic emissions, these can be treated, paradoxically, by giving the patient aspirin (which normally induces tinnitus) (Penner & Coles, 1992). Aspirin attenuates action of OHC, which are responsible for spontaneous otoacoustic emissions and which are involved in tinnitus (Jastreboff, 1990; Jastreboff & Jastreboff, 2001, 2003a). A more detailed discussion of somatosounds is presented in Ch. 6.

1.8 Components of decreased sound tolerance

Tinnitus is frequently accompanied by decreased sound tolerance. Decreased sound tolerance is a complex phenomenon.

Decreased sound tolerance includes more than one phenomenon (Jastreboff & Jastreboff, 2001a,b, 2003a). In the past, we have used two terms: *hyperacusis* and *phonophobia*. Hyperacusis was used to describe patients experiencing discomfort to sound resulting from abnormally high activation occurring within the auditory system. Phonophobia was used to describe patients expressing a fear of certain sounds, or all sounds, resulting from abnormal activation of the limbic and autonomic nervous systems.

Consideration of the auditory system alone cannot lead to an accurate definition of decreased sound tolerance, as in clinical practice the limbic and autonomic nervous systems are always involved to a greater or lesser extent and they are necessary to assess the overall implications of decreased sound tolerance.

Hyperacusis is an abnormally strong reaction to sound occurring within the auditory pathways.

Hyperacusis can be defined as an abnormally strong reaction to sound occurring within the auditory pathways (Jastreboff, 2000; Jastreboff & Jastreboff, 2003a). At a behavioral level, it is manifested by a patient experiencing physical discomfort as a result of exposure to sound (quiet, medium or loud). The same sound would not evoke a similar reaction in the average listener. The strength of the reaction is controlled by the physical characteristics of the sound, for example its spectrum and intensity. Consequently, patients would react in the same way to sounds with similar physical characteristics in different situations.

Many patients, previously labeled as phonophobic, are not really afraid of sound, but rather they simply disliked sound; this aversive reaction is not related to the functioning of the auditory system. The use of the term *phobia* frequently meets with objections from patients because of the implied existence of a fear of sound, the existence of a phobia, and, therefore, a purely psychological basis for their problem. It is obvious that the negative reaction to a sound can be driven by various emotions, and not only by fear. The task was to find a term that would be sufficiently general to encompass these various emotions, while being specific enough to describe the situation in an adequate manner. To describe this situation, we use "dislike of" or "aversion" to sound. The word *misophonia* translates into "strong dislike of sound." As such, it is close to the patients' description of their symptoms and can encompass a variety of negative emotions generated by the sounds in question (Jastreboff & Jastreboff, 2003a).

Phonophobia is still a valid term, but it describes a specific type of misophonia, when fear is the dominant emotion involved in the dislike of the sound. The majority of patients with decreased sound tolerance have misophonia, but only some of them are phonophobic. A common reason for phonophobia is the fear that sounds, frequently normal environmental sound, may damage the ear or make symptoms worse. This can result in patients spending much time and effort trying to avoid sound exposure. Misophonic patients simply dislike these sounds without necessarily fearing them; this dislike, in turn, induces negative emotional responses. We have already found the term misophonia to be very helpful in our clinical practice.

Misophonia and phonophobia are abnormally strong reactions of the limbic and autonomic nervous systems resulting from enhanced connections between the auditory and limbic system without abnormal activation of the auditory pathways. Phonophobia describes a specific type of misophonia, when fear is the dominant emotion involved in the dislike of the sound.

Misophonia and phonophobia can be defined as abnormally strong reactions of the autonomic and limbic systems resulting from enhanced connections between the auditory and limbic systems. Importantly, misophonia and phonophobia do not involve a significant activation of the auditory system. At a behavioral level, patients have a negative attitude to sound (misophonia) or are afraid of sound (phonophobia). In cases of misophonia and phonophobia, the strength of the patient's reaction is only partially determined by the physical characteristics of the upsetting sound. It is also dependent on the patient's previous evaluation and recollection of the sound (e.g., sound as a potential threat and/or the belief that the sound can be harmful), the patient's psychological profile and the context in which the sound is presented.

Hyperacusis, misophonia and phonophobia do not have any relation to hearing thresholds. Patients with these problems may have normal hearing, or they may be hearing impaired.

Please note that hyperacusis, misophonia and phonophobia do not have any relation to hearing thresholds. Patients with these problems may have normal hearing, or they may be hearing impaired.

There are few data available regarding the prevalence of decreased sound tolerance. Nonetheless, our research indicates that hyperacusis and tinnitus frequently coexist in the same ear. Approximately 40% of tinnitus patients exhibit some degree of decreased sound tolerance, with 27% requiring specific treatment for hyperacusis. Conversely, a study of 100 patients with hypersensitivity to sound showed that 86% of them suffered from tinnitus.

Hyperacusis and tinnitus frequently coexist, but hyperacusis can be an exclusive problem.

It is possible to extrapolate that significant hyperacusis probably exists in at least 1–1.5% of the general population based on clinical observation that approximately 27% of tinnitus patients required treatment for hyperacusis (Jastreboff, 1999a; Sheldrake, Hazell & Graham, 1999), 86% of patients with hyperacusis reported tinnitus (Anari et al., 1999) and approximately 4–5% of the general population have clinically significant tinnitus (Jastreboff & Jastreboff, 2000a) (Davis & El Refaie, 2000).

In the majority of patients, the etiology of hyperacusis is unknown. Hyperacusis has been linked to sound exposure (particularly short, impulse noise), head injury, stress and medications. The lack of strong epidemiological data, and the lack of an animal model for hyperacusis, prevents us from proving the validity of any theory of the mechanisms responsible for hyperacusis.

It is impossible at present to prove the validity of any theory of the mechanisms responsible for hyperacusis because animal models and strong epidemiological data are lacking.

Decreased sound tolerance can exist as an independent medical diagnosis, or it may be associated with more complex problems. Medical conditions previously linked to decreased sound tolerance include tinnitus, Bell's palsy, Lyme disease, Williams syndrome, Ramsay Hunt syndrome, stapedectomy, perilymphatic fistula, head injury, migraine, depression, withdrawal from benzodiazepines, increased cerebral spinal fluid pressure and Addison's disease (Adour & Wingerd, 1974; Fallon *et al.*, 1992; Fukaya & Nomura, 1988; Gopal *et al.*, 2000; Henkin & Daly, 1968; Jastreboff, Jastreboff & Sheldrake, 1999a; Klein *et al.*, 1990; Lader, 1994; McCandless & Goering, 1974; Nields, Fallon & Jastreboff, 1999; Oen *et al.*, 1997; Vingen *et al.*, 1998; Waddell & Gronwall, 1984; Wayman *et al.*, 1990).

Most frequently, significantly decreased sound tolerance results from a combination of hyperacusis and misophonia/phonophobia. It is important to assess the presence and the extent of all these phenomena in each patient, as misophonia/phonophobia needs to be treated differently from hyperacusis.

While there is no consensus regarding a method for the evaluation of decreased sound tolerance, loudness discomfort levels (LDLs) provide a reasonable estimation of the problem.

While there is no consensus regarding a method for the evaluation of decreased sound tolerance, there appears to be general agreement that LDLs provide a reasonable estimation of the problem. A detailed pre-test interview is needed with each patient to determine the relative contribution of hyperacusis, misophonia and phonophobia to decreased sound tolerance, reflected in the decreased behavioral LDLs. Note that the acoustic reflex threshold is not predictive for loudness perception (Olsen, 1999; Olsen *et al.*, 1999).

1.9 Involvement of hearing loss in tinnitus

Tinnitus and hearing loss frequently coexist.

The concepts and definitions of hearing loss are widely discussed in the literature, and even though we will not discuss these in this text some basic definitions are included in the Glossary. The only point we would like to make is the distinction between sensory (resulting from missing outer hair cells – OHC), and neural (damage of inner hair cells – IHC or neurons of the auditory pathways) hearing loss. In the majority of patients, there is no sensorineural hearing loss but only sensory hearing loss. This distinction plays an important role in counseling tinnitus patients. Consequently, we are against the use of the term sensorineural when there is no clear indication that both types of hearing loss are indeed present.

1.10 Summary

The following definition will be used throughout this book: *Tinnitus is the perception of a sound that results exclusively from activity within the nervous system without any corresponding mechanical, vibratory activity within the cochlea, and unrelated to external stimulation* (Jastreboff, 1995). As such, tinnitus is equivalent to *phantom auditory perception*. We are not excluding various types of hallucination, including auditory imagery, from being defined as tinnitus. However, somatosounds of various origins and also any auditory sensations resulting from external stimulation (e.g., cochlear implants, direct magnetic stimulation of the auditory cortex, etc.) are excluded from the definition of tinnitus.

As the proposed definition in this book restricts tinnitus to phantom auditory perception, consequently, both the theory and clinical practice of tinnitus focuses on the nervous system, with the cochlea and the periphery of the auditory system playing a secondary role.

Except when specifically stated, the word *tinnitus* will be used in this book to describe tinnitus perceived as a formless sound (different from auditory hallucination), since this is by far the most common experience of tinnitus.

Decreased sound tolerance, with its components hyperacusis and misophonia, plays a significant role in both theory and clinical practice. These components can exist independently from tinnitus; however, they frequently accompany tinnitus. In some cases, hyperacusis and tinnitus might be closely linked and reflect two manifestations of the same mechanism of enhanced gain within the auditory pathways.

2

The neurophysiological model of tinnitus and decreased sound tolerance

The neurophysiological model of tinnitus is the essential basis and frame of reference for understanding tinnitus, hyperacusis and misophonia, as well as for the specific clinical approach based on the model. The main postulate of this model is that a number of systems in the brain, other than the auditory system, are involved in the phenomenon of tinnitus. Particularly the interactions between the auditory system and the emotional (limbic) and autonomic nervous systems are of crucial importance in clinically significant tinnitus. The difference between people who merely experience tinnitus and those who suffer because of it depends on the presence of these connections. By modifying these interactions, and altering the central processing of tinnitus-related neuronal activity, habituation of tinnitus can be achieved.

There are two types of tinnitus habituation, habituation of reaction and habituation of perception. Habituation of reaction occurs when tinnitus no longer evokes any emotional or autonomic response, whereas habituation of perception occurs when the subject is no longer aware of tinnitus, except when focusing attention upon it. To achieve habituation, it is crucial to demystify tinnitus, to understand its correct mechanism according to the model and to change its classification from something bad or unpleasant to that of a neutral signal.

Habituation is further facilitated by the use of sound, the main role of which is to weaken the tinnitus signal at both perceptual and subconscious levels. This can be provided by enriching environmental sounds and, in the majority of patients, by wearable sound generators. Hearing aids can also be used to remove the "straining to hear" phenomenon and to amplify enriched background sound. The adding of appropriate sounds (with or without amplification by hearing aids) rather than using any particular device is fundamental.

The specific implementation of the neurophysiological model of tinnitus is known as Tinnitus Retraining Therapy (TRT) and has been shown to provide significant improvement in tinnitus in about 80% of patients. This therapy can also be used effectively to treat decreased sound tolerance, both hyperacusis and misophonia, and somatosounds. The information presented in this chapter is used during the TRT counseling sessions.

2.1 Development of the neurophysiological model of tinnitus

Over thousands of years, during which time tinnitus has been identified as a problem, many different treatments have been tried without any consistent success.

Tinnitus has been identified as a problem for thousands of years and many different treatments have been tried without any consistent success. With the rapid advances in medical science during the twentieth century, new methods were introduced. Chapter 6 reviews some of the most frequently discussed treatments, including medications. The failure to achieve a consistently successful outcome with tinnitus treatment has discouraged many professionals and has left tinnitus patients without help. In addition, tinnitus was also a rare topic of research or discussions during scientific meetings. The neurophysiological model of tinnitus and decreased sound tolerance has created a new dimension for both research and clinical endeavors (Jastreboff, 1990; Jastreboff & Jastreboff, 2003a).

The neurophysiological model of tinnitus and its clinical implementation (TRT) were created by the work of P. J. Jastreboff in the mid 1980s.

In order to understand the neurophysiological model of tinnitus, it is helpful to follow the reasoning and path that led to its development.

Perception of tinnitus is very prevalent but only about 20% of people with tinnitus have a problem with it.

The starting point for developing the model was the clinical findings that characterized a population of tinnitus patients combined with selected, well-established facts from neuroscience. P. J. Jastreboff had the advantage of no preconceived clinical knowledge of tinnitus before starting experimental work on animal models of tinnitus in 1983. During a literature survey, it became obvious that perception of tinnitus is very prevalent, affecting approximately 17% of the general population around the world, although figures ranging from 6% to 30% were reported depending on country and methodology. At the same time, epidemiological studies revealed that only approximately 4% of the general population really have a problem with tinnitus (anon., 1981a; Coles, 1984; McFadden, 1982). Further data have fully confirmed these observations (e.g., Davis & El Refaie, 2000). So the question was why, of all the people who experience tinnitus, do less than a quarter have a problem with it to the extent that they seek medical attention.

There is no difference in the psychoacoustical characterization of tinnitus between "experiencing" and "suffering" groups.

Many research studies have focused on the psychoacoustical properties of tinnitus and have showed that there is no difference in the characterization of tinnitus between "experiencing" and "suffering" groups. That is, its loudness pitch and the lowest amount of noise to suppress tinnitus (the minimal suppression, or "masking" level (MSL)) were, on average, the same in both groups (Hazell *et al.*, 1985a; Henry & Meikle, 2000).

Clinical and research data strongly suggested that there is no vibratory mechanical activity within the cochlea that could be related to tinnitus perception.

The unusual masking properties of tinnitus, and lack of phase-related phenomena (such as beating with external sounds), strongly suggested that there is no vibratory mechanical activity within the cochlea that can be related to tinnitus perception (see Ch. 1 for details). This observation, combined with knowledge of neurophysiological mechanisms of perception, provided the crucial concept of the model tinnitus as a phantom perception.

Severity of tinnitus and its impact on life do not correlate with its psychoacoustical characterization.

In other words, tinnitus is not represented in the cochlea by any mechanical vibration, but rather it reflects neuronal activity within the auditory pathways. It, therefore, cannot obey the rules of psychoacoustical masking, the suppression effects are frequency independent and can be as effective contralaterally as ipsilaterally. Furthermore, the severity of tinnitus and its impact on life do not correlate with its characterization (Hazell *et al.*, 1985b; Henry & Meikle, 2000).

The obvious conclusion from these data was that the psychoacoustical characterization of tinnitus (e.g., its pitch, loudness, suppressibility) is not really important from a clinical point of view, as they were neither correlated with tinnitus severity nor with treatment outcome. A later research study reanalyzing the same data fully confirmed this conclusion and, in addition, showed that the initial description or measurement of tinnitus has no value in predicting whether or not a person is going to be helped by a currently available treatment ("partial masking" combined with counseling) (Jastreboff, Hazell & Graham, 1994). The conclusion was that systems other than the auditory system are responsible for the severity of tinnitus and determine whether a subject suffers because of tinnitus or merely experiences it.

Other systems, separate from the auditory system, are responsible for the severity of tinnitus and determine whether a subject is suffering because of tinnitus or merely experiencing it.

The auditory system is connected to many systems and centers in the brain.

For years, an oversimplified view of how the auditory system functions was widely accepted. The connections between the inner ear, where sound is changed into electrical impulses, and the cortex, where sound is perceived, were viewed as simple cables, transmitting signals but without processing the signal. In reality, the neuronal centers (neuronal networks) between the inner ear and cortex are performing complex tasks, enhancing some signals and suppressing others (Fig. 2.1). Furthermore, it was not commonly appreciated that the auditory

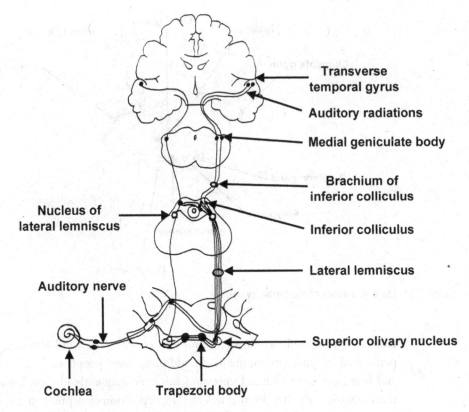

Figure 2.1   Main structures and connections of the auditory system.

system is connected with many other non-auditory systems and centers in the brain. Incoming sounds are constantly activating many areas of the brain and evoke a variety of reactions. Noticing and stressing the role of non-auditory centers in the brain was a crucial point, which created the base for the neurophysiological model of tinnitus.

The majority of patients have a problem with attention, sleep, concentration and activities that are performed in quiet environments; furthermore, many people experience anxiety and lose enjoyment of life.

In the early stages of development of the neurophysiological model of tinnitus, two important questions arose. First, which systems in the brain, other than the auditory systems, are responsible for the problems created by tinnitus. Second, what are the mechanisms involved in tinnitus perception and in tinnitus-induced disturbances? The literature provided insight into these issues. Clinical papers describing the most common complaints related to tinnitus showed that the majority of

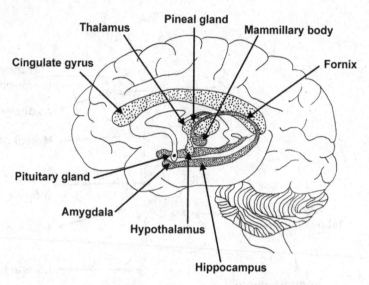

Figure 2.2   Main structures of the limbic system.

patients have a problem with attention, sleep, concentration and activities that are performed in quiet environments. In addition, many people experience anxiety and lose enjoyment of life. Depression was very frequently observed, and there was discussion whether tinnitus was causing depression or depression was causing tinnitus.

Frequently, patients became obsessive about their tinnitus and went to enormous lengths to find a cure for it. It was not unusual to encounter a patient who went to 30 or 40 of the best specialists in the country and spent tens of thousands of dollars in their search for a cure for tinnitus. Patients were trying bizarre treatments, even if they were a hazard to their health and life quality.

In clinically significant tinnitus, in addition to the auditory systems, two systems are involved: the limbic and the autonomic nervous systems.

Based on the literature it was also clear that a large number of medications and procedures had been tried, but none was effective in suppressing or eliminating tinnitus in a significant proportion of patients (see Ch. 6).

The problems consistently described by patients suggested that two systems have to be involved in clinically significant tinnitus; the limbic system (Fig. 2.2), which controls our emotions, and the autonomic nervous system, which is responsible for controlling all the automatic functions in the brain and the body. These systems are crucial for normal functioning of the brain and body, and changes in their activity have profound health and behavioral impact.

> The limbic system controls our emotions.

The limbic system controls our emotions, both positive and negative.[1] Fear, thirst and hunger, as well as joy and happiness, are controlled and mediated by this system. Experiments on animals and observations on humans provide us with extensive information on how this system works. It has been shown that by stimulating a specific region, the nucleus of amygdala (a crucial part of the limbic system), it is possible to induce fear; when this nucleus is destroyed, fear can no longer be evoked or experienced, in either animals or humans (Bast, Zhang & Feldon, 2001; Buchel & Dolan, 2000; Davis & Whalen, 2001; Goosens & Maren, 2001; Sprengelmeyer *et al.*, 1999).

> The limbic system is strongly connected with all sensory systems.

The limbic system is strongly connected with all sensory systems, such as smell, vision and the auditory system. Consequently, certain stimuli, sounds, pictures or smells, are able to evoke very strong positive or negative reactions. For example, if someone points a gun at a person, or the sound of a rapidly approaching car is heard, fear is induced and the limbic system is strongly activated. In extreme cases, the situation is labeled as "fight or flight." These reactions involve the activation of the sympathetic part of the autonomic nervous system.

> The autonomic nervous system controls all the automatic body functions.

The autonomic nervous system, which is closely connected to the emotional system, controls all the automatic body functions such as heart rate, breathing, muscle tone, bowel function, levels of hormones and sexual activity.[2] Most people do

---

[1] The limbic system is a heterogeneous array of brain structures at or near the edge (limbus) of the medial wall of the cerebral hemisphere and includes the olfactory cortex, hippocampal formation, cingulate gyrus and subcallosal gyrus, which are all cortical structures, and the amygdala, septum, epithalamus, hypothalamus (habenula), anterior thalamic nuclei and parts of basal ganglia, which are all subcortical structures. The limbic system exerts an important influence upon the endocrine and autonomic motor systems. These, in turn, control multifaceted behavior, including emotional expression, seizure activity, memory storage and recall, and motivational and mood states (Swanson, 1987).

[2] The autonomic nervous system, one of the two main divisions of the nervous system, provides the motor innervation of smooth muscle, cardiac muscle and gland cells. It controls the action of the endocrine glands; the functions of the respiratory, circulatory, digestive and urogenital systems; and the involuntary muscles in these systems and the skin. It also has a reciprocal effect on internal secretions, being controlled to some degree by the hormones and exercising some control, in turn, on hormone production.

The autonomic nervous system consists of two physiologically and anatomically distinct, mutually antagonistic components: sympathetic (thoracicolumbar), and parasympathetic (craniosacral). The sympathetic division stimulates the heart, dilates the bronchi, contracts the arteries, inhibits the digestive system and prepares the organism for physical action (in the extreme, fight and flight). The parasympathetic division has the opposite effect, it prepares the organism for feeding, digestion and rest (Brooks, 1987).

The sympathetic and parasympathetic systems are functionally connected in a reciprocal manner, each inhibiting the other. As a result, the autonomic nervous system tends to function in one of two states, with either sympathetic or parasympathetic control being dominant. When the sympathetic system is sufficiently activated, the parasympathetic system is suppressed; the internal feeling of reward or pleasure is inhibited and the positive aspects of life are no longer enjoyed.

(*continued overleaf*)

not have direct control over this system and its functions; however, where a situation requires a fast reaction (e.g., a threat), the system is automatically stimulated in preparation for physical or mental activity. Activation of the sympathetic part of the autonomic nervous system results in mobilization of the whole body, making it ready for quick action.

The limbic (emotional) and autonomic nervous systems are normally activated by both pleasant and unpleasant stimuli, and their action is essential for our well-being and effective function.

It is important to realize that the limbic (emotional) and autonomic nervous systems are normally activated by both pleasant and unpleasant stimuli, and that their action is essential for our well-being and effective function. Activation of the limbic system is also needed for any learning process, including retraining of the brain, as happens during TRT. In the tinnitus patient, the limbic and autonomic nervous systems might previously have been functioning entirely within normal limits. A problem only arises when they are highly and inappropriately activated by a neutral stimulus, such as tinnitus.

In the next part of this chapter, we address the issues of mechanisms involved in tinnitus perception and the problems induced by it. Specifically, we examine the hypothesis that perception of tinnitus reflects compensation of the auditory pathway to changes, modifications or damage occurring within the auditory system. The tinnitus signal itself is innocent and is not causing any harm. The problem develops when tinnitus becomes associated with something negative or unpleasant and, as a result, produces strong reactions in the limbic and autonomic nervous systems. This sets up a vicious circle involving these three interconnected systems (auditory, limbic and autonomic nervous systems). Once arousal of the limbic and autonomic nervous systems is sufficiently high, the stimulus linked to this activation will dominate all other brain functions.

(*continued*)
    For both divisions, the pathway of innervation consists of a synaptic sequence of two motor neurons, one of which lies in the spinal cord or brainstem as the preganglionic neuron. The thin but myelinated axon (preganglionic or B fiber) emerges with an outgoing spinal or cranial nerve and synapses with one or more of the postganglionic neurons composing the autonomic ganglia; the unmyelinated postganglionic fibers, in turn, innervate the smooth muscle, cardiac muscle or gland cells. The preganglionic neurons of the sympathetic part lie in the intermediolateral cell column of the thoracic and upper two lumbar segments of the spinal gray matter; those of the parasympathetic part compose the visceral motor (visceral efferent) nuclei of the brainstem and, with the cranial nerves (particularly the vagus and accessory nerves), pass to ganglia and plexuses within the various organs. The lower part of the body is innervated by fibers arising from the lateral column of the second to fourth sacral segments of the spinal cord. Impulse transmission from preganglionic to postganglionic neuron is mediated by acetylcholine in both the sympathetic and parasympathetic sections; transmission from the postganglionic fiber to the visceral effector tissues is classically said to be by acetylcholine in the parasympathetic part and by norepinephrine in the sympathetic part. Recent evidence suggests the existence of a further class of non-cholinergic, non-adrenergic postganglionic fibers (Brooks, 1987).

2.2 Mechanisms of tinnitus signal generation

2.2.1 Tinnitus perception as a by-product of a compensatory action by the auditory system

High levels of random spontaneous activity of neurons within the auditory pathways are not perceived as a sound.

Study of electrical activity of single neurons within the auditory pathways has shown that their spontaneous activity is at a relatively high level, about 50 discharges per second. This activity is random and is not perceived as a sound. It is possible to think of it as a "code for silence," although its characteristic feature is the absence of any systematic pattern. This random activity fluctuates, since nothing in the central nervous system is completely stable; however, as our brain is adjusting to these fluctuations all the time, there is no perception of sound. When we are exposed to some external sound, neuronal activity increases and becomes more regular. At the same time, the auditory pathways are continuously filtering and suppressing spontaneous neural activity so that activity does not reach cortical areas involved in awareness, and there is no perception of sound.

We are reacting not to the absolute strength of the stimulus but rather to its relative strength compared with the background.

Another observation comes from psychological experiments and everyday experience. A weak sound in a quiet room (e.g., a ticking clock) appears relatively loud and clear. If exactly the same clock is put in a room with increased background noise, although it is still audible it would appear to be much softer.

This observation reflects a general principle for all the senses: we react not to the absolute but to the relative strength of the stimulus compared with the background (Fig. 2.3). Our hearing and vision are adjusting all the time to the average level of sound or light around us, illustrating the principle of automatic gain control. For instance, a small candle will appear to be very bright in a darkened room but is hardly visible in broad daylight.[3]

In a reduced sound environment, gain or amplification increases at all levels within the auditory system, resulting in an overall increase in loudness perception of all sounds.

When the background sound level is low, hearing becomes more acute than when moderate sound levels are present. Moreover, in a quiet situation, sounds are perceived as much louder than they would be in normal everyday background noise. What will happen if we purposefully and significantly decrease the level of

---

[3] The adaptation of the eye is partially responsible for this phenomenon, but even taking adaptation into account, the light will still be perceived as brighter in the darkness.

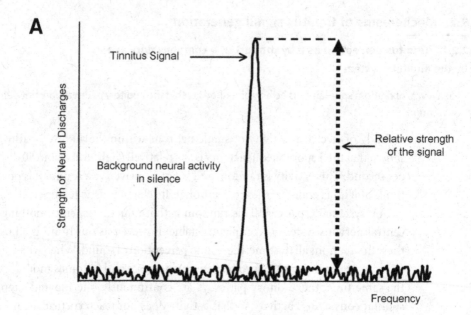

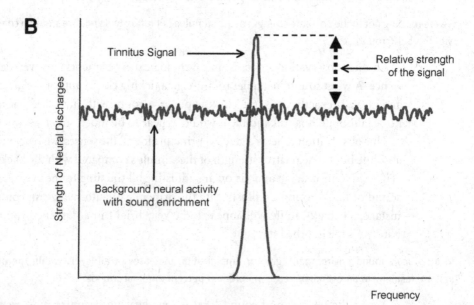

Figure 2.3   Tinnitus signal versus background neuronal activity. The strength of the signal depends on
the difference between the signal and the background neuronal activity. By increasing the
background it is possible to decrease effectively the strength of the tinnitus signal.

background noise? Such an experiment has been performed by Heller and Bergman (1953). A group of 80 subjects were placed one by one in a sound-proofed room. During the first few minutes of being in this room, subjects start hearing their heartbeat, breathing and every small sound caused by normal body function. These sounds quickly became loud, very clear and really dominant. The most interesting observation was that within five minutes, 94% of these subjects heard sounds identical to those described by tinnitus sufferers (e.g., hiss, buzz, ring, hum, roar, whistle, crickets, steam, sea shell), which disappeared after they left the sound-proofed room.

Emergence of tinnitus and increase of the loudness of sounds can be explained by studies of electrical activity from the auditory pathways in animals. Experiments with reduced input to the auditory pathways showed an increased sensitivity of auditory neurons (Boettcher & Salvi, 1993; Gerken, 1992, 1993; Salvi, Wang & Powers, 1996). When there are less than normal levels of sound in our environment, and the ears are relatively understimulated, gain, or amplification, increases at all levels within the auditory system, resulting in an overall increase in loudness perception of all sounds. Consequently, even the small variations of spontaneous activity in the auditory pathways, mentioned above are perceived as sound. In this special situation – the sound-proof room experiment – almost everybody perceives tinnitus.

Taking a high dose of aspirin or entering a sound-proofed room evokes tinnitus in practically everybody.

Another conclusion from this experiment is that the perception of tinnitus itself is not pathological but rather is a physiological response of central auditory pathways to signals (or their absence) coming from the auditory periphery. It is generally known that everybody can experience a temporary perception of tinnitus, and that taking a high dose of aspirin (or entering a sound-proofed room) evokes tinnitus in practically all subjects. Why, then, do some people have tinnitus in a normal sound environment and some do not? Why do some people have distress from tinnitus and others not? Clearly there is a difference between tinnitus sufferers and those experiencing tinnitus during the sound-proof room experiment. What are the mechanisms involved in the continuous perception of tinnitus?

Lateral inhibition describes the situation when a neuron exerts an inhibitory effect on adjacent neurons. The tinnitus-related neuronal activity, created by any mechanisms, will be enhanced by lateral inhibition while being processed within the auditory pathways.

Lateral inhibition is a common phenomenon throughout the nervous system and describes the situation when a neuron exerts an inhibitory effect on adjacent neurons. This mechanism, as presented in Fig. 2.4, was first proposed by von Bekesy.

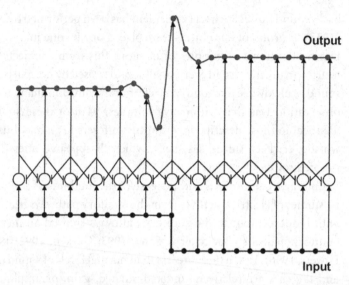

Figure 2.4   Lateral inhibition. Length of arrows represents the strength of the signal coming to a cell or its output (every other cell and its connections are shown). Note enhancement of the output at the edge of the signal. The layer of cells may represent cells in any nucleus of the auditory pathways receiving tonotopically organized signals.

It results in enhancement of changes, or edges, within the spatial distribution of the signal in the neuronal networks. This basic mechanism was proposed as a mechanism for the emergence of tinnitus by Liberman and Kiang (1978) and further expanded and elaborated by Gerken (1996). The principle of lateral inhibition can be applied to one or many layers of neurons. Note that the lateral inhibition principle enhances any heterogeneity of activity within the neuronal network, independent of its initial source. Therefore, the tinnitus-related neuronal activity, created by any mechanisms, will be enhanced by lateral inhibition while being processed within the auditory pathways.

2.2.2   Discordant dysfunction theory of tinnitus production

There are many hypotheses attempting to explain the mechanisms of the source of tinnitus; however, none has yet been proven.

There are many hypotheses attempting to explain the mechanisms of the source of tinnitus (e.g., Brummett, 1995; Eggermont, 1990; Feldmann, 1992; Gerken, 1996; Jastreboff, 1990, 1992; Kaltenbach, 2000; Lenarz et al., 1993; Moller, 1984, 1995; Pujol, 1992; Tonndorf, 1980; Zenner & Ernst, 1993). The hypothesis that seems to explain a number of the puzzles of tinnitus was proposed by P. J. Jastreboff in 1990 and is known as a discordant dysfunction/damage theory. The theory proposes that differential damage or dysfunction of OHC and IHC at a given portion of basilar membrane in the cochlea will give rise to discordant activation of type I and type II auditory nerve fibers, which are innervating IHC and OHC, respectively. Except in a very few situations, OHC are damaged more than IHC; this, in turn, results in disinhibition of neurons in the dorsal cochlear nuclei. All clinical and experimental results strongly support the postulate that tinnitus emerges when activity of the OHC system is disturbed (e.g., with large doses of aspirin, quinine, cisplatin, noise exposure).

This hypothesis was initially known as the discordant damage theory, but as discordant activation occurs when hair cells are damaged or, in a more general sense, dysfunctional, "discordant dysfunction" is a better descriptor. This theory has been described in detail elsewhere (Jastreboff, 1990, 1995), and only the main points are presented below.

Discordant dysfunction (damage) theory postulates that the tinnitus signal originates from the inner ear when OHC are more damaged than IHC.

The discordant dysfunction (damage) theory postulates that the tinnitus signal originates in the inner ear when one type of sensory cell, OHC, is more dysfunctional than the other type of sensory cells, IHC, at the same area of the basilar membrane in the cochlea. The damage can be caused by excessive noise, viral infection, exposure to certain drugs or just the normal process of ageing (Fig. 2.5).

IHC are the true receptor cells for sound transduction. They convert mechanical vibrations of the structures within the inner ear (resulting from sound reaching the cochlea) into electrical impulses in the auditory nerve, which finally result in sound perception. Most of the fibers in the auditory nerve (95%) connect with IHC and convey these electrical impulses to the brain. OHC work as mechanical amplifiers within the cochlea, enhancing the detection of weak sounds by providing up to 50 dB of amplification. This amplification is achieved by physical vibrations of the OHC and can be evaluated by measurement of otoacoustic emissions. As external sound levels increase, the level of amplification gradually reduces.

When neurons in the dorsal cochlear nuclei receive excitation from IHC but not from the damaged OHC, then an imbalance occurs at this level of the auditory system. This, in turn, causes abnormal activity in the form of bursts of high-frequency neuronal discharges, which, after amplification within the auditory system, are perceived as tinnitus.

When there is any kind of damage to the cochlea, OHC are damaged first and adjacent IHC later (Chen & Fechter, 2003). Signals from both types of hair cell converge on the same group of neurons in the dorsal cochlear nucleus. When neurons

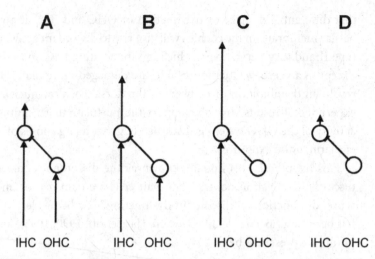

Figure 2.5   Discordant dysfunction (damage) theory. The following scenarios are shown. (A) Undamaged OHC and IHC; (B) partially damaged OHC and intact IHC; (C) totally destroyed OHC and intact IHCs and (D) totally destroyed OHC and IHC systems. The size of the arrows represents the signal from IHC and OHC and strength of neuronal activity of the cells in dorsal cochlear nucleus (DCN) in the brainstem. Arrowheads indicate excitation and flat bars inhibitory connections. Note the presence of an inhibitory interneuron in the path of the signal coming from OHC, which is inhibiting the output cell of the DCN. Note enhancement of the signal parallel with increased damage of OHC system, and only a low level of spontaneous, intrinsic activity present when both systems are equally damaged.

in the dorsal cochlear nucleus still receive excitation from IHC but not from the damaged OHC, then an imbalance is created at this level of the auditory system. This, in turn, causes abnormal activity in the form of bursts of high-frequency neuronal discharges; after amplification within the auditory system, these discharges are perceived as tinnitus. Increased spontaneous activity has been recorded in association with tinnitus in the dorsal cochlear nucleus (Kaltenbach & Afman, 2000) and the inferior colliculus of the brainstem (Chen & Jastreboff, 1995; Jastreboff & Sasaki, 1986; Kwon *et al.*, 1999) (Figs. 2.6 and 2.7). Furthermore, bursts of spontaneous activity, correlating with the extent of tinnitus perception, have been shown in the inferior colliculus (Jastreboff *et al.*, 1999b; Kwon *et al.*, 1999).

At least two mechanisms might act as a source of tinnitus-related neuronal activity, either independently or together: first, increased gain at any level in the auditory pathways may result in enhancement of natural fluctuations of spontaneous activity to the extent that these fluctuations are detected and perceived as sound (tinnitus). Second, a potential source occurs when some (even very slight or local) dysfunction or damage of the OHC system is created.

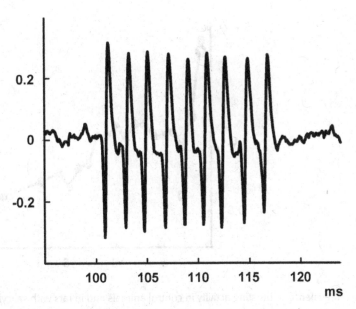

Figure 2.6   Bursts of neuronal activity from the inferior colliculus in rats. A recording of a single neuron spontaneous activity from a rat with salicylate-induced tinnitus. This is a very high frequency, prolonged activity normally observed only in epilepsy. Tinnitus most probably results from the perception of this neuronal activity. (Modified from Chen & Jastreboff, 1995.)

At least two mechanisms might act as a source of tinnitus-related neuronal activity, either independently or together. First, increased gain at any level in the auditory pathways may result in enhancement of natural fluctuations of spontaneous activity to the extent that these fluctuations are detected and perceived as sound (tinnitus). The sound-proof room experiment (Heller & Bergman, 1953) indicated that this can indeed happen. Second, a potential source occurs when some, even very small or local, dysfunction or damage of the OHC system is created, which might not be detectable on a standard hearing test such as the pure tone audiogram and of which the individuals themselves would be completely unaware.

An imbalance of neuronal activity caused by tinnitus-related changes affects type I and type II fibers of the auditory nerve differently, and this results in bursting activity at the dorsal cochlear nuclei level. After further amplification within the auditory pathways, this may be perceived as tinnitus.

The resulting imbalance of neuronal activity between type I and type II fibers of the auditory nerve generates bursting activity at the dorsal cochlear nuclei level, which, after further amplification within the auditory pathways, may be perceived as tinnitus. Because of the tonotopic organization of the cochlea and the auditory pathways, localized dysfunction will result in the perception of sounds, the pitch of

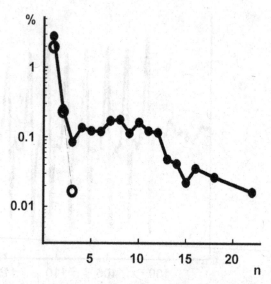

Figure 2.7   Prevalence of bursting activity in control animals and in rats with salicylate-induced tinnitus. Vertical axis shows the ratio of the number of trains of discharges of a given length to the total number of intervals recorded from a group of cells responding to tones with frequencies corresponding to the perceived pitch of tinnitus. Horizontal axis shows number of intervals in a train. Note that in control animals (open circles and dashed line) only short bursts are present (no longer than 4 time intervals) and their probability decreases rapidly. In animals with salicylate-induced tinnitus (full circles and solid line), it is possible to observe bursts up to 23 intervals, occurring quite frequently. The data are consistent with the postulate that disinhibition is the mechanism responsible for the tinnitus-related neuronal activity. Modified from Chen & Jastreboff, 1995.

which reflects the affected area of the basilar membrane. When several areas of the basilar membrane are affected, then any resulting perception can be very complex and will reflect contributions from all the individual sources.

It is likely that a combination of these two factors creates a perception of tinnitus. Experiments on animals show that temporary or permanent hearing loss (involving OHC dysfunction) gives rise to a measurable increase in the sensitivity of a high percentage of neurons in the auditory pathway (Gerken, 1979; Gerken, Saunders & Paul, 1984). Decreased or distorted auditory input to the auditory system results in compensation within neuronal pathways. Recent reports support the suggestion that the extent of OHC damage is related to tinnitus (Kaltenbach *et al.*, 2001; Mitchell & Creedon, 1995).

The discordant dysfunction hypothesis helps to explain a number of observations. For example, why the perceived pitch of tinnitus is typically localized near the bottom of the slope of hearing loss on the audiogram. This is the area in the cochlea that has the largest difference between damaged OHC and normally functioning IHC.

Approximately 20% of patients with tinnitus have normal hearing. This is because changes too small to be detectable on a standard audiogram, if localized, can result in heterogeneity and trigger compensatory reactions of the auditory system, resulting in tinnitus.

Why then does 20% of tinnitus occur in those with normal hearing (Davis & El Refaie, 2000)? This group may not have any hearing defect detectable on a traditional audiogram but could still have microchanges in their OHC system. These changes can be detected by tests such as the distortion product otoacoustic emission, which measures the functional property of the OHC system in an objective manner. Even small changes, if localized, can result in heterogeneity, triggering compensatory reaction of the auditory system and resulting in tinnitus.

Tinnitus does not occur in 27% of totally deafened people, because when both types of hair cell are totally damaged the resulting imbalance is smaller than when the one type, IHC, still functions.

Why do 27% of totally deafened people not have tinnitus (Hazell, McKinney & Aleksy, 1995)? If both systems (IHC and OHC) are totally damaged, the resulting imbalance is actually smaller than when one system still functions while the other is not providing any signal (Fig. 2.5d).

In the majority of patients, tinnitus is a side effect of a normal compensatory action of the auditory system.

In conclusion, in the majority of those affected, tinnitus is simply a side effect of a normal compensatory action by the auditory system. This system is constantly attempting to restore homeostasis[4] and trying to provide the best possible hearing.

The auditory pathways attempt to compensate for a decrease of input and to correct heterogeneity of signals corresponding to adjacent frequencies; this generates and enhances the tinnitus-related neuronal activity.

In a situation where there is an inadequate signal coming from the cochlea to the brain, with or without disorder of cochlear function as described above, the auditory pathways always attempt to compensate for a decrease of the input and to correct heterogeneity of signals corresponding to adjacent frequencies. While this may provide better hearing, it generates and enhances the tinnitus-related neuronal activity.

[4] Homeostasis is defined as the state of equilibrium (balance between opposing forces) in the body with respect to various functions and the chemical compositions of the fluids and tissues. The term is also used to describe the processes through which such bodily equilibrium is maintained. The term physiological homeostasis is used to describe the set of mechanisms responsible for the cybernetic adjustment of physiological and biochemical states in postnatal life.

2.3 Decreased sound tolerance

The model predicts that a relatively high percentage of tinnitus patients should exhibit decreased sound tolerance.

The model predicts that a relatively high percentage of tinnitus patients should exhibit increased sensitivity to an external sound, that is decreased sound tolerance. This is what one would expect from the increased auditory gain, or the combination of an increased gain and some even minor dysfunction of the inner ear. At the time the model was first presented (Jastreboff, 1990), this concept was not supported by most data in the published literature, which claimed that only a small percentage (0.3%) of tinnitus patients exhibited decreased sound tolerance (Vernon, 1987). When we started measuring sensitivity to external sounds in our population of tinnitus patients, both in the USA and the UK, it transpired that about 40% of patients showed a degree of increased sensitivity to environmental sound (Hazell & Sheldrake, 1992; Jastreboff, Gray & Gold, 1996). As our practice of TRT progressed and we systematically evaluated patients for any decreased sound tolerance, it became increasingly evident that a high proportion of patients (25–30%) were seeking help because of hyperacusis, which may be even more of a problem to them than their tinnitus. Decreased sound tolerance was even less recognized than tinnitus, and patients frequently were blaming tinnitus for the problems they experienced, being unaware of the true reason.

2.4 Relationship of tinnitus to hearing loss

Hearing loss and tinnitus are only indirectly related.

Another important implication of this model is that hearing loss and tinnitus are only indirectly related. As hearing loss increases sensitivity of neurons within the auditory pathways (Gerken et al., 1985), it could be expected that people who have some hearing loss might be more prone to tinnitus. This observation is confirmed by epidemiological data. As people with sensory hearing loss typically have damage to OHC, there is a higher likelihood of an imbalance between IHC and OHC systems. The incidence of tinnitus in a hearing-impaired population is approximately twice that of the population with normal hearing (Coles, 1987). At the same time, 20% of people with tinnitus have normal hearing (Davis & El Refaie, 2000) and 27% who are totally deaf do not have any tinnitus (Hazell et al., 1995). Furthermore, if we compare average audiograms from a population of people attending a tinnitus clinic with those from a normative population study, the audiograms are basically identical (Hazell & McKinney, 1996). The finding that hearing loss, specifically of a high frequency in the worse ear, approximately doubles the risk that a person will have tinnitus predicts that the ratio of tinnitus patients with normal hearing to those without hearing loss should be about 2 to 1. The finding in clinical practice that about 30% of tinnitus patients do not have a hearing loss fits this prediction. The hypothesis of discordant dysfunction provides an explanation for this apparent paradox. If tinnitus emergence depends on a dysfunction of the OHC system, then this dysfunction can be very localized, very discrete, not reflected in the audiogram and not noticed by the patient.

> In the vast majority of patients, tinnitus is not related to any on-going pathological process; in only a very small percentage will tinnitus be related to some medical problem, such as Ménière's syndrome (disease), otosclerosis or compression of the auditory nerve.

In the vast majority of those affected, tinnitus is not related to any on-going pathological process. It is not an indication of progressive hearing loss, nor a predictor that a person is more susceptible to hearing loss. In only a *very* small percentage will tinnitus be related to some medical problem, such as Ménière's Syndrome (disease), otosclerosis or compression of the auditory nerve by a slowly growing benign tumor. Such conditions should be screened for at the initial routine evaluation of a patient by the otolaryngologist and treated appropriately.

2.5 Phantom perception

> The perception of tinnitus results from the detection of an activity within the auditory pathways without an external sound corresponding to the tinnitus. Consequently, tinnitus perception does not obey the same rules as perception of external sounds.

The very real perception of tinnitus results from the detection of modification of spontaneous activity within the auditory pathways, and there is no external sound corresponding to the tinnitus. In other words, tinnitus is a phantom sound, similar to phantom pain or the phantom limb phenomenon (Jastreboff, 1990; Moller, 1997; Muhlnickel *et al.*, 1998). Consequently, perception of tinnitus does not obey the same rules as perception of external sounds; for example, its suppression is governed by totally different principles. Even if the signal itself is very weak, it may be heard in the presence of high levels of environmental sound. It can be persistent and irritating, simply because it is an unusual signal, and unlike perception generated by external sounds.

2.6 Natural habituation

> More than three-quarters of people who experience tinnitus naturally habituate to it.

Notably, more than three-quarters of people who experience tinnitus can naturally habituate to it (Davis & El Refaie, 2000; McFadden, 1982). The recognition of habituation can be linked to Pavlov (Konorski, 1948):

When a stimulus is repeatedly presented without being followed by any arousal-producing consequences, these effects are gradually attenuated and some of them may be eventually totally abolished. This phenomenon, originally denoted by Pavlov as "extinction of orientation reaction," is now usually called "habituation."

More recent wording offers the same meaning (*Stedman's Concise Medical Dictionary*, 1997):

The method by which the nervous system reduces or inhibits responsiveness during repeated stimulation

or (American Heritage Dictionary, 1994):

The decline of a conditioned response following repeated exposure to the conditioned stimulus

Adaptation involves a peripheral sensory organ while habituation occurs within the central nervous system.

Contrary to adaptation, which involves a peripheral sensory organ, habituation occurs within the central nervous system.

Habituation of tinnitus means that the tinnitus-related neuronal activity is blocked from reaching the limbic and autonomic nervous systems and consequently there are no negative reactions to tinnitus (habituation of reaction). Moreover, the auditory system is capable of blocking this tinnitus-related neuronal activity, preventing it from reaching higher cortical areas and thus being perceived (habituation of perception).

Habituation of tinnitus means that the tinnitus-related neuronal activity is blocked from reaching the limbic and autonomic nervous systems and consequently there are no negative reactions to tinnitus (habituation of reaction). Moreover, the auditory system is capable of blocking this tinnitus-related neuronal activity, preventing it from reaching higher cortical areas and thus being perceived (habituation of perception). Individuals who naturally habituate are unaware of the presence of tinnitus, except at times when they consciously focus their attention on it. The role of natural habituation was noticed by Stephens, Hallam & Jakes (1986). These authors, however, did not propose a specific or effective protocol for inducing and sustaining habituation, which is necessary for clinical success of a treatment. Such a protocol, aimed at inducing and sustaining habituation, is an integral part of TRT.

2.7 The process by which tinnitus becomes a problem

A novel sound induces a new pattern of activity within the auditory pathways and subawareness centers allowing this activity to reach the cortex. After reaching the highest cognitive centers, sound will be perceived and further evaluated.

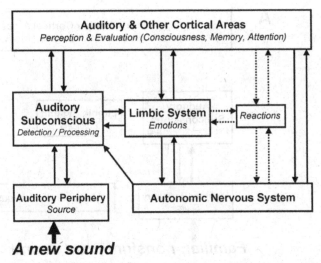

A new sound

Figure 2.8   Activation of various systems evoked by a new sound. In this and subsequent figures, the thickness of the arrows and darkness of the boxes represent the strength of activation. Note a low-level activation evoked by a new sound.

To understand why the perception of tinnitus might create a problem, we can start by studying what is happening in the brain when it is exposed to any new sound. The novel sound induces a new pattern of activity within the auditory pathways. This activity in groups of nerve fibers will increase and become regular, rather than being random as nerve activity is in the absence of signal. While the pattern of activity is new and not previously experienced, subawareness centers allow this activity to reach the cortex. These centers are also responsible for our selective hearing by blocking unimportant auditory information. The new sound-induced pattern will be compared with that stored in memory patterns representing other sounds. If this pattern does not find a match in auditory memory, then it is passed to the highest cognitive centers, where it will be perceived and evaluated further (Fig. 2.8).

Sounds can be classified in three general categories: neutral (not significant), having some positive (pleasant) meaning, and having a negative (unpleasant) association or meaning. During this process, with every new sound, the limbic and the autonomic nervous systems are activated to some extent (Fig. 2.8). This results in an orientation reaction (startle reflex[5]) in which the head may be turned in the direction of a sound to learn more about it. Meanwhile, our autonomic nervous system is preparing our body to an appropriate reaction should it be needed.

---

[5] The startle reflex involves a quick, involuntary movement, frequently contraction of the limb and neck muscles, in response to some sudden and unexpected stimulus.

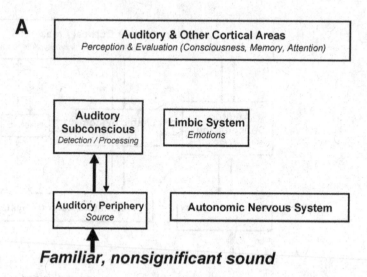

Familiar, nonsignificant sound

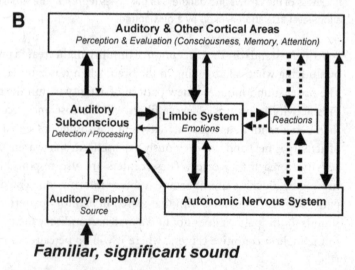

Familiar, significant sound

Figure 2.9   Activation evoked by a new sound. (A) An unimportant non-significant, familiar sound does not activate the limbic and autonomic nervous systems nor the higher cortical areas responsible for sound awareness. These signals are not inducing reactions (habituation of reaction) and are not perceived (habituation of perception). (B) By comparison, a familiar, significant sound will result in a high level of activation of the limbic and autonomic nervous systems and of higher level cortical areas.

If the new sound is judged to be of no particular importance it will induce little activation of the limbic and autonomic nervous systems. With repetitive appearance of this particular sound, the subcortical pathways will block it, and there will be no awareness of the sound. This is the process of habituation of perception.

The initial response from the limbic and autonomic nervous systems is relatively mild. If the new sound is judged to be of no particular importance, for example the sound of a truck passing on a highway some distance from the house, then, each time the sound reappears, it will induce less and less activation of the emotional and autonomic nervous systems (Fig. 2.9a). With repetitive appearance of this particular sound, the subcortical pathways will block it, and the individual will be unaware that the sound is present. This is the process of *habituation of perception*. If the sound is familiar but significant, its repetitive appearance will result in strong activation of the limbic and autonomic nervous systems every time a subject is exposed to it. Consequently, the strength of the reflex arc and resulting reaction will gradually increase (Fig. 2.9b).

2.7.1 Selective perception

Only one task can fully occupy our focus of attention at a given time and it is impossible to perform more than one task that requires full attention. Therefore, we may have to switch rapidly between one attentional focus and another, while carrying out other tasks automatically.

The mechanism of selective perception reflects one important limitation of the brain: the fact that only one task can occupy our focus of attention at a given time. Consequently, it is impossible for us to perform more than one task that requires our full attention at the same time. This problem is partially solved by rapid switching of an attentional focus between tasks (Kimberg, Aguirre & D'Esposito, 2000). For example, it is impossible to read a book and write a letter at the same time, or even read a book and listen attentively to music. One way of dealing with this limitation is by making some tasks automatic by the subconscious processing of information related to these activities, which do not require our full conscious attention. For example, when driving a car, the brain is continuously performing complex tasks while blocking the majority of sensory signals from reaching awareness. It is sometimes an alarming experience to arrive at a familiar destination without much memory of the journey!

The selection process, deciding if an incoming sound is neutral and can be ignored or important and requiring perception, has to take place at a subconscious level.

We are not aware of the vast majority of sounds arriving at our ears, which are of no significance to us. The crucial factor is that the selection process, deciding if the incoming sound is neutral and can be ignored, or important and requiring conscious perception, has to take place at a subconscious level. Otherwise a process of conscious selection would occupy all the resources of the brain, and we would not be able to perform any other task or activity. The process of habituation to non-important stimuli allows us to concentrate on more important, and novel tasks. The question is, how does the brain decide what is important to us and how is the selection process organized?

If we are paying attention to all incoming stimuli, we are obliged to deal first with those that suggest something bad might happen. In most instances, it is more important to avoid an unpleasant situation than to experience something pleasant. Since avoiding disturbing situations frequently requires fast reactions, it occurs on a reflex basis, before we are able to analyze the situation consciously. We cannot afford the time to debate the issue before acting, and consequently we do not have much control over these reflex reactions. A car's brake-light illuminating just in front of us will evoke a reflex reaction of foot hitting brake.

Once we associate a stimulus with something negative, we are unable to remove this association easily because it is a part of a conditioned reflex.

Once we associate a stimulus with something negative, or we are simply annoyed by it, we are unable to remove this association easily because it has become part of a conditioned reflex. An example would be trying to hold a conversation in the presence of a untethered wild animal. Our attention would be drawn to the animal, and it would be very difficult, or just impossible, to carry on a conversation. Concious attempts to control this monitoring process will be unsuccessful, as we have no means of directly controlling or altering these reflex-based reactions. In this case, the reflex reactions involved in observing a wild animal are necessary for self-protection. Our attention would be preoccupied with the negative event, and this would prevent us from engaging in any other activities.

2.7.2 Suppression of positive emotions

Negative and positive emotions oppose each other. If we are afraid of something, or under significant stress or unhappy, then we are unable to feel positive emotions and cannot, at that time, appreciate anything that otherwise would be a pleasant experience. For example, if we are waiting at a dentist's office and we know that we are shortly going to have a painful root canal procedure performed, and at the same time someone is offering us the most delicious meal, most of us would probably not be able to touch it, and if we tried to eat the meal, we would not enjoy it. This principle of opposing action of negative and positive motivations is very well established. It is actually used in psychological experiments to measure the extent of fear (Estes & Skinner, 1941), as well as in the animal model of tinnitus (Jastreboff et al., 1988).

> Many of those with persistent tinnitus have no enjoyment of life and become very frustrated and depressed.

Consequently, when the patient is focusing attention on tinnitus, which has now assumed a dominant role, it becomes impossible to perform other tasks requiring attention, even things that normally would be enjoyed. It is not surprising that many patients with persistent tinnitus have no enjoyment of life, cannot see a positive future and become very frustrated and depressed.[6]

2.7.3 Sleep impairment

> Approximately 50% of tinnitus patients have disturbed sleep.

According to population studies, approximately 50% of tinnitus patients have disturbed sleep (Tyler & Baker, 1983). This observation can be explained by the fact that problem tinnitus results in stimulation of the sympathetic part of the autonomic nervous system and keeps high levels of activation during both day and night. This is possible because the auditory system is very active at subconscious levels during sleep, and there is a known anatomical connection between the auditory and limbic systems at this level. Keeping the sympathetic autonomic nervous system at a higher level of activation can be positive if we have to get up early, but otherwise results in a poor night's sleep with very little rest. If it

---

[6] From the point of view of tinnitus, it is important that the limbic system is involved in all aspects of life involving motivation, mood, and emotions, and that it activates the endocrine and autonomic nervous systems. A highly activated limbic system results in mood swings (a person being controlled by emotions), potential changes in hormone levels (with all its consequences) and, through activating the autonomic nervous system, influences on all body functions. Typically, patients exhibit syndromes indicating a dominance of the sympathetic division of the autonomic nervous system, which stimulates the heart, inhibits the digestive system and in general prepares the body for physical action. This, in turn, leads to problems with sleep, which is very common among tinnitus sufferers (Coles, 1996). Abnormally high activation of these systems results in stress, anxiety and loss of well-being. These patients are extremely annoyed by their tinnitus, which, as it is argued in Ch. 2, continues to get worse because of the feedback loop connecting the auditory, limbic autonomic nervous systems.

Please note that a high level of activation of the limbic and autonomic nervous systems by any factor, even without tinnitus present, will result in the same syndromes as described by tinnitus patients. Sleep deprivation itself can account for many behavioral and psychological changes reported by patients (such as inability to concentrate, mood swing, problems with logical decision, rapid illogical reactions to encounter problems; see Holgers et al. (1999) and Ch. 6). The difference is that when the external factors go away (stress induced by overwork, personal relationship problems, etc.) activation of the limbic and autonomic nervous systems decreases to the normal level. However, in those with tinnitus, the tinnitus signal (i.e., tinnitus-related neuronal activity) is still present. Once the conditioned reflex arcs are established, activation of both the limbic and autonomic nervous systems increases and is maintained. If this occurs for a sufficiently long period, then physiological exhaustion is reached with all the negative behavioral consequences associated with tinnitus.

Another crucial issue reflects the physiological fact that a high level of activation of the sympathetic part of the autonomic nervous system, for any reason, activates the fight or flight reaction and suppresses or even eliminates positive emotions, resulting in decreased ability to enjoy life. In those with severe tinnitus, it is frequently observed that patients no longer enjoy activities previously pleasant to them, and life ceases to offer joy. This, in turn, leads to depression.

happens occasionally, it does not have negative impact, but if it happens regularly it results in chronic sleep deprivation.[7]

Sleep deprivation affects concentration and attention; it creates mood swings and irritability. There are a lot of similarities between the complaints of those sleep deprived in other ways, and those suffering from tinnitus.

Sleep deprivation has a profound impact on brain metabolism as well as on general behavior. The influence of tinnitus on sleep may be responsible for many of the behavioral changes observed in tinnitus patients. The rapid eye movement (REM) phase of sleep is particularly affected (Culebras, 1992). REM sleep is necessary for the restoration of normal brain activity, and serious changes in the biochemistry of the brain occur in subjects who are deprived of REM sleep (Basheer *et al.*, 1998; Cirelli & Tononi, 1999; Sallanon-Moulin *et al.*, 1994).

The study of people who are sleep deprived but who do not have tinnitus provides interesting insight. These people have a problem with concentration; they are more susceptible to emotional fluctuations and are less able to think logically. Their rapid swings of emotions are unpredictable and they may be described as "having a short fuse" and being "likely to explode." People with sleep deprivation may have problems with work of any kind as well as having problems with attention and not being able to relax and enjoy life. It is obvious that there are many similarities between the complaints of sleep-deprived people and those of people suffering from tinnitus. Many problems experienced by tinnitus patients, especially in the early stages, arise from the fact that they are not getting a sufficient amount of sleep.

Tinnitus may make falling asleep more difficult as the whole brain is in an alert state from overactivation of the limbic and autonomic nervous systems. Tinnitus effects on sleep are particularly profound in preventing continuation of sleep. We all sleep in cycles of approximately 90 minutes going through different stages of sleep (McKenna, 2000). In each cycle, there is a period of time when we are in very shallow sleep, perhaps even waking for a few seconds. When waking in the middle of the night, as the normal sleep pattern dictates, tinnitus will be noticed immediately and perceived as being loud, because background sound during the night is typically low. This perception of tinnitus will evoke a further higher level of autonomic activity, causing anxiety and annoyance. Consequently, the individual

---

[7] Trying to sleep with distressing tinnitus is similar to trying to sleep with a live snake moving around in the same room. In both situations, the sound is disturbing. The problem with sleep is that tinnitus creates a high level of anxiety, putting the body into "alert" or even "flight or fight" mode. In such a state, sleep is entirely inappropriate. This is illustrated by the "early morning flight syndrome." Imagine that you have to catch a flight at 4 o'clock in the morning, which you simply cannot afford to miss. After setting three or four alarm clocks and asking the family, including the dog, to wake you up, you eventually fall asleep but proceed to wake up every hour, and at least 10 minutes before the alarms start ringing. You are absolutely ready to jump out of bed and run for the plane, wide awake and ready for action. You will get to airport on time, but this sleep will not provide rest.

will experience much more difficulty in getting back to sleep, spending long periods in the night awake and listening to troublesome tinnitus.

2.8   The components of the neurophysiological model

2.8.1   Main systems involved in the model

The auditory system provides the source of a signal, tinnitus, which through inappropriately created functional connections causes activation of the limbic and autonomic nervous systems, resulting in annoyance and distress.

The auditory system provides the source of a signal, tinnitus, that creates inappropriate functional connections with, and causes activation of, the limbic and autonomic nervous systems, resulting in annoyance and distress.

It has been puzzling why and how tinnitus becomes such a strong and dominant signal when the source can be relatively weak; also why even loud tinnitus does not bother some people at all, and weak, nearly inaudible tinnitus causes major problems for other people. Let us analyze what neurophysiological mechanisms are involved when clinically significant tinnitus develops.

If tinnitus perception is associated with high levels of emotional distress, conditional reflexes are created causing the tinnitus-related neuronal activity (conditioned stimulus) to evoke high levels of activation of the limbic and autonomic nervous systems (conditioned reaction).

On many occasions, tinnitus emerges very rapidly, particularly when its perception is triggered by loud sounds (discos, shotguns). New, or rapidly changing, signals are always perceived and attract attention. If perception of a signal is associated with high levels of emotional distress, conditioned reflexes are created, causing the tinnitus-related neuronal activity (conditioned stimulus) to evoke high levels of activation of the limbic and autonomic nervous systems (conditioned reaction). Because of the presence of feedback loops between the auditory, limbic and autonomic nervous systems, and also because of brain plasticity, once tinnitus acquires a negative connotation and starts to induce activation of the autonomic nervous system, it initiates a cascade of events. As a result, there is stronger and stronger activation of the limbic and autonomic nervous systems, through a conditioned reflex arc, even when the tinnitus signal remains unchanged. This phenomenon, commonly labeled as a vicious cycle, is illustrated in Fig. 2.10.

A conditioned reflex arc can also be created automatically if some abnormality in the auditory system already exists (or has recently developed) concurrently with high levels of emotional stress. The emotional stress provides the negative reinforcement needed to create the link in the conditioned reflex arc. Once tinnitus acquires this negative association, an aversive conditioned response is established, and is responsible for the persistence of tinnitus.

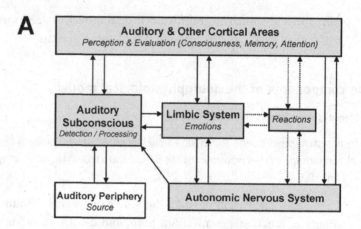

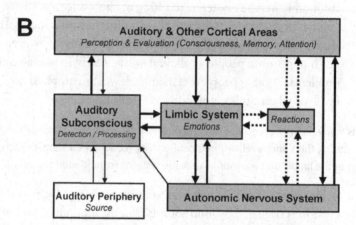

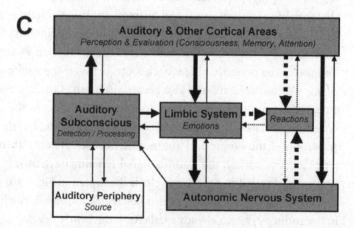

Figure 2.10 Development of a vicious cycle. The thickness of the lines and darkness of the boxes reflect the extent of activation. Note the gradually increasing activation of the limbic and autonomic nervous systems (stages A, B, C), which becomes dominant in the final stage C.

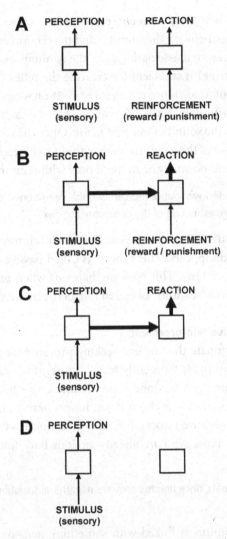

Figure 2.11 Development and extinction of conditioned reflexes. (A) Initial temporal coincidence of sensory stimulus and reinforcement occurs. (B) A conditioned reflex link is created. (C) Consequently, the sensory stimulus alone induces the reaction previously evoked by reinforcement. (D) Continuous repetition of the sensory stimulus without reinforcement results in disappearance of the conditioned reflex (passive extinction).

2.8.2 Conditioned reflexes

Many body reactions result from conditioned reflex arcs. Importantly, the temporal association of stimulus and reaction is sufficient to create a reflex, without the necessity for a causal relation.

Many body reactions, and particularly those requiring a fast response, result from the conditioned reflex arcs (Fig. 2.11). A reflex is created when a sensory stimulus is associated with reinforcement (punishment or reward). Although typically there is a causal link between the stimulus and the reinforcement in creating a conditioned reflex, a temporal association (i.e., the stimulus and reinforcement happening at the same time) is sufficient for creating the reflex (Konorski, 1948; Fig. 2.11a,b). Examples of conditioned reflexes are salivation when we see delicious food, stopping at a red traffic light, hitting the brake when the car ahead of us brakes suddenly, or turning to the sound of our first name. Once the conditioned reflex is established, the presence of the stimulus, even without reinforcement, results in a full reaction, which would normally be induced only with reinforcement (Fig. 2.11c).

If the stimulus is repeated without reinforcement, the conditioned reflex gradually disappears. This process is called passive extinction of the conditioned reflex.

If a neutral stimulus is repeated without reinforcement, the conditioned reflex gradually disappears. This process is called passive extinction of the conditioned reflex (Fig. 2.11d). This typically happens when reflexes result from a temporal association only, without a causal link between the stimulus and reinforcement.[8]

2.8.3 Effect of negative reinforcement

It is unfortunate that anyone seeking professional advice about the new experience of tinnitus is frequently met with negative counseling. People are typically told "nothing can be done about tinnitus, you have to learn to live with this," or even worse, "let us check if you have a brain tumor." Even those who had no particular negative associations with their tinnitus frequently and quickly develop them, and those who are already anxious have their worst fears confirmed and enhanced.

As with all negative signals, once tinnitus acquires negative associations, it becomes constantly monitored.

Once tinnitus is linked with something negative, it acquires a warning label indicating that "there might be something wrong." Furthermore, even if there is no specific negative association, tinnitus can simply be annoying by its continuous presence, and through this alone acquires a negative connotation. The negative link ensures that there is activation of limbic and autonomic responses whenever the tinnitus signal is detected. As with all negative signals, once tinnitus acquires negative associations, it becomes constantly monitored.

---

[8] These types of reflex were labeled by Konorski "superstitious reflexes". They are surprisingly common in everyday life. For example, such a reflex is created if an extremely unpleasant emotional situation develops and persists during a learning period. During this period, negative associations can develop to any events, names, places, experiences occurring at that time, resulting in the triggering of an aversive reaction whenever they are encountered in the future.

At the same time, our autonomic nervous system is automatically activated to prepare us for physical or mental activity and, in extreme conditions, a "fight or flight" response. This evokes a strong desire to run away or to fight in order to attempt to destroy the source of the problem. However, we cannot run away from tinnitus, though some sufferers get out of bed in the night and run out of the house in an attempt to do so. We cannot fight or destroy tinnitus, but patients frequently describe attempts to "fight it" and "not let it beat them." Such attempts attract even more attention and importance to tinnitus and consequently increase stress, anxiety and frustration.

2.8.4 Feedback loops

The reactions of the autonomic nervous system provide the main negative reinforcement for conditioning the response to tinnitus.

The reactions of the autonomic nervous system provide the main negative reinforcement for conditioning the response to tinnitus, and this in turn enhances the strength of the negative association. Consequently, the more unpleasant the symptoms resulting from tinnitus-related autonomic activation, the stronger the link between tinnitus and those responses, resulting in enhancement of monitoring of tinnitus. In other words, because tinnitus seems important and acquires negative associations, more time is spent on checking the status of tinnitus. The tinnitus becomes more noticeable (greater loudness, awareness), inducing further activation of the limbic and autonomic systems and increasing unhappiness, fear, concern, stress, anxiety, tension and other negative emotions. This, in turn, further enhances the need for monitoring of tinnitus. The reactions of the autonomic nervous system lead to "tuning up" of the auditory networks to enhance the tinnitus signal, which results in a still stronger stimulation of the autonomic nervous system. As a result, another loop of enhancement of tinnitus-induced reaction is created.

The feedback interaction consists of two loops: conscious, involving the cortical awareness level (Fig. 2.12a), and subconscious, involving subconscious centers (Fig. 2.12b). For both loops, a small initial negative association that remains unchallenged can grow with the aid of this feedback mechanism and result in a high level of anxiety, stress and dysfunction. The situation is similar to a small ball of snow rolling down a hill, gathering momentum and growing to an avalanche. However, activation of the conscious loop requires perception of tinnitus, which is not needed for activation of the subconscious loop. Thus, the tinnitus-related neuronal activity can activate the limbic and autonomic nervous systems either with or without conscious perception of tinnitus.

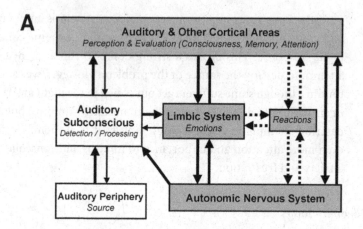

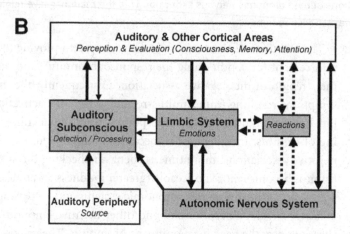

Figure 2.12 Conscious and subconscious systems. (A) Loops involving awareness and cognitive processes of tinnitus. (B) Loops acting at subconscious levels.

A constant state of alertness causes tinnitus patients to become exhausted and complain of lack of sleep. They are be unable to focus attention on anything else but tinnitus and experience overall loss of life quality.

The signal is present all the time in clinically significant tinnitus, causing continuous activation of the autonomic nervous system; this, in turn, serves as negative self-reinforcement. Consequently, the conditioned reflexes get stronger, and their spontaneous extinction is prevented (Fig. 2.13). At a behavioral level, this results in a constant state of alertness (being ready for any danger), having much greater effects than those evoked by other negative experiences, which tend to be relatively transitory in nature. Tinnitus patients are exhausted and complain of lack of sleep, an inability to focus attention on anything else but tinnitus and overall loss of life quality.

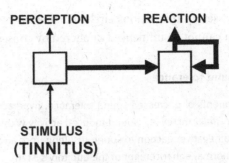

Figure 2.13 Mechanism hindering spontaneous extinction of conditioned reflexes in tinnitus: the continuous presence of the tinnitus signal and the reaction of the autonomic system acts as self-reinforcement.

2.8.5   Irrelevance of the strength of the tinnitus signal

The initial strength of tinnitus signal is irrelevant.

The initial strength of a tinnitus signal is irrelevant (it can be weak or strong), as the final strength of reaction and severity of distress caused by tinnitus results from the strength of the feedback loops within the model (Figs. 2.10, 2.11 and 2.13). The final level of reaction will depend on the intrinsic properties of the limbic and autonomic nervous systems. Even a very weak, low-level, very soft tinnitus can result in a high level of anxiety and annoyance when modified by powerful feedback loops. Imagine the sound of a creaking floorboard in the middle of the night, when we are afraid that someone has broken into the house and we are in danger. The signal is very weak, but it causes a very strong reaction. Much louder, but neutral signals, like the sound of a thunderstorm, might not cause any reaction at all. The sound of creaking floorboards during the day evokes no response, as it does not have the same negative association – it is to a large degree expected – and so it will not trigger activation of the limbic or autonomic nervous systems.

The development of a vicious circle involves processes at both conscious and subconscious levels and follows the principle of conditioned reflexes. Once the conditioned reflex is created, it cannot be influenced or altered by conscious thoughts alone.

The process of creating and strengthening these feedback loops, popularly referred to as a vicious circle, involves processes at both a conscious and a subconscious level and follows the principle of conditioned reflexes. Conscious thinking, involving words and beliefs, are secondary to the subconscious reflex-based processes. Although beliefs about tinnitus may facilitate or create initial associations (for example, fear that there may be a brain tumor), they are not needed to set up this vicious circle. Furthermore, once the conditioned reflex is created, it cannot be influenced or altered by conscious thoughts alone.

2.8.6 Decreased sound tolerance

There are two components of decreased sound tolerance: hyperacusis and misophonia. In hyperacusis, there is an abnormally increased, sound-induced activity within the auditory pathways. In pure misophonia, there is a negative reaction to sound resulting from an enhanced limbic and autonomic response, without abnormal enhancement of the auditory system.

A significant proportion of those complaining about tinnitus are also affected by decreased tolerance to external sounds, as discussed in Ch. 1. There are two components of decreased sound tolerance: hyperacusis and misophonia. In hyperacusis, there is abnormal increased sound-induced activity within the auditory pathways. As a result, sounds that are non-intrusive, or unnoticed by the general population, are uncomfortable to people with hyperacusis. Abnormal enhancement of sound-evoked neuronal activity occurs within the auditory pathways and causes only secondary activation of the limbic and autonomic nervous systems (Fig. 2.14a). This enhancement may involve both peripheral (cochlear) and central auditory pathways.

In pure misophonia, a negative reaction to sound results from an enhanced limbic and autonomic response, without abnormal enhancement of the auditory system (Fig. 2.14b). As a result, sound may induce a strong dislike of sound, as well as produce changes in body functions and feelings of discomfort. The term "misophonia" (dislike of sound) is used to describe this phenomenon (Jastreboff & Jastreboff, 2003a). Phonophobia, a specific form of misophonia, is seen when fear is the principal component of a patient's emotions. In misophonia or phonophobia, the reaction to sound depends not only on its physical characteristics but also on other aspects such as past associations, beliefs about specific sounds (or sounds in general) and the psychological status of the patient.[9]

Recruitment, defined as an abnormally high slope of loudness growth, is a necessary outcome of sensorineural hearing loss.

All these phenomena are independent of recruitment, defined in audiology as an abnormally high slope of loudness growth. Recruitment is an inevitable outcome of sensorineural hearing loss and results from a reduction in the OHC population

---

[9] Examples of misophonia include people who are reacting to the sounds of childrens' voices (as they do not like children) or a dislike of other people eating or chewing. Examples of phonophobia include general fears that sounds will be gradually destroying the cochlea or the fear that they will be exposed to sound which will permanently make their symptoms worse.

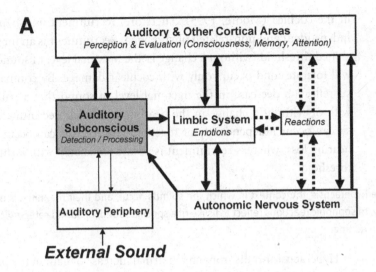

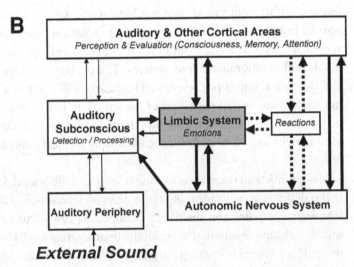

Figure 2.14 Mechanisms of decreased sound tolerance. (A) In hyperacusis, the external signal undergoes abnormal enhancement/amplification within the subconscious auditory pathways (marked by gray color) and only secondarily activates the limbic and autonomic nervous systems. Note that the connections between the auditory and other systems are normal and that the increase of stimulation of the limbic and autonomic nervous systems results from stronger signals coming from the auditory system. (B) In misophonia, activity within the auditory pathways is normal, but connections between the auditory and limbic and autonomic nervous systems are enhanced, causing high levels of activation of the limbic and autonomic nervous systems.

in the cochlea (Moore, 1995). Therefore, recruitment and hyperacusis are two independent and non-related phenomena. Recruitment is an inevitable result of a shifted threshold (without a change in the maximal level of sound that the patient will tolerate) and occurs only with cochlear damage. By comparison, hyperacusis reflects a decrease in the maximal level of sound that a patient will tolerate with or without a change in the hearing threshold. Recruitment and hyperacusis can occur independently or together. Hyperacusis can occur with or without hearing loss, whereas recruitment is always associated with a shift in the hearing threshold.

In pure hyperacusis, the context in which the sounds occur, and their meaning, is not relevant. Conversely, misophonic reactions reflect a dislike of a specific sound, or sound category, that is dependent on its meaning.

Hyperacusis results from an abnormal increase of gain in the peripheral or central parts of the auditory system. Regardless of the specific mechanism, patients feel discomfort from sounds that would be within comfortable listening levels for normal individuals. In pure hyperacusis, exposure to these sounds will create a very high level of activation within the auditory system, and only secondarily in the limbic and autonomic nervous systems. The context in which the sounds occur, and their meaning, is not relevant. The patient will react in a very similar manner to the same sound regardless of the situation. For example, the reaction will be the same whether the sound is presented at home, in a cinema while watching a favorite movie, or as sounds made during medical evaluation in the doctor's office.

Misophonic reactions reflect a dislike of a specific sound, or sound category, that is dependent on its meaning rather than on its acoustic characterization (e.g., frequency spectrum and intensity). Misophonia can occur to certain classes of sound, for example sounds that are louder than a certain level. For pure misophonia, the auditory system is working normally and does not exhibit any abnormally high activity when stimulated by these sounds. In misophonia, however, such sounds will cause feelings of dislike, and consequently a strong reaction from the patient through powerful activation of the limbic system.

Once misophonia is established, reactions to the specific sounds are governed by the principles of conditioned reflexes.

Once misophonia is established, reactions to specific sounds are governed by the principles of conditioned reflexes. Reaction to the sound will be very fast; once the reflex is set, the person will react without thinking about the meaning of the sound, or the validity of the belief that it is bad or dangerous. Another aspect of misophonia is that reaction to the sound may depend on the context. That means the same sound will evoke a different reaction depending on the place and context in which the sound is heard.

In a clinical situation, hyperacusis, misophonia and phonophobia can coexist or can be present as individual problems. Their action results in decreased sound tolerance, the term used to describe the presence of one, any or all of these phenomena. Decreased sound tolerance can have an extremely strong impact on a patient's life. It can prevent people from entering loud environments, from working, interacting socially and from enjoying many everyday activities. In extreme cases, patients do not leave their homes, and their lives and the lives of their families are completely controlled by the issue of sound avoidance.

In any patient with significant hyperacusis, some misophonia is automatically developed, as normal sounds will evoke discomfort and, therefore, the dislike or fear that sound in general may be harmful or distressing. Misophonic patients may also develop hyperacusis from prolonged overprotection of hearing with earplugs and muffs. Both issues are important in the practical treatment of patients, and this will be discussed below. Note that the mechanisms of tinnitus, hyperacusis and misophonia involve the same centers in the brain, are governed by similar rules and provoke similar symptoms, because of the consistent involvement of the limbic and autonomic nervous systems.

In hyperacusis, the goal is to desensitize the auditory system by systematic exposure to a variety of sounds.

However, because of the differences in the mechanisms of hyperacusis and misophonia, different treatment approaches are needed. In hyperacusis, the goal is to desensitize the auditory system by systematic exposure to a variety of sounds. We are using very basic physiological processes to eliminate hyperacusis, with mechanisms that do not involve conditioned reflexes and conscious thinking. As a result, in pure hyperacusis, it is irrelevant whether or not patients are paying attention to the sound being used, and their beliefs and understanding of the process of desensitization and the neurophysiological model of tinnitus is not as crucial.

The most effective way of reversing the conditioned reflexes in misophonia is to associate the sounds with something positive.

Misophonia and phonophobia, by comparison, involve the process of conditioned reflexes, as the sounds are linked with some negative meaning. The most effective way of reversing these reflexes is to associate the sounds with something positive (a procedure known as the active extinction of conditioned reflexes). The details of how to apply the appropriate protocol will be presented in Ch. 3.

In clinical practice, decreased sound tolerance nearly always consists of a variable mixture of hyperacusis, misophonia or phonophobia, and each of these components needs to be addressed appropriately.

2.9   The mechanism of tinnitus habituation and the neurophysiological basis for TRT

In designing an effective treatment for tinnitus and sound sensitivity, there are four critical questions.

1. Is it possible to reverse or nullify the conditioned reflex arc?
2. Is it possible to detach perception of tinnitus (or external sound) from the reflex reaction set up by it?
3. Is it possible to block perception of tinnitus?
4. What treatment protocol is required to achieve this?

All conditioned reflexes can be reversed: body reactions to any stimulus can be reversed and the brain is able to learn throughout life. Natural habituation of various stimuli is continuously taking place.

Neuroscience provides us with the necessary information to answer these questions. First, all conditioned reflexes can be reversed; consequently, everything which we have been trained to do can be retrained. Second, reactions of our body to any stimulus can be reversed. Third, our brain is able to continue learning throughout life. Fourth, natural habituation of various stimuli is continuously taking place.

Habituation of tinnitus-induced reactions reflects the decrease of tinnitus-induced activation of the autonomic nervous system.

From the diagram of the neurophysiological model of tinnitus (Fig. 2.10c) and principles of reinforcement of conditioned reflexes involved in tinnitus (Fig. 2.13), it is clear that the crucial factor is whether we can detach the reaction of the autonomic nervous system (which is causing annoyance and other negative reactions evoked by tinnitus) from the tinnitus signal (Fig. 2.15a). In other words, if we can produce habituation of the tinnitus reaction, then the patient will not be bothered in any way by tinnitus. This, in itself, would be a fundamental achievement that would create major relief for the tinnitus sufferer, as all the important distressing symptoms we have discussed would disappear.

Habituation of tinnitus perception takes place when tinnitus-related neuronal activity is identified, blocked by the auditory neuronal networks and is not allowed to reach the area of the cortex where conscious perception of the tinnitus sound occurs.

Following habituation of the reaction, another important process takes place automatically but slowly. This is the habituation of perception (Fig. 2.15b). In this

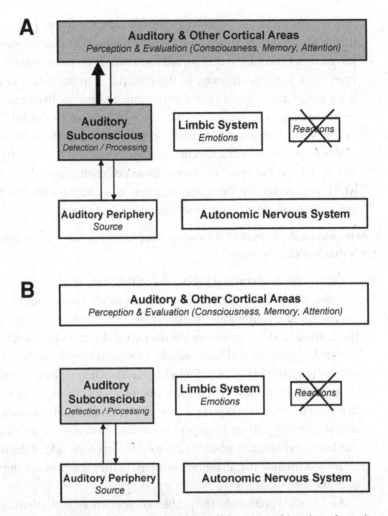

Figure 2.15 Mechanisms of habituation of reaction and perception. (A) Habituation of reaction reflects the disappearance of activation of the limbic and autonomic nervous systems. (B) Habituation of perception prevents the signal from reaching higher cortical areas involved in signal awareness.

case, tinnitus-related neuronal activity is identified, blocked by auditory neuronal networks and not allowed to reach the area of the cortex where conscious perception of the tinnitus sound occurs. As a result, the patient will no longer be aware of the tinnitus.

Habituation is not a "cure" for tinnitus. Tinnitus can still be perceived when attention is focused on it, but there is no reaction to tinnitus and awareness is greatly reduced.

Note that habituation is not a "cure" for tinnitus. Tinnitus can still be perceived when attention is focused on it, almost always softer, but occasionally its perception may remain the same.[10] Tinnitus loudness match, pitch and the ability to suppress it with sound may be unchanged by habituation. The crucial point is that there is no reaction to tinnitus following full habituation, and awareness is greatly reduced. Even when patients are aware of tinnitus, this is unimportant to them because it is no longer associated with any annoyance or distress. In conclusion, the clinical goal is to achieve habituation of the reaction induced by tinnitus, which will then be followed automatically by habituation of tinnitus perception.

While this sounds attractive, the question remains of how it can be achieved. How can we retrain the brain to reverse these powerful conditioned reflex responses, which are created by the initial negative associations with tinnitus and further enhanced by the vicious circle we have described above?

Plasticity of the brain is the basis of all learning and memory; it is needed for continuous adjustment to constantly changing circumstances.

One of the fundamental properties of the brain is its ability to undergo plastic changes. Plasticity of the brain is the basis of all learning and memory, and it is needed for the continuous adjustment to constantly changing circumstances in the outside world. These adjustments occur at a conscious level (e.g., learning a foreign language) as well as at a subconscious level involving the acquisition of new reflexes (e.g., driving a car, riding a bicycle, dancing, playing a musical instrument or golf). To keep these reflexes working properly, for example to keep your golf handicap down, it is necessary to practice techniques and continuously to enhance and strengthen reflexes by repetitive action. If necessary, we can actively adapt our learned reflexes, as when we drive on the opposite side of the road in a foreign country; consequently, all reflexes involved in the process of driving will be changed to fit the new situation.

As discussed previously, the problems experienced with tinnitus result from the creation of inappropriate reflex arcs between the auditory system and the limbic and autonomic nervous systems. Certain structures in the brain have been trained to react both very strongly and in a defensive manner to what is, in fact, a harmless signal (tinnitus-related neuronal activity).[11]

Even if the patient becomes totally convinced that tinnitus is harmless, these conditioned reflexes will remain for some time. To dissociate tinnitus from the

---

[10] With prolonged full TRT treatment, about 20% of patients will be unable to perceive tinnitus for some period of time, even when focusing on it (Sheldrake, Jastreboff & Hazell, 1996). While this is not permanent habituation, it can be considered as total.

[11] For example, if a subject participates in an experiment in which short presentations of a sound occur in a random and unpredictable manner a few times a day, each followed by a very unpleasant electrical shock, this will rapidly result in the development of a strong reaction whenever subsequent sounds are presented, even if they are not accompanied by a shock. Any kind of sound can result in a similar strong reaction if used with this protocol. Similarly, any kind of tinnitus sound can result in a very strong reaction of the autonomic and limbic nervous system, regardless of how it is perceived.

reflex responses induced by its negative associations, it is necessary purposefully to retrain these reflexes so that the strong link between tinnitus-related neuronal activity and the limbic and autonomic nervous systems is abolished.

Dissociation can occur at two levels. First, we might block the activation of the autonomic nervous system resulting from tinnitus-related activity (Fig. 2.15a). On achieving this, the patient will still perceive the sound of tinnitus with unchanged awareness, but this will no longer be followed by reaction of the autonomic nervous system and the patient will not be annoyed or bothered by tinnitus. At this stage, tinnitus will have the same lack of meaning as the sound of a refrigerator in the kitchen, and it can be heard without any feelings of unpleasantness. This habituation of reaction follows the classical definition of habituation, in which the reaction to the stimulus gradually disappears with repeated exposure to a stimulus, and without any positive or negative reinforcement (Thompson, 1987). We refer to this phenomenon as *habituation of reaction* throughout this book.

The second type of habituation, *habituation of perception*, occurs when the tinnitus-related neuronal activity is constrained from reaching the cortical level of awareness (Fig. 2.15b). In this situation, tinnitus-related activity will not reach the level of the cortex at which its conscious perception would occur; as a result, the patient will not be aware of the presence of tinnitus. It is sufficient to achieve a state in which the patient is not aware of the presence of tinnitus the majority of the time, and when awareness does occur for short periods, it does not lead to annoyance. Consequently, the tinnitus ceases to have any impact on the patient's life.

The habituation approach can be used to treat tinnitus regardless of its etiology.

An important consequence of this treatment approach is that, since the level of the brain where habituation occurs is above the source of tinnitus, the etiology or initial trigger of tinnitus is irrelevant. Therefore, the same treatment can be used for tinnitus from any cause. It is irrelevant whether tinnitus emerges after damage of the inner ear induced by loud sounds, aminoglycoside antibiotics, infection or an ear operation, and whether it occurs in a patient with normal hearing or hearing loss. The approach based on habituation of tinnitus can be applied and be an equally effective treatment in every patient regardless of its etiology; consequently, there is no need for preselecting patients for the treatment.

2.10   A clinical approach to induce habituation of tinnitus

Any stimulus, providing that it does not have negative associations, can be habituated. As long as a stimulus is related to danger, is inducing fear or is simply causing a high level of activation of negative emotions for whatever reason, habituation cannot occur or can progress only at a very slow rate. Therefore, to achieve habituation of tinnitus, the patient must be convinced that its perception is not related to a disease, but it is rather a harmless side effect of compensation within the auditory system. Presenting and discussing data supporting this concept are crucial in initiating habituation of tinnitus. Many patients arrive with a strong, preconceived idea that tinnitus is linked to some disease, injury, hearing disorder or unspecified health problems.

Even when the patient totally believes that tinnitus is harmless, the reactions of the limbic and autonomic nervous systems, resulting from a conditioned response, will still cause the brain and body to respond as in the past. Therefore, there is a need to change the reflexes responsible for the tinnitus-induced reactions. Working on beliefs about tinnitus, while an important part of the treatment in some cases, is not sufficient on its own to remove the reaction of the limbic and autonomic nervous system that occurs as the result of a conditioned reflex reaction.

2.10.1 TRT counseling

Counseling/teaching sessions aim to reclassify tinnitus into the category of neutral stimuli, remove the negative connotation from tinnitus and thus allow habituation to occur.

The first stage of our habituation-based treatment is teaching the patient about tinnitus; to convey the message that tinnitus by itself is harmless and does not reflect a serious health hazard. At this moment, we cannot reach the limbic system and its connections directly, so the counseling/teaching sessions are the method of choice to reclassify tinnitus into a category of neutral stimuli, remove the negative connotation from tinnitus and thus allow habituation to occur. In doing this, we are reclassifying tinnitus from an important "necessary to monitor" problem to something neutral, which can be potentially controlled and blocked. One of the consequences of counseling is reduced activation of the limbic and autonomic nervous systems from the level of the cortex (Fig. 2.16). The goal is to create a situation where tinnitus achieves a neutral status and the brain starts to reduce and subsequently block spreading of tinnitus-related neuronal activity to the limbic and autonomic nervous systems. This will result in decreased activation of these systems, facilitating habituation.

"Demystification" of tinnitus is an important part of the process of inducing habituation.

"Demystification" of tinnitus is an important part of the process of inducing habituation. It is based on the observation that the reaction of the autonomic nervous system and its effect on our body is much smaller to a known than to an unknown event. The same is true about a situation that is predictable, in contrast to one that is not. With tinnitus, even when the patient is still thinking

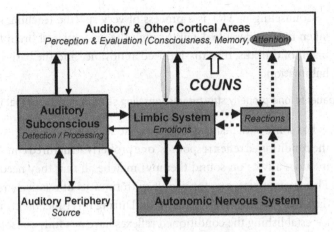

Figure 2.16 Effects of TRT counseling alone. Counseling (*COUNS*) affects cortical areas and may decrease descending connections from cortex to subcortical centers (indicated by the open arrow). Thickness of arrows and darkness of the boxes indicates the strength of the signal and activation of the given system. Note that the activation of limbic and autonomic nervous systems may remain the same, as the signal from the subcortical centers is not changing. Some decrease of the activation of the autonomic nervous systems might occur through the positive effect of tinnitus reclassification into a category of non-significant stimuli.

of it as unpleasant and negative, the effect of understanding the mechanisms by which tinnitus is generated is quite profound. Once it is understood that it is not the tinnitus sound itself that is responsible directly for the high level of annoyance and anxiety, but instead functional connections between tinnitus and reactions, this understanding typically leads to a rapid decrease of tinnitus-induced distress.

Tinnitus distress arises from the correct reaction to the wrong stimulus.

Tinnitus reclassification is achieved by giving the patient new concepts about the mechanisms of tinnitus and the distress caused by it. The perception of tinnitus results from a side effect of compensation in the auditory system to otherwise frequently irrelevant changes (e.g., small patches of missing OHCs; see Ch. 1). Reaction of the brain and body reflecting activation of the limbic and autonomic nervous systems would be appropriate if there really was a problem. So tinnitus distress arises from the correct reaction to the wrong stimulus.

Counseling in TRT is a very specific teaching method in which patients are taught the principles of brain function, the mechanisms of tinnitus and of tinnitus-induced annoyance, and the basis for achieving tinnitus habituation.

Counseling in TRT is a process of very specific teaching in which patients are taken in considerable detail through the principles of brain function, the mechanisms of tinnitus, tinnitus-induced annoyance and the basis for achieving tinnitus habituation.

For some patients, one properly structured counseling session may be all that is needed.

For some patients, depending on the severity of the tinnitus and the strength of the conditioned reflex responses, one properly structured counseling session (which includes advice on sound therapy) may be all that they need (Ch. 3, category 0). This is often also true for people with tinnitus of relatively recently onset, within days or a few weeks of the first visit. During this time, the connections responsible for establishing the conditioned reflexes have not fully consolidated and can more easily be changed.

2.10.2   Sound therapy

Sound therapy is the second component of TRT. Its main goal is to decrease the strength of the tinnitus signal within the brain.

Sound therapy is the second component of TRT. It should be noted that sound therapy alone is not effective and must be accompanied by proper counseling. The main goal of sound therapy is to decrease the strength of the tinnitus signal within the brain. There are several features that characterize the processing of neuronal signals in the brain and the mechanisms of perception.

If the level of environmental sound decreases, then amplification within the auditory system increases.

It has been shown that practically everybody experiences temporary tinnitus if put into a quiet environment (Ch. 1; Heller & Bergman, 1953). As a rule, patients with tinnitus find that their tinnitus seems much louder and more intrusive in a quiet room. These observations reflect two mechanisms involved in controlling the auditory system. First, if the level of environmental sound decreases, then amplification (including enhancement of pattern recognition) increases within the auditory system. As a result, even weak sounds can cause strong excitation of cortical areas and be perceived as loud. In a silent environment, the auditory gain increases to the point where natural fluctuations of background spontaneous activity could be perceived as tinnitus.

Our senses react not to the absolute value of a stimulus but to the difference or contrast between stimulus and background.

The second factor reflects the fact that our senses react not to the absolute value of a stimulus but rather to the difference or contrast between stimulus and background.

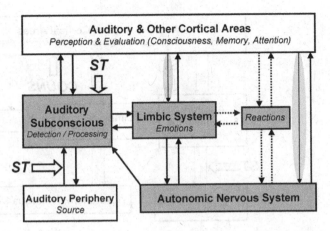

Figure 2.17 Effects of sound therapy alone. Sound therapy (*ST*) decreases the signal reaching, and the level of excitation in subcortical auditory centers, cortical areas and consequently in the limbic and autonomic nervous systems. Since tinnitus remains classified as an important signal, the initial decrease of reaction is reversed by feedback loops and any potential improvement cannot be maintained.

The same signal – sound, light or temperature – can be perceived as strong or weak depending on the background level present. The light of a small candle is perceived as very bright in a darkened room but appears much weaker in full sunshine. The noise of a moving chair in a busy restaurant is scarcely noticed while in a quiet classroom it will create a significant disturbance. Consequently, tinnitus appears to be much louder and more intrusive when the patient is in a quiet environment, even if the source of tinnitus remains unchanged. Additionally, because of enhanced pattern recognition, tinnitus can be detected even with higher levels of other competing signals. Consequently, tinnitus can be heard not only in a quiet environment but also detected in high levels of environmental sound.

By enhancing environmental sound, we can effectively decrease the strength of the tinnitus signal and reduce activation of the limbic and autonomic nervous systems.

The difference between signal and background can be used in a positive manner to facilitate habituation of tinnitus. By enhancing the environmental sound to which the patient is exposed, we can effectively decrease the strength of the tinnitus signal as it passes from the auditory periphery up to the cortex. This will, in turn, reduce activation of the limbic and autonomic nervous systems (Fig. 2.17) and decrease annoyance which acts as a negative reinforcement. Therefore, all patients are advised to avoid silence.

Once the tinnitus signal becomes weaker, the process of habituation will be facilitated. Gradual reduction of the conditioned reflexes involved in creating reactions

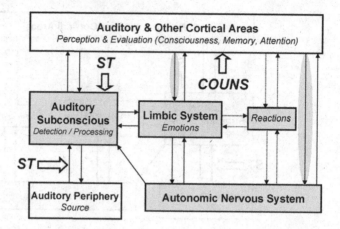

Figure 2.18 Combined effect of counseling (*COUNS*) and sound therapy (*ST*). Under this condition, all connections will weaken, and activation of all centers involved will lessen. This will promote a final blockage of connections between the auditory system and the limbic and autonomic nervous systems (habituation of reaction), and of the connections between the subconscious and conscious levels of the auditory system (habituation of perception).

to tinnitus and its perception will follow, as described above. The combined effects of counseling and sound therapy are shown in Fig. 2.18.

2.10.3 Active continued promotion of habituation

Within the neurophysiological model of tinnitus, there is continuous counteraction of two opposing forces, tinnitus-induced aversive reaction and habituation (Fig. 2.19). Once established, the tinnitus-induced conditioned reflexes enhance activation of the limbic and autonomic nervous systems, resulting in annoyance and leading to increased awareness and severity of tinnitus. The process of habituation works in the opposite direction. If the conditioned response is dominant, then tinnitus will persist and become stronger (moving the balance toward persistent tinnitus and induced reactions). If habituation is dominant, then the balance moves towards weakening of the tinnitus. Consequently, continuous promotion of habituation is needed during the treatment. This is achieved by active follow-up contacts, during which counseling promoting habituation is performed. Compliance with specific treatment protocol, including systematic follow-up contacts, assures the successful outcome of TRT.

2.11 Summary of the model

The essential feature of the neurophysiological model of tinnitus is its postulate that systems outside the auditory pathway are responsible for the severity of tinnitus. The difference between someone simply experiencing tinnitus and someone being

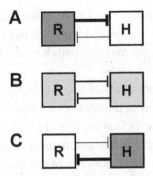

Figure 2.19 Tinnitus-induced reaction versus strength of habituation. Reactions induced by tinnitus (R) are a manifestation of the strength of conditioned reflexes connecting the auditory with the limbic and autonomic nervous systems. Habituation (H) is aimed at weakening and finally removing these reflexes. The systems involved in enhancement and weakening are connected reciprocally in an inhibitory manner; as a result the systems tend to remain in one of two stages, with one of the subsystems being dominant (like a light switch). (A) The reactions are dominant (darkened block), inhibiting potential spontaneous habituation of tinnitus and resulting in a strong reaction to tinnitus. Active decrease of the tinnitus signal (by sound therapy) and of the limbic and autonomic nervous system reactions (by counseling to explain tinnitus and allow its reclassification as neutral stimuli) brings both forces towards a balance. To sustain this balance a continuous effort is needed by procedures aimed at inducing habituation. (B) When the action of both systems is equal, the tinnitus-induced reactions will be further automatically decreased by inhibitory feedback loops in the system, without the need for active intervention. (C) Eventually, the reactions are effectively attenuated. As all these processes require plastic changes to occur within the nervous system, the timescale of treatment is measured in weeks and months in order to establish a new, stable state with permanent habituation of tinnitus.

annoyed or distressed by it depends exclusively on the activation of the limbic and autonomic nervous systems. The limbic system plays a crucial role by preventing habituation of the tinnitus signal, enhancing its perception and altering the activity of the autonomic nervous system, which is responsible for the majority of the patient's symptoms. The activity of the limbic and autonomic nervous systems is influenced by both subconscious connections and a pathway involving (cortical) awareness, which is involved in conscious verbalized thinking, and concerns about tinnitus. The initial negative associations of tinnitus results in increased activation of both the limbic and autonomic nervous systems.

All the systems involved in tinnitus are cross-connected, creating the possibility of feedback loops/vicious circles. One of these vicious circles involves attention to tinnitus. Any stimulus that has a negative meaning will, as a general rule, attract attention proportional to its significance. The increased attention results in enhanced significance of this particular stimulus: increased significance results in increased awareness, creating self-enhancing feedback loop. This effect is further strengthened by our limited ability to pay attention to more than one thing at a time. Consequently, many patients have the impression that they are aware of their tinnitus 100% of the time.

Similar enhancements of tinnitus happen at a subconscious level through the direct connections of the auditory and extra-auditory systems involved. Both conscious and subconscious centers are governed by the principles of conditioned reflexes: as such, they occur automatically and are difficult to reverse without appropriate retraining. In the absence of retraining, this reflex tends to strengthen with ever increasing levels of limbic and autonomic activity. This can reach a level of saturation, when the patient is constantly aware of, and distressed by, the tinnitus (the "worst case scenario").

When the final level of activation of the limbic and autonomic nervous systems is reached, and thence the annoyance and anxiety created by tinnitus peak, the initial perception of tinnitus, which reflects the strength of the tinnitus-related neuronal activity, is of secondary importance. The mechanisms responsible for creating and sustaining reactions are based on self-enhancing conditioned reflex loops. Subconscious levels of the brain are dominant in this process. Patients have no direct control of these processes any more than it is possible to alter directly blood pressure or other automatic body functions by thinking.

All mechanisms involved in emergence of tinnitus perception and tinnitus-evoked distress represent the natural defense of the individual to potential danger and should not be interpreted as a psychological or psychiatric malfunction. However, certain psychological states, such as obsessive behavior or somatic anxiety, may favor the development of tinnitus distress.

The neurophysiological model outlined in this chapter leads directly to TRT, which is described in more detail in subsequent chapters. The information in this chapter is used when the principles of the model are explained to patients. The summary of the neurophysiological model of tinnitus and of TRT are presented in several recent publications (Jastreboff & Jastreboff, 2001c, 2003a,b).

3

Tinnitus retraining therapy (TRT): clinical implementation of the model

In the previous chapter, the theoretical basis of the neurophysiological model and its clinical implications were presented. This chapter is devoted to the practical implementation of the model in the form of TRT, stressing the points that are crucial for successful treatment. Forms for initial and follow-up interviews are attached in the appendices. This chapter contains the information necessary to treat straightforward cases of tinnitus and hyperacusis. Both theory and practical information are shown, as presented to the patient during counseling sessions. For successful implementation of TRT, the professional must have a complete knowledge of the mechanisms of tinnitus as described in the neurophysiological model of tinnitus and, consequently, should not confine reading to this chapter. As with any other clinical method, TRT cannot be learned from reading material alone; specific training and practice are needed to achieve proficiency.

3.1 Outline of tinnitus retraining therapy

The clinical implementation of the neurophysiological model of tinnitus in TRT is based on two fundamental properties of brain function: its plasticity (the ability to learn new reflexes and relearn previously acquired ones) and its natural tendency to eliminate (habituate) reactions to irrelevant stimuli and any perception induced by them. Therefore, once we remove the negative associations of the tinnitus signal, gradual habituation should occur.

Once we remove the negative associations of the tinnitus signal, gradual habituation should occur.

With tinnitus and misophonia, habituation involves separate brain systems. First, there is habituation of the reactions to tinnitus (autonomic nervous system) and, second, there is habituation of perception (blocking of the tinnitus-related neuronal activity within the auditory pathways before it reaches the level of awareness). Since we do not have a means of direct control over subconscious areas of the brain, the only way to bring about change is to remove negative associations gradually, by providing patients with knowledge about the mechanisms involved in the generation of their tinnitus and its distress. Typically, the main reason for developing negative associations about tinnitus is the patient's lack of knowledge about tinnitus mechanisms, converted into concerns and fears by negative counseling provided by some professionals or visits to Internet tinnitus groups. This results in a build up of fear about an unknown danger or a sense that tinnitus is indeed something to be feared or concerned about. Naturally, these will induce stress and anxiety.

The etiology, cause or trigger of tinnitus is totally irrelevant, and tinnitus retraining can be used in every tinnitus sufferer.

It should be stressed that TRT is aimed at modifying neuronal connections in centers that are separate from the centers responsible for the generation of tinnitus-related neuronal activity (the tinnitus source). Consequently, the etiology, cause or trigger of tinnitus is totally irrelevant, and TRT can be used in every tinnitus patient without need for any preselection of patients.

TRT consists of two principal components: retraining counseling and sound therapy.

Sound therapy facilitates tinnitus habituation by decreasing the strength of the tinnitus signal.

TRT consists of two principal components: TRT counseling and sound therapy.

3.1.1 Principles of retraining counseling

Retraining counseling is aimed at reclassification of tinnitus by the patient into a category of neutral, or only mildly negative, signals to enable habituation of tinnitus.

Retraining counseling (teaching sessions) is an indispensable and crucial part of TRT. By teaching patients the components of the neurophysiological model of tinnitus, patients are encouraged to reclassify their tinnitus as a neutral or only mildly negative signal. During this session, tinnitus is explained and converted into a phenomenon that has predictable behavior and consequences. Furthermore, the principles of the treatment are explained on the basis of the model, including habituation, as a way of taking tinnitus under control. A significant part of counseling is devoted to the role of sound in the therapy, the mechanisms of sound action in facilitating habituation and the specifics of various sounds (e.g., sound of nature, music, speech) on brain function and behavior. Last but not least, specific and realistic expectations are discussed.

3.1.2 Sound therapy

Sound therapy is always included in TRT but does not necessarily involve the use of instrumentation. Sound therapy facilitates tinnitus habituation by decreasing the strength of the tinnitus signal. In practice, this is achieved by instructions to the patient to avoid silence and to enrich the background sound environment, for example by the use of table-top sound machines or, frequently, by wearable sound generators. For patients with significant hearing loss, the enriched background sound is further amplified by hearing aids.

Supplemental therapies aimed at stress reduction or improvement of well-being are helpful but not a required part of TRT.

3.1.3 The basic protocol

TRT is a structured approach, involving assessment, treatment categorization, specific counseling and sound therapy, over an extended period.

TRT is a structured treatment comprising an initial visit and follow-up appointments. An introductory contact with the prospective patient is important to help in making decisions about engaging in the complete TRT protocol. The initial visit consists of taking the tinnitus history, audiological evaluation, medical evaluation, TRT counseling and fitting of instruments, where appropriate. Follow-up contacts are important for monitoring the progress of treatments and introducing modifications if needed. In most patients, treatment is closed during the first 18 months from the initial visit.

TRT may be divided into the following stages:

1. Introductory contact
2. Initial visit
    i. taking history of tinnitus, decreased sound tolerance and hearing loss
    ii. audiological evaluation
    iii. medical evaluation
    iv. assessing the category for treatment
    v. giving appropriate TRT counseling including introduction to sound therapy
3. Fitting of instruments (where appropriate) and counseling regarding their role and use
4. Follow-up visits: evaluation of the patient's status and further counseling
5. Closing the treatment.

3.2 Initial visit and evaluation

Distressed tinnitus patients have a tendency to seek information everywhere, search the web, read literature, participate in various bulletin boards and contact available centers where they believe help might be found. Therefore, it is necessary to be prepared for lengthy telephone calls, letters, faxes, e-mails, etc. Personnel should be trained to identify and handle separately seriously distressed patients, who might require an urgent appointment or even intermediate referral for psychological or psychiatric treatment. Specially prepared written materials are sent to the prospective patient containing general information about TRT, the treatment center, the personnel involved, a questionnaire and appointment forms. Patients are asked to read the material and we encourage patients to visit our web pages (www.tinnitus-pjj.com and www.tinnitus.org) to get further information before making any decision about enrolling in the treatment. If they decide to follow the treatment with us, all that is needed is to fill in the forms and send them back to us. Only then is the appointment scheduled. In every interaction with a prospective patient, it is essential to avoid any negative statements (potential negative counseling) and to convey the message that an effective treatment is available, without attempting to provide specific counseling, as this, without proper evaluation, could bring additional anxiety and confusion.

3.2.1   Initial interview and taking a history

A detailed interview is crucial for proper diagnosis and consequently treatment. Results of medical and audiological evaluation, while needed, will be insufficient for this purpose on their own. A sufficient amount of time and resources needs to be committed to this process.

Before meeting personally with a patient, the general medical and tinnitus questionnaires received back from the patients are reviewed. This allows for basic evaluation of a patient's status and helps in the first personal contact with the patient. The questionnaires save time during an initial visit as well, since past medical history, medications and their dosage need only to be checked, rather than thoroughly investigated. It is easier for patients to answer questions in the privacy of their own home, without any of the time restriction or stress that might be induced by an office visit. Moreover, patients will feel less of a need to describe a detailed history of their problems during the office visit, as they know they have already supplied the information, and time can be devoted to investigating the points of importance for diagnosis.

Taking a proper history, using TRT interview forms, is essential in selecting the correct treatment category.

During an open discussion with the patient, general information related to tinnitus is gathered. This discussion follows a structured interview form (Appendix 1), on which the interviewer records the patient's responses. The initial interview helps to evaluate the patient's problem and the degree of distress caused by it. Together with the outcome of the medical assessment and results of the audiological evaluation, the interview provides crucial information needed for choosing the appropriate protocol for treatment, as well as indicates the proper direction for counseling. Additionally, interview forms contain data that serve as a reference for future assessment of the treatment outcome. The questions are asked in a neutral manner, using carefully chosen words. Specific questions are provided in the legend of the interview form (see Appendix 1) and Henry *et al.* [2003], which contains detailed instructions.

There is no evidence that tinnitus and hyperacusis are inherited disorders, although this is possible. A pattern of tinnitus experience and reaction to it in another family member, with attendant anxiety and other emotional behavioral responses, can be a learning environment for patients; consequently recording this information is useful, especially for counseling. It is important to identify any factors that may enhance or attenuate tinnitus or hyperacusis. Often these will be emotional or stress factors, but the cyclical behavior of tinnitus may also be related to exposure to certain sounds or it simply reflects the natural circadian rhythm of the body.

Part of the problem with tinnitus is that some patients have unfounded negative thoughts about tinnitus: tinnitus will get worse; tinnitus will go on forever; tinnitus is a physical disease; there is no treatment available for tinnitus; sleep deprivation is likely; increasing deafness will result; it will make me go mad; it may be caused by a tumor; my ability to cope will be severely affected; my family life will be severely affected; I will permanently lose the enjoyment of silence. These worries induce anxiety. They almost always prove to be unfounded, but their presence has a powerful effect in promoting the problem and enhancing symptoms.

The patient's concerns may be assessed by various methods. One approach is to ask the patient to say why tinnitus is a problem for them, or what their concerns are, and to list all the negative associations that they can think of. It is important not to be too directive in this questioning because it can lead to a bias in the answers and misdirect subsequent counseling. This approach avoids suggesting to patients negative thoughts and associations that they did not have already.

Additionally, many patients have tinnitus-induced annoyance, without any fear or association that they are able to put into words. It is important to remember that the severity of tinnitus does not relate to the number of negative concepts about tinnitus. A single negative belief, if very powerful and strongly held, can have a profound effect on tinnitus and its severity.

It is a common practice of professionals working with tinnitus patients to focus on the etiology of the tinnitus or its triggering factors, usually concentrating on those related to the cochlea. It was shown, however, that the onset of clinically relevant tinnitus in 75% is related to emotional or stress factors experienced by the patient, rather than something related to their ears (Hazell & McKinney, 1996). This further supports the postulate that clinically relevant tinnitus is related to the activation of systems other than the auditory system, particularly emotional centers. In TRT, triggering factors are secondary and do not significantly affect the treatment.

In 75% of those with tinnitus, the triggering factor is not related to the ear or hearing.

In those with hyperacusis, the trigger is commonly one of acute exposure to loud sound. While it is not clear if this itself is a crucial factor, this episode frequently initiates a practice of extreme overprotection of hearing, so that earplugs and ear defenders or muffs are worn even in an environment of social noise. While temporarily helpful, this approach greatly enhances the development of hyperacusis. It is usual for these patients to believe that there has been serious damage to their ears, whether or not this proves to be the case. They frequently exhibit a strong misophonic or phonophobic state as well. To plan an effective treatment, it is essential to assess the degree of misophonia that is present in each patient.

Acquiring a complete and detailed history of tinnitus, and other related problems such as decreased sound tolerance and hearing loss, is very important. It gives us information about the patient's experience of tinnitus, its progress and the various aspects of tinnitus problems particularly bothersome to the patient. It allows us to develop an assessment of the personality of the patient, which will have an impact on the TRT approach. Skilled clinicians will detect the presence of psychological disturbance, which may need separate management by appropriate specialists. It is crucial during this session to establish contact, rapport and a feeling of mutual trust between the patient and those who will be involved in TRT during the treatment period. TRT counseling, which is performed later on, is highly specific to each individual patient and requires personal adjustment for its optimal outcome.

Psychological disturbance may require separate management.

With the exception of measuring pure tone thresholds and loudness discomfort levels, taking an adequate history is the single most important step in making a proper categorization of the tinnitus or hyperacusis, in deciding the appropriate treatment strategy and in creating a firm basis for effective counseling. Therefore sufficient time (at least 30 minutes) must be allowed for this stage.

Subjective description of tinnitus and decreased sound tolerance

It is a common observation that patients like to talk about the sounds they experience. They typically believe that detailed description of these sounds is important for success of the treatment. Frequently they search their environment for the tinnitus sound, or for sounds that are similar; in reality, psychoacoustical characterization of tinnitus has no bearing on the treatment and its outcome. However, starting with this information helps to initiate discussion and shows a real interest in the patient's complaints.

Discussion about the character of tinnitus and decreased sound tolerance opens and facilitates dialog with a patient.

The onset and emergence of tinnitus (e.g., whether sudden or gradual) and progress to its present state are recorded, together with fluctuations of loudness or perceived pitch, any periods of remission that may occur, the various sounds perceived and their apparent localization. Enquire whether the sounds appear to be grouped and acting as one entity, or whether they change independently of each other. The main reason for collecting this information is that sounds which are highly fluctuating may be more difficult to habituate to than those that are stable. Any reduction in tinnitus perception that has already taken place may indicate that spontaneous habituation is occurring already. Take notes of any reported hypersensitivity to environmental sounds. Patients may report that some external sounds are more troublesome than others. Some patients have decreased sound tolerance before tinnitus starts (Hazell & Sheldrake, 1992); in addition, these two symptoms commonly coexist. Decreased sound tolerance may be experienced to loud sounds such as traffic but also to relatively quiet sounds such as kitchen noises or conversation. Create an inventory of sounds that cause discomfort and those which do not trouble the patient. Inquire about the use of ear protection; in which situations and how frequently it is used. Ask in detail about the auditory environment in which the patient works and lives. It is important to establish how much time during an average week the patient is in an environment with very low level sound, in a quiet environment (e.g., where speech may be heard without raising the voice) or in a noisy environment. This is helpful later when advising about sound enrichment.

Misophonia and phonophobia often reflect the concern that external sound may damage the ear or the hearing. This concept is common in patients whose symptoms may have been initially triggered by exposure to a loud noise (even when no damage has actually occurred). The sounds disliked or feared do not have to be very loud but simply belong to the same category of sound (such as loud music, a slammed door, etc.) that was initially thought to be responsible for the onset of symptoms.

Almost all patients with hyperacusis have some degree of misophonia.

Almost all patients with hyperacusis have some degree of misophonia, particularly patients who experience hyperacusis for a long time (Jastreboff & Jastreboff, 2002). As the treatments for hyperacusis and for misophonia are different, the proper diagnosis is crucial. Since loudness discomfort levels (LDLs) are not sufficient to discriminate between hyperacusis and misophonia, a detailed interview is vital for proper diagnosis.

Effects of tinnitus on daily life

It is important to establish the effects of tinnitus and decreased sound tolerance on the individual's life. Patients are asked what specific activities are interfered with by tinnitus and by decreased sound tolerance (when applicable). Tinnitus may be affecting concentration at work or it may be less noticeable during these periods when attention is focused away from the symptoms. In the worst situation, the patient may be unable to work and is on disability leave. During the interviews, we ask about specific activities prevented or interfered with by tinnitus and by hyperacusis (Appendix 1). Note that this standard list of activities is an open list, with options, to encourage the patient to identify any activity with which the tinnitus problem interferes. These questions are of particular importance, as they are part of the criteria for evaluating treatment outcome and reflect on the patient's quality of life.

Assessing the effects of tinnitus on daily life is essential in evaluating the severity of symptoms as well as treatment outcome.

Sleep disturbance is a common and particularly pronounced early experience of tinnitus. It may affect getting off to sleep or getting back to sleep on waking during the night. Tinnitus does not on its own wake an individual, nor is it commonly experienced during dreaming. Prolonged sleep disturbance is very stressful and exhausting and may produce a number of secondary effects (problems with concentration, emotional stability, irritability, etc.) that enhance tinnitus persistence and severity. In addition, tinnitus may be greatly enhanced following sleep, even short cat naps, and this is an issue that needs to be addressed later during counseling. In the elderly, periods of wakefulness are more frequent because of a natural decrease in the duration of the sleep cycle. This might contribute to increased reports of night-time tinnitus in the elderly.

Information about the patient's basic background and basic psychological profile are helpful during counseling. Therefore, inquire about depression, anxiety, panic attacks and phobic or aversive reactions, noting if they have occurred before or after the tinnitus or hyperacusis started. These questions must be posed with great sensitivity. Ask the patient whether they think these feelings are the cause or result of the tinnitus or decreased sound tolerance. Establish areas of stress that may be present in the patient's work or social environment. Ask about their educational background, occupation and hobbies. In some cases, interference by tinnitus and hyperacusis with quiet recreational activities and hobbies may have more of an impact on the quality of life than problems created at work.

Establishing the patient's own assessment of the interrelation of tinnitus and hearing loss

The majority of patients have some hearing loss in addition to tinnitus and decreased sound tolerance. Frequently, these patients come with the misconception that the tinnitus is actually responsible for the problems with hearing, that tinnitus masks their hearing and if the tinnitus was removed then their hearing would be normal.

These patients should be clearly identified and the issue discussed in detail during the counseling sessions. There is experimental evidence showing that tinnitus does not act as a masker of external sounds (Levi & Chisin, 1987) and cannot interfere in this way with hearing.

Scoring of tinnitus, decreased sound tolerance and hearing loss

In our interview form (Appendix 1), we invite patients to score important variables in a specific manner. Patients are asked to estimate the percentage of waking hours when they are aware of tinnitus and the percentage of waking hours when tinnitus is annoying or creates anxiety. This helps to differentiate between the perception of and the reaction to tinnitus. In describing tinnitus awareness, we ask not only how much of the time the patient is aware of tinnitus but also what percentage of the time the patient is annoyed by it. This gives an indication of whether some degree of habituation is already occurring. It is useful to know whether the tinnitus is getting better or worse, and whether there are certain times of day when it is worse.

Next, the severity of tinnitus, its annoyance and effect on life are ranked on a scale from 0 to 10, where zero represents an absence of the measured parameter and 10 indicates as great an effect as the patient can imagine. Nearly all patients automatically assume that severity and perceived loudness are the same. Since the interview is conducted before the counseling session, when the validity of this assumption will be challenged, patients are asked "how loud or severe is your tinnitus?" This phrasing is easier for patients to understand and avoids confusion. We fully realize that their responses in reality are related to the perceived loudness of their tinnitus.

Multilevel scales are used in the assessment of each parameter.

Almost identical sets of questions are asked about decreased sound tolerance, modified to reflect the differences between these two phenomena. For example, in the case of severity, zero indicates that the patient can tolerate all normal sounds and 10 that they cannot tolerate any sounds. The list of activities is similarly qualified.

The absolute values of these scores provide only a broad approximation of the severity of the assessed problems. In our practice, we see patients whose quality of life is severely affected (as evident from the interview) but who give answers with very low scores. On the other extreme, there are patients with minimally affected daily life who report all parameters to be "10." Of significance is the observation that, while there is a substantial variability of assessed severity and reported scores, the majority of patients are very consistent in their estimation of a given parameter from one visit to another. Note, that we are not revealing to patients their responses given in the past. It is typical that while patients are not improving they give practically the same numerical response as at the initial interview; once they start improving, then scores gradually change in a systematic manner.

When tinnitus or hyperacusis are enhanced by external sounds, it is crucial to obtain a reasonable estimate of the time taken for the tinnitus or hyperacusis to return to the pre-exposure level. This helps to identify patients who require a separate approach. It has been found that patients with prolonged symptoms after noise exposure (persisting after a good night's sleep) seem to have a less promising prognosis and require a specific approach to their treatment (category 4 patients).

As hearing loss will be assessed by a standard auditory evaluation in the next stage, the interview focuses on a subjective judgement of the extent of hearing loss and its interference with life. Patients are also asked if they have used hearing aids in the past, and to describe their experiences.

Finally, we ask patients to rank the importance, as a problem, of tinnitus, hearing loss and decreased sound tolerance. This ranking is helpful in deciding on the proper emphasis of treatment. If patients have a problem deciding the relative importance of these factors, we invite them to choose which they need most help with, if only one of these problems could be solved.

Since 1999, these questionnaires have been used for the evaluation of all patients in our clinics for initial visits and follow-up contacts.

3.2.2 Audiological evaluation

Audiological evaluation plays an important role, allowing for assessment of basic hearing status. In conjunction with the initial interview, it helps to determine the extent of hyperacusis and misophonia. It is also crucial when amplification is recommended as a part of therapy.

The audiological evaluation provides an assessment of the basic functions of the auditory system. In Ch. 2 it was argued that the auditory system is of secondary importance in tinnitus; however, changes in its activity can contribute to tinnitus enhancement and it is crucial in the development of hyperacusis. The audiological tests performed can be divided into crucial (needed for diagnosis and for carrying out treatment in an optimal way), useful but not necessary, and superfluous, which are performed because of historical, legal or other reasons.

Out of four measurements used for the classification of the patients (presented in detail further below), two involve audiological evaluation: the presence of hyperacusis and subjectively significant hearing loss. Consequently, the following audiological tests are crucial: Loudness discomfort level (LDL), for hyperacusis, and a pure-tone audiogram plus speech discrimination, for hearing loss. Note that these audiological tests alone are not sufficient for making the diagnosis; a detailed interview is essential, particularly to discriminate hyperacusis from misophonia. However, these tests, together with the initial interview, are sufficient for diagnosis and proceeding with TRT.

Pure tone audiometry and LDLs must be performed on each patient.

Distortion product otoacoustic emission (DPOAE) assessment is useful but not a necessary test. Its main usefulness is for counseling, where it is very helpful discussing the potential mechanisms of initiating the tinnitus signal, particularly when the function of outer hair cells (OHC) and their role in the emergence of tinnitus perception is discussed. On some occasions, it may indicate the presence of a peripheral component of hyperacusis. The threshold, most comfortable level and discomfort level for speech, while not necessary, provide quick approximations of potential hearing loss and decreased sound tolerance.

There are a number of tests that do not have a direct bearing on the management of tinnitus but are recorded because of their importance in audiological diagnosis or because of their traditional value as a tinnitus measurement. These include pitch matching, loudness matching and minimal suppression level (MSL: previously referred to as minimal masking level (MML)).

Tinnitus loudness and pitch bear no relationship to the severity of tinnitus, to its diagnosis or to the outcome of treatment.

Tinnitus loudness and pitch bear no relationship to the severity of tinnitus, to its diagnosis or to the outcome of treatment; consequently the details of their evaluation are not presented here. While MSL do not have a predictive value for the diagnosis and treatment outcome, they exhibit changes in group data related to habituation of perception (Jastreboff *et al.*, 1994). They indicate de-tuning of the neuronal networks that are involved in the detection of tinnitus-related neuronal activity (Jastreboff *et al.*, 1994). It is crucial to stress that measurements of MSL are irrelevant in treating individual patients by TRT: an equally successful outcome is experienced by patients regardless of whether their tinnitus can be suppressed by external sounds. Therefore, we will not discuss this measurement either. If desired, any generally accepted method can be used for measurements of tinnitus pitch, its loudness match and MSL (e.g., Tyler, 2000).

Many "tinnitus tests" have historical interest only and little validity.

Other tests for tinnitus may be used during counseling to provide a patient with a more detailed analysis of their tinnitus characteristics, but they are not useful otherwise. They might be required if the patient is involved in litigation. Acoustic impedance, as a routine audiological test evaluating the middle ear function, may be performed, but if DPOAE are present this test is redundant. We do not recommend doing acoustic reflexes as a routine, because approximately half of our patients exhibit decreased sound tolerance, and approximately 25–30% require specific treatment for hyperacusis. The reflexes, and particularly reflex decay, are performed when there is a suspicion of vestibular schwannoma. Acoustic impedance testing is most useful in counseling a patient with inappropriate beliefs about middle ear pathology, but it should always be performed after LDLs have been established and must never exceed these levels. We are not recommending auditory brainstem responses as these have not been shown to provide useful information about tinnitus and do not provide sufficient information to detect or reject the presence of vestibular schwannoma.

We have abandoned the test of residual inhibition (i.e., the change in tinnitus loudness after exposure to sound, typically for one minute at 10 dB above MSL, originally described by Feldmann (1971)) because this has not been found to have any clinical or scientific value. Although at one time there was an expectation that such an effect might have some therapeutic value, this was never achieved. From a neurophysiological standpoint, this phenomenon simply reflects the rebound effect, well-recognized in the neuroscience, in which the activity of neurons decreases below the level of spontaneous activity after a period of strong stimulation.

In practice, the following protocol is followed in our centers. All procedures are performed assuming the presence of decreased sound tolerance until proven otherwise. This approach prevents unintentional overstimulation of patients during testing, which could worsen their symptoms and make future interaction more difficult, because of loss of trust. Information from the initial interview allows appreciation of the potential for decreased sound tolerance. Careful otoscopic examination of the ears is needed; if significant wax accumulation is present, this should be removed. Precautions have to be taken, however, to ensure that the patient is not exposed to unnecessary loud sound during this procedure as this can aggravate symptoms or evoke hyperacusis or misophonia.

First the threshold, most comfortable listening level and the discomfort level for conversational running speech are evaluated, using 5 dB steps (smaller steps if hyperacusis is a concern, as evident from the initial interview). This step, while not essential, saves time by indicating the ranges of sound levels for pure tone audiogram and LDL. Next, a pure tone audiogram is obtained (air and bone conduction, when indicated) for both ears. We are recommending comprehensive audiometry with a wider frequency range and routine testing of the interoctaves: testing at 125, 250, 500 Hz, 1, 2, 3, 4, 6, 8 and 12 kHz. In addition to other factors, this expanded frequency range and increased frequency resolution is helpful for assessing the presence and extent of misophonia (Jastreboff & Jastreboff, 2000a).

Speech discrimination is performed at the most comfortable level and provides useful information when hearing aids are recommended. The perception of speech in noise by tinnitus patients is an interesting issue, though its potential is not yet clarified. It provides an indication of potential problems within central auditory processing. Interestingly, a proportion of patients with a central processing disorder, where patients have difficulty hearing speech in noise but have normal pure tone audiometric thresholds, also report tinnitus (Higson, Haggard & Field, 1994). There are no clear data, however, linking the presence of tinnitus to problems with central auditory processing.

Measurement of LDLs are essential for accurate treatment categorization.

Testing of LDL is of fundamental importance in classifying patients into treatment categories. LDLs reflect all components of decreased sound tolerance; that is, it presents a sum of the effects of hyperacusis and misophonia. As we are interested in differentiation between misophonia and hyperacusis, our protocol attempts to reduce the effect of misophonia on LDL measurements, so they reflect predominantly the effects of hyperacusis. Furthermore, care is taken to prevent overstimulation of the patient and to avoid inducing or enhancing misophonia. Since there are different ways of evaluating LDL, and there is no consensus on how they should be performed, it is advisable to follow the specific protocol that we are recommending. The protocol is as follows.

Testing is done with an intermittent test tone, which should be presented no faster than one per second to allow for enough time for consistent response (particularly important for elderly or highly anxious patients). Begin at the most comfortable level for running speech and increase in 5 dB steps (smaller steps if hyperacusis is a concern), testing for all frequencies for which the audiogram was evaluated. Patients are instructed that this is a test of tolerance for sound, so they should achieve as high a level as possible yet respond whenever the sound is uncomfortable. Patients should be assured that this is not an endurance test. All frequencies are tested twice to determine an accurate LDL (i.e., testing is performed for all frequencies and then repeated), and the second set of numbers is recorded on the audiogram. The specific instructions are given to patients: "We want to get past 'too loud' to where it would actually be uncomfortable;" "This is not an endurance test;" "I will stop immediately when you tell me that it is enough;" "Try to hold on as long as possible;" "This test cannot do any permanent damage to your hearing, or permanently make your tinnitus worse." The procedure should not alarm the patient or cause anxiety. The patient must at all times be relaxed and confident while doing this test. Do not perform the test if the patient specifically requests you not to do so. In almost all cases, even anxious patients become compliant when they understand the importance and relevance of the test. In some cases, this may not happen until after discussion of the neurophysiological model.

The issue of frequency dependence of the dynamic range (pure tone threshold subtracted from LDL) is particularly important for patients with hyperacusis and hearing loss. Because they have both an elevation of the threshold and a decrease in the maximal level of sound tolerated, typically the dynamic range is more reduced at high frequencies. Consequently, hyperacusis patients often complain about discomfort for sounds containing high-frequency components such as rattling cutlery, children's voices, distorted sound from loudspeakers. This is because with a very narrow dynamic range at high frequencies these sound create discomfort as soon as they are perceived.

LDLs can be assessed safely in all patients provided proper instructions and adequate counseling is given first, and the tester is aware of potential decreased sound tolerance.

Impedance audiometry is performed provided that the test will not exceed LDL values. Reflexes are performed routinely by Hazell and when needed by Jastreboff but only after measuring LDL. DPOAE assessment is performed last. The assessment uses 65/55 dB SPL primaries, 500 to 12 kHz frequency range, with 10 points per octave. In Hazell's clinic transient evoked otoacoustic emissions and audioscans (or Bekesy audiometry) are routinely performed as well.

3.2.3 Medical evaluation

The main purpose of medical evaluation is to detect any medical problems which may cause, contribute to or have an impact on the treatment of tinnitus. This is essential in creating the basis for reassurance that there is nothing medically wrong, requiring separate treatment, that can be linked to tinnitus or decreased sound tolerance.

The purpose of medical evaluation is to detect any medical problems which may impact on the treatment of tinnitus. A description of these problems, and an approach to their treatment, are presented in Ch. 6.

Medical evaluation is an important part of TRT protocol. As TRT can be provided by various professionals, it is necessary to have a definitive statement from an otolaryngologist, if not part of the team, that there are no medical problems which could be linked to tinnitus. If a medical problem is detected (such as vestibular schwannoma, Ménière's syndrome, etc.), it should be treated appropriately. Treating tinnitus with TRT but without an appropriate medical evaluation may remove tinnitus as a syndrome and delay/prevent proper treatment of an underlying condition.

A full medical evaluation is essential to exclude, or otherwise treat, any underlying tinnitus-related pathology, and to enable reassurance during counseling.

Medical evaluation consists of taking a history (general, social, otological, characterization of tinnitus and hyperacusis), a physical examination and assessing other medical conditions; further referrals (e.g., psychological, psychiatric, neurological, etc.) are made if needed. A significant part of taking the tinnitus/decreased sound tolerance history is performed during the initial audiological evaluation.

Therefore, depending on the degree of the physician's involvement in future treatment, this part can be less detailed and left in the hands of the audiologist. However, the medically relevant parts of the initial evaluation are necessary in order to exclude otological and other medical problems requiring attention or referral. They may also be relevant in legal cases. The questionnaire that the patient fills before a visit, with questions regarding medical history, is also helpful during the medical evaluation.

In the verbal description of tinnitus, attention is paid to whether the tinnitus is constant or pulsatile. If pulsatile, whether it is synchronous with the heartbeat and whether it varies with exertion. A synchrony of tinnitus with the heartbeat might indicate the presence of a somatosound, rather than tinnitus. Note, that synchronization alone is not sufficient to diagnose the somatosound.

Recently accumulated data show that tinnitus can be evoked or modulated by stimulation of the somatosensory system (e.g., by pressing in the head and neck area, performing a variety of movements or by looking in a certain direction) (Cacace *et al.*, 1999a,b; Levine 1999; Sanchez *et al.*, 2002). While the clinical relevance of this phenomenon at the moment is uncertain, its presence should be noted to provide proper information during counseling. Otherwise, the ability to modulate tinnitus in this way in some patients can give rise to the fear that they have a neurological disease, or it may initiate a search for treatment involving manipulation of joints etc. (e.g., jaw joint therapies, chiropractics, etc.). In a number of cases, these treatments can actually make tinnitus, and the patient, worse.

Past treatments can affect the patients' reaction to TRT. For example, if the patient was advised in the past that just using hearing aids will help tinnitus, then special counseling is needed to explain the difference between just wearing hearing aids and using them as a part of sound therapy. The examiner should determine what prior treatments have been tried and their outcome. These may include psychiatric treatments, antidepressants or antianxiety drugs, hearing aids, maskers, biofeed-back, hypnosis, acupuncture or herbal agents such as ginkgo. Finally, the general level of knowledge about tinnitus, sources of information (e.g., the web, magazines, the American Tinnitus Association, self-help group, other patients) and the type of information is checked.

A thorough otolaryngological examination is performed, including examination of the ears with an otoscope or microscope. The presence of middle ear fluid, inflammation, negative pressure or abnormal vascular masses is determined. In examining the oropharynx and nasopharynx, one may see subtle evidence of palatal myoclonus. Auscultation of the neck for carotid bruits is done and auscultation around the temporal bones may reveal other somatosounds. Palpation of the temporomandibular joint areas may show crepitus, muscle spasm or tenderness. In patients with pulsatile tinnitus, one should assess the effect of compression over the internal jugular vein (jugular outflow syndrome). A neuro-otologic examination assesses cranial nerves, cerebellar function and balance.

The majority of patients are very focused on medications for tinnitus and on drugs that might cause its enhancement. If patients definitely see a worsening of their tinnitus after taking a certain drug, they are advised to avoid it and to discuss careful withdrawal from this drug with the specialist who prescribed it. Note that warnings in the Physician Desk Reference/Pharmacopeia overstate the risk of a causal relation between drugs and tinnitus. Many patients are already taking medications prescribed specifically for treatment of tinnitus or depression. If they are taking antidepressants or benzodiazepines for a separate pre-existing problem with depression or an anxiety disorder, the medication should be continued under the guidance of their primary-care physician or psychiatrist. If the medication has been given for tinnitus, patients are advised that it may not be necessary to continue. It is best not to make changes in medication until the patient begins to see improvement in their tinnitus from TRT. Then patients should be gradually weaned off medications (especially those used for treating anxiety, depression and insomnia) to avoid withdrawal effects. This process should always be done under the supervision of a physician. Treatment for unrelated medical conditions should be continued. Use of innocuous agents such as ginkgo or vitamins or other herbal agents can be continued if the patient feels they derive some benefit from them.

The withdrawal of unnecessary psychotropic medication needs to be performed very gradually and under proper supervision.

The identification of associated or contributing psychiatric problems is important in managing tinnitus patients. If a patient has a significant problem with depression, anxiety disorder, somatization disorder or obsessive–compulsive disorder, they need to be under the care of someone who can expertly manage these problems. The physician treating tinnitus needs to communicate with these professionals to coordinate care and share, which will make patient management easier and more effective.

While somatosounds (sounds created by the body) are common, they only very occasionally indicate conditions requiring surgical intervention.

Somatosounds are worth exploring, as on some rare occasions they provide an opportunity for removing the source of the sound by surgical intervention. They might result from various sources, which generate different sounds. The most frequently encountered are given in Table 3.1.

In the majority of our patients with somatosounds, there is no pathology detectable, as the body sounds being heard are part of normal physiological

Table 3.1 Sources of somatosounds

Source	Sound
Vascular blood flow arterial or venous pulsations	Whooshing sound
Glomus tumor	Pulsatile humming
Benign intracranial hypertension	Pulse synchronous noise
Patent eustachian tube	Roaring airflow with breathing
Palatal or middle ear muscle myoclonus	Clicking
Spontaneous otoacoustic emissions	Ringing
Temporal mandibular joint abnormalities	Clicking or Crunching

function. In many cases where pathology is found, surgery is frequently not indicated, or is potentially dangerous, and in any case these patients can achieve effective control of their somatosounds with TRT.

In some subjects a simple decrease of the auditory input is sufficient to evoke tinnitus or enhance it to the extent of annoyance. This phenomenon is a repetition of the classical experiment in which subjects start to perceive tinnitus when placed for a few minutes in a very quiet environment (Heller & Bergman, 1953). Obviously hearing loss of any type will result in a decrease of the auditory input and may promote tinnitus. This is regularly observed in those with conductive hearing loss, resulting from wax impaction, otitis media, ossicular stiffness/discontinuity and otosclerosis. These conditions offer the possibility, and frequently the need, for intervention. Caution is recommended when suction is used for cerumen removal, as this procedure can be noisy and should not be performed on patients with decreased sound tolerance.

Other medical conditions, such as Ménière's syndrome and vestibular schwannoma, are not common within the large population of tinnitus patients. Note that all patients being referred for magnetic resonance imaging must be advised about the need for hearing protection, as this examination involves quite high levels of sound. In those with severe decreased sound tolerance, it should be considered that the scan is delayed until significant improvement is noted. It is possible to use TRT concurrently with treatment for Ménière's syndrome. Before embarking on specific therapies, patients should be advised that tinnitus might persist after successful treatment of the condition but can still be successfully treated by TRT.

It is of uttermost importance during medical evaluation that negative counseling is avoided, and a positive view of the future is created. A medical opinion has a larger impact on the patient than that obtained from other sources, and negative counseling given by doctors is, therefore, particularly powerful and damaging in its effects.

3.3 Diagnosis and patient categories

3.3.1 Basis for classifying tinnitus

The classification of patients into treatment categories has to be approached with flexibility and an open mind, realizing that there is a continuous spectrum of clinical manifestations of tinnitus and decreased sound tolerance, and that each patient should be treated individually. However, it is very helpful to assign patients to one of several categories. For all categories, the treatment involves repeated counseling sessions and instruction to enrich auditory background and avoid silence. There are common elements in the treatment for all categories; however, each category has its own specific features. As symptoms improve, patients may need to be assigned to a different category.

Patients seeking help for tinnitus and decreased sound tolerance present a wide spectrum of problems and, therefore, require a varied implementation of TRT. Based on the similarities and differences between patients and the potential neurophysiological mechanisms involved, five classes or categories of patients are proposed (Jastreboff, 1998). These categories have distinct features and are designed to serve as a method of assessing a patients' problems and guiding a suitable treatment protocol. It should be remembered that there is a continuous spectrum of clinical features and each patient should be assessed for their particular needs. Note that patients can move from one category to another as they progress through TRT.

All patients are placed in one of five categories, which may be changed during the treatment. These categories depend on the severity of symptoms, the presence or absence of hyperacusis, the significance of subjectively assessed hearing loss and the exacerbation of symptoms by sound exposure.

Patients are assigned to a given category on the basis of the following factors:
• severity and/or duration of tinnitus
• presence and extent of hyperacusis
• subjective significance of hearing loss
• prolonged exacerbation of symptoms following sound exposure.
Note that hyperacusis should not be confused with misophonia or phonophobia; the latter can exist in any category and are treated concurrently with other problems by a separate protocol. Table 3.2 illustrates this classification.

At this point we present a very brief outline of this classification, which will be discussed later in more detail. For all categories, the common elements of the treatment are counseling intended to reclassify tinnitus (and/or perception of external

Table 3.2 Classification of tinnitus problems

Category	High level of tinnitus severity	Hyperacusis	Hearing loss[a]	Prolonged sound-induced worsening
C0	No	No	No	No
C0/2	No	No	Yes	No
C1	Yes	No	No	No
C2	Yes	No	Yes	No
C3	Yes/no	Yes	No	No
C3/2[b]	Yes/no	Yes	Yes	No
C4[c]	Yes/no	Yes/no	No	Yes
C4/2[c]	Yes/no	Yes/no	Yes	Yes

All terms defined in the text. If both hyperacusis and misophonia are present then misophonia is treated when some improvement in hyperacusis is observed, or concurrently when hyperacusis is relatively mild. If misophonia exists without hyperacusis, it can be treated from the beginning of the treatment.

[a] Patients with hearing loss accompanying other problems belong to a modified category.

[b] In C3/2, sound therapy was performed initially with sound generators followed by hearing aids. Now it is possible to use combination instruments while still following the general principles of a two-stage protocol.

[c] In category C4, either tinnitus or hyperacusis must exhibit prolonged worsening after sound exposure.

sounds, in case of misophonia) into a neutral signal, and enrichment of the auditory background.

Tinnitus retraining counseling covers all aspects of tinnitus and decreased sound tolerance: its origin, symptoms and rationale for the habituation-based approach.

The aims of counseling are to convey the following concepts.

1. Tinnitus/hyperacusis do not reflect medical problems but they are side effects of compensatory action within the auditory pathways.
2. Misophonia results from enhanced functional connections between the auditory and limbic systems.
3. Problems caused by tinnitus, or misophonia, reflect activation of the autonomic nervous system, which, by attempt to prepare us for (unnecessary) action, evokes neuronal and hormonal changes perceived at a behavioral level as anxiety, stress, annoyance, etc.
4. Auditory and the limbic and autonomic nervous systems typically are working normally. The problem results from incorrect functional connections between these systems, resulting in a proper reaction to an improper stimulus.

5. These connections are created, and work, following the principles of conditioned reflexes.
6. It is possible to retrain these reflexes, once tinnitus is reclassified to a category of neutral/slightly negative stimuli, to achieve habituation of the reactions induced by tinnitus and to achieve habituation of its perception.
7. The process of habituation is facilitated by enrichment of the auditory background, which by increasing background neuronal activity weakens the tinnitus signal.

3.3.2 Categories of treatment

The characteristic features of TRT for each treatment category are outlined below.

Category 0

Category 0 patients show a low level of tinnitus severity, and tinnitus has relatively little impact on life. This category also includes patients with a very recent experience of tinnitus who have not received negative counseling.

Patients classified as belonging to category 0 present with a low level of tinnitus severity, and tinnitus has relatively little impact on their lives. This category also includes patients with a very recent experience of tinnitus (measured in days or a few weeks) who have not received negative counseling or created strong negative associations with their symptoms.

For these patients the functional connections between the auditory, and limbic and autonomic nervous systems are relatively weak, and one session of simplified general counseling combined with basic instruction of sound use is often sufficient for achieving tinnitus control. Follow-up visits are still needed to make certain no more problems develop and that habituation of tinnitus occurs. Patients are also instructed to return if their symptoms do not rapidly improve, at which point they can be reassigned to one of the other categories.

Category 1

Category 1 patients have tinnitus of high severity as their predominant complaint and do not have other hearing-related problems.

Category 1 patients have tinnitus of high severity as their predominant complaint and do not have hyperacusis, subjectively significant hearing loss or prolonged exacerbation of tinnitus from sound exposure.

These patients will be treated with detailed counseling focused on tinnitus and are fitted with wearable sound generators set to a level close to the "mixing point."

Category 2

Category 2 patients have tinnitus coexisting with a hearing loss.

Category 2 patients have tinnitus coexisting with a hearing loss, which has a significant effect on the patients' life. These patients do not have significant hyperacusis, and sound exposure has no prolonged effect on tinnitus.

These patients receive appropriate counseling and sound therapy, involving the fitting or refitting of appropriate hearing aids. As is discussed below, the primary purpose of a hearing aid fitting in this category is to provide patients with an enhanced sound input rather than improving their communication skills. However, hearing aids are important in removing the "straining to hear" effect and in improving their life quality. These patients are instructed to provide an enriched auditory background while using the hearing aid as an amplifier. Providing hearing aids alone, without any background sound enrichment, will have no impact on tinnitus except possible short-term suppression effects, which amplified environmental sound provides in some patients.

Category 3

Category 3 patients exhibit significant hyperacusis, with or without significant tinnitus.

Category 3 patients exhibit significant hyperacusis with or without significant tinnitus. Neither tinnitus nor hyperacusis exhibit prolonged exacerbation following sound exposure. Note that hyperacusis is the characteristic feature in this category. Misophonia can also be present, as in any other category; however, it is to be expected that misophonia will be more prevalent in this category. If in doubt, it is recommended that it is always assumed that hyperacusis is present and the treatment is conducted accordingly. It is of secondary importance whether tinnitus or hyperacusis is the dominant problem. In the initial stage, the treatment approach is identical regardless and is aimed at removing hyperacusis.

In this group, the aim is to desensitize the patient, first using wearable sound generators set at a level below any discomfort. More stress is placed on the *continuous* use of sound generators.

Because patients with significant hyperacusis and hearing loss may not tolerate amplification, in the past we have recommended treating hyperacusis with sound generators alone, and we have deferred TRT until the hyperacusis was under control. Only then was a full program of auditory rehabilitation introduced, paying careful attention to compression of gain to avoid overstimulation of an auditory system, which still might not be responding with normal activation to external sounds. The recent appearance on the market of high-quality digital combination instruments, which bring together an independently controlled digital hearing aid and a sound generator built into one shell, allow an alternative approach. In this case, hyperacusis is still treated first, but some modest amplification is introduced at the early stage of the treatment. These instruments are now used with success by P. J. Jastreboff since they were introduced in the USA in 2001.

Category 4

Category 4 patients are most difficult to treat; hyperacusis is the dominant complaint, with tinnitus secondary or absent. They experience the exacerbation of symptoms for prolonged periods of time as a result of noise exposure.

Category 4 patients are the most difficult to treat but they represent the smallest group. Typically, hyperacusis is the dominant complaint, with tinnitus secondary or absent. The crucial feature is the exacerbation of symptoms for prolonged periods of time as a result of noise exposure. While most patients report an increase in tinnitus or hyperacusis following any kind of noise for minutes or hours, the characteristic feature of patients in this category is that the worsening of symptoms persists at least until the following day and may last for weeks. As relatively low levels of sound may trigger this enhancement, these patients are difficult to treat with sound therapy in the normal way and require a protocol based on very slow desensitization. Specifically, treatment commences using wearable sound generators but without switching them on for a few days. They are next set at the threshold of hearing, and their loudness is very gradually increased under the constant control of the TRT professional.

3.3.3 Allocation of patients to categories

Treatment for each category of patients involves a different and specific approach, both for counseling and for implementation of sound therapy. Wrong classification and hence treatment can make symptoms worse.

Assigning the patient to the correct category of treatment is essential for successful therapy because inappropriate treatment could make symptoms worse; this is a common source of claims that TRT "does not work with everyone." During treatment, a patient often moves from one category to another as the situation changes. Successful patients will reach category 0 before final complete habituation.

Patients from all groups are instructed to practice enrichment of the auditory background and to avoid silence.

Patients from all groups are instructed to practice enrichment of the auditory background. All patients are told to maintain a constant background level of sound using any source that does not produce annoyance or attract their attention. The important message, which is repeated on several occasions, is to "*avoid silence.*"

Patients should be taught during counseling that sounds are helpful in improving their symptoms while silence can be harmful.

3.4 Counseling (retraining) sessions: common features

It is stressed that tinnitus and hyperacusis are a side effect of normal compensatory mechanisms in the brain. It is stressed that the perception of tinnitus is of secondary importance, and that the severity of tinnitus results from activation of the limbic and autonomic nervous systems. While we cannot eliminate the source of tinnitus, it is possible to use the naturally occurring mechanisms of plasticity in the brain to achieve habituation of physiological reactions to tinnitus and, subsequently, habituation of its perception. Although tinnitus might have the same loudness and pitch at the end of treatment as at the beginning, it will no longer produce negative reactions. Following habituation of reaction to tinnitus, which is the primary goal, habituation of perception will occur, to a varying degree. Counseling should be adjusted to the individual patient, bearing in mind the individual's needs and their general psychological status. The similarity of mechanisms for tinnitus and misophonia are pointed out, while for hyperacusis stress is placed on the mechanisms controlling gain within the auditory pathways, the properties of automatic gain control and desensitization.

The following sections describe non-specific general counseling, selected components of which are used for a given category of patients. Non-specific counseling includes the basic elements of the model, common for all categories of patient. The final version of counseling, for each specific patient, consists of selected elements of this non-specific counseling expanded by additional information. The extent of emphasis of these elements of non-specific counseling, and selection of additional parts, are related to the specifics of the individual patients and their diagnostic category. Consequently, each counseling session is individualized and optimized for the needs of each patient, while it still preserves the core of basic information. The coherence of explanation must be maintained so that the logic and relevance can easily be followed. At the same time, the problems that are not part of the classification process (e.g., misophonia or sleep problems) are treated in a very similar manner in each treatment category, modified only by the specific personal needs of the patient.

Counseling in TRT has a special meaning. It involves the teaching of the neurophysiological model, tailoring the explanation to the precise needs of an individual patient.

Counseling in TRT has a specific meaning. It describes teaching patients about the mechanisms of hearing, the basics of brain function and the specifics of the neurophysiological model of tinnitus. Interaction with the patient is always on a one-to-one basis, with the aim of demystification of tinnitus and/or decreased sound tolerance. As this process involves transferring information from counselor to patient, it falls into the broad term "directive counseling," as defined in psychological literature. Part of the process also involves listening to the patient's experiences and answering questions on the basis of the neurophysiological model. We have used the term "directive counseling" in the past to describe our interaction with patients in TRT. However as TRT counseling has a number of additional features, the term TRT counseling, or "teaching session," is more appropriate, and we use these terms now. It is also useful to describe the patient's on-going activity in TRT as a "study" of the neurophysiological model and other information. Many of the concepts enshrined in the neurophysiological model are difficult understand, and to teach, reflecting the complexity of the brain itself. That is why we recommend the use of illustrative stories, or parables, to make the model an understandable everyday experience, which every patient can easily relate to and comprehend (see Appendix 2 for examples). Their increasing knowledge and understanding is paralleled by improvement, and habituation of reaction and perception of tinnitus. Nevertheless, traditional counseling skills and strategies are still useful in dealing with tinnitus patients.

We cannot directly alter the activity of the autonomic and limbic systems, which results in the annoyance produced by tinnitus. We can only use an indirect approach, based on the neuropsychological principle that a situation associated with a known danger induces a smaller reaction of the autonomic nervous system than one associated with an unknown danger. Therefore, much of TRT counseling is devoted to demystifying tinnitus: teaching patients about the mechanisms involved in its emergence and those responsible for its impact on life and its annoyance. TRT counseling should not be a series of didactic statements about tinnitus but should present logically linked information. The therapist must bear in mind different educational backgrounds and pay special attention to providing patients with everyday examples with which they may easily identify, while illustrating the main principles of the neurophysiological model. It is important that the patient receives consistent information from all team members and those involved in administrative support.

Removal of tinnitus annoyance is by an indirect approach, starting with the demystification of its mechanisms.

Each counseling session is tailored to fit a particular patient, taking into account all the information gathered so far. The counseling sessions can be divided into several subtypes depending on a patient's category. Each counseling session contains, however, certain common elements, which are described in more detail in the following sections.

1. Explanation of the results of audiological testing
2. Presentation of the basic functions of the auditory system
3. Presentation of the basic rules of perception including the impact of contrast on signal strength

4. Presentation of the basics of brain function and the interactions of various different systems of the brain
5. Relating these basic concepts to the specific patient: explaining why tinnitus and decreased sound tolerance create such profound problems
6. Explanation of the theoretical basis of habituation and how it can be achieved
7. Discussion with the patient about proposed treatment(s), including discussion regarding the role and utilization of sound
8. Answering any additional questions that the patient may have on the basis of the neurophysiological model.

Explanation of the results of audiological testing

When discussing the results of audiometric testing, the patient is taught how to interpret an audiogram, pointing out the frequency range corresponding to speech perception, the importance of LDLs and the normal dynamic range of the ear. A graphic representation of tinnitus is marked on the audiogram (pitch and loudness, if measured) and briefly discussed. The vast majority of patients have a tinnitus loudness match within 15 dB of the threshold of hearing at the perceived pitch of tinnitus. It is pointed out that if tinnitus was an external sound of such a low intensity it would be masked almost all the time by other external sounds. This reflects the fact that tinnitus perception differs from that of external sounds.

MSL are briefly mentioned, pointing out that they have no predictive value for the treatment outcome. If LDLs are decreased, then the relevance and meaning of these measurements are discussed with the patient, together with the meaning of the altered dynamic range. Where LDLs are reduced, decreased sound tolerance and its appropriate components are discussed. Hyperacusis is presented as a physiological lowering of tolerance to external sound, reflecting overamplification within the auditory system. Misophonia is also discussed, where there is dislike or negative reaction of the individual to a specific sound or sounds.

If hearing aids are indicated as a part of the treatment, then hearing loss and difficulty in speech discrimination are discussed in detail. With hearing in noise difficulty, the "cocktail party effect" is explained, together with its relevance to high-frequency hearing loss and sound localization. Normal impedance measurements and auditory reflexes are almost always present and are useful in counseling the patient that any middle ear and nasal symptoms do not contribute towards the tinnitus (a commonly held misconception). The discussion of the DPOAE results is deferred until the function and role of OHC are presented.

Explanation of the basic functions of the auditory system

A description of the basic function of the auditory system starts with a presentation of the anatomy and properties of the external and middle ear, liberally illustrated by appropriate charts and drawings. These are available in any audiological or otolaryngological office. In most cases, these parts of the ear will be normal. Some patients are convinced that their symptoms, particularly ear pain, are related to physical injury or inflammation of the external and middle ear, and they will require strong reassurance based on an understanding of the outcome of audiological measurements, together with a thorough otological examination.

The function of the peripheral auditory system is explained to the patient with diagrams and copies of the patient's test results.

An explanation of the function of the auditory system proceeds in the following manner. The normal ear collects sound in the external meatus; the sound vibrates the eardrum and this vibration is then transmitted through the ossicular chain to the cochlea. Sound waves pass through the cochlear fluids to vibrate the basilar membrane in a tonotopic fashion (high-frequency sounds exciting the basal tone of the cochlea and low-frequency sounds, the apex). The tonotopic organization of the cochlea is explained with respect to its mechanical properties, using an analogy of the strings of a piano, and stressing that each point on the cochlea, and each associated group of hair cells, has its own characteristic frequency to which it responds best. Accordingly, dysfunction of a small area of the cochlea results in hearing loss for this particular frequency. Stimulation of a narrow part of the cochlea by sound results in the perception of a pure tone or narrow band of noise.

Next, illustrations of the organ of Corti by scanning electron micrographs are presented showing normal and noise damaged ears. This helps to show that with most events which are traumatic to the ear, such as noise exposure, ototoxic drugs, infections, as well as in ageing and genetic deafness, OHC are predominantly affected and reduced in number in a frequency-specific manner. However, 95% of the fibers of the auditory nerve connect to the IHC and conduct messages from them to the brain. When OHC are totally damaged, by whatever cause, there is only approximately a 50 dB flat hearing loss. When all the IHC are damaged, regardless of whether the OHC remain, there is a total hearing loss, and this loss corresponds to the frequency region in the cochlea where the damage occurs.

The different function of OHC and IHC was a puzzle until the early 1990s. Recent research shows that the IHC are the transducers converting vibration on the basal membrane into nerve impulses, which are finally perceived as sound. The OHC act as mechanical amplifiers enhancing vibrations of the organ of Corti for low levels of sound.

OHC are most susceptible to any kind of damage and, once destroyed, they are not capable of regeneration in humans. However, temporary changes in the cochlea are common after exposure to loud sounds (e.g., pop concerts, discos). Typically OHC are affected, and their recovery then takes place over a few days but can be delayed up to a few months in some cases (Cardinaal *et al.*, 2000; Emmerich *et al.*, 2000; Stopp, 1983).

The OHC system exhibits a high degree of redundancy. This allows for up to 30% diffuse loss of OHC without affecting the audiogram (Bohne & Clark, 1982; Chen & Fechter, 2003). Consequently, since OHC are dying at approximately 0.5% per year from the first years of life, the appearance of a hearing loss is not usually expected before the end of the fifth decade, providing that there are no other factors such as noise exposure, ototoxic drugs, genetic predisposition, etc. Small patchy areas of degeneration may not result in detectable changes in the hearing threshold because of compensation provided by adjacent healthy hair cells. However small areas of OHC degeneration, which can be detected by DPOAE, may play a significant role in tinnitus emergence.

Discordant dysfunction theory provides a frame of reference for interpretation of distortion product otoacoustic emission measurements and for explanation of the role of hair cells in tinnitus.

Results of the DPOAE examination of the patient are discussed and related to their audiogram. The discussion about DPOAE is particularly useful in tinnitus patients with normal hearing. This allows for the demonstration of how small areas of dysfunctional OHC, as documented by DPOAE, may lead to emergence of tinnitus, following the theory of discordant dysfunction of OHC and IHC systems (presented in Ch. 2).

The neural pathways leading from the cochlea to the cortex are quite extensive. These pathways act as a number of highly complex, interconnected computer systems processing sound-evoked neural activity through the auditory pathways. These neural networks are processing information, extracting important patterns and filtering out and suppressing irrelevant activity. The process of recognition of patterns and filtering out other information is performed by extensive networks of interconnected nerve cells. Each nerve cell is capable of acting as a complex processing unit, which converts, processes and alters information coming from many other units.

The connections between neurons are changing all the time, can be either excitatory or inhibitory and can enhance or suppress the activity of a target neuron. When the contribution of a connection between neurons increases, then the same signal from the first neuron will have a larger impact on the activity of the target neuron. Because of their complexity, these neuronal networks are capable of processing many different signals at the same time, strongly enhancing some and suppressing others.

The experience of tinnitus by all in very quiet situations (the soundproofed room experiment) can be explained in terms of adaptive mechanisms in the auditory system.

The auditory system is also able to control its overall gain: the degree to which it enhances external sounds. At the level of the cochlea, gain can be achieved by the amount of mechanical amplification within the cochlea from the activity of the OHC. Central to the auditory nerve, the properties of neuronal networks can change to provide increased enhancement of incoming signals. The gain increases automatically when the level of external sound decreases, and it returns to lower values when sound level increases.

An important example of this adaptive property of the auditory system with relevance to tinnitus was shown by the experiment performed by Heller and Bergman in 1953. They placed 80 normally hearing people without tinnitus in a soundproofed room for five minutes with instructions to record any sound that they might hear. Tinnitus was experienced by 94% as a result of being in a low level of sound. This demonstrates that the perception of tinnitus is inherent in the auditory system and not necessarily the result of a pathological process.

On the physiological level, this experiment may be explained in the following manner. Spontaneous neuronal activity in the auditory nerve fibers, which occurs in the absence of sound, has a high rate of 50–100 impulses per second. This activity is random, and each neural spike occurs independently of others. In the presence of sound, the average activity increases and becomes more regular. In auditory nerve fibers, the patterns of neural activity reflect the sound waves that have previously arrived in the ear canal. At this stage, there is little processing and classification of the auditory information. This activity then undergoes extensive processing at several levels in the subcortical auditory pathways before it reaches the auditory cortex, where sound is finally perceived. As a part of this processing, the spontaneous random activity is filtered out, and we do not perceive this as sound under normal circumstances. When, however, gain within the auditory system increases because of decreased auditory input, then fluctuations of spontaneous activity are perceived as tinnitus.

Presentation of the rules of perception

Neuronal networks in the brain are trained to detect important sounds automatically.

In audiology, much emphasis and attention are placed on threshold measurements of auditory function: for example, the quietest sound that can be detected, the smallest change in frequency, etc. Typically, these measurements are performed in quiet. However, real-life situations involve the detection of a complex signal in the presence of other competing sounds. The auditory system is able to discriminate one complex pattern from others occurring at the same time. This ability is acquired by training the neuronal networks to detect a specific pattern of activity with great accuracy. The training is achieved by repeated exposure to a sound, recognized as being important. A classical example of this is the ability to hear the sound of our own first name, even in a high level of competing background noise and when we are not expecting it. Because of the repeated presentation of our first name throughout our life, and its significance to us, our auditory system becomes tuned to this complex pattern, and we are able to detect this even in a noisy environment.

The identical scenario happens in tinnitus. The initial signal, once recognized and evaluated as important because of its continuous presence, causes tuning of the neuronal networks to its pattern, and the auditory system can easily recognize it, even in the presence of other signals.

Loudness perception depends on the contrast of signal against background.

The perception of signal strength, whether it is auditory, visual, tactile, or temperature etc., is not dependent upon the absolute physical strength of the signal but is based on a comparison with the level of the background surrounding it. By changing the background, it is possible to make the same signal weaker or stronger. A good example of this is provided by the perceived intensity of a birthday candle seen under different conditions. In the first instance, walking into a totally darkened room, a single candle lit in the far corner will be seen as a brilliant light and cannot be ignored. Once lights in the room are turned on, the light from the candle will be perceived as much weaker and might easily be overlooked. If the blinds on the window are now opened, allowing brilliant sunshine to illuminate the corner with the candle in it, the candlelight will be barely noticeable. Similarly, the sound of a car radio being played at a comfortable listening level while driving along a busy street may seem to become uncomfortably loud once the car has been parked in the owner's garage.

Even if tinnitus-related neuronal activity does not change, tinnitus will appear much louder while going to sleep in a quiet bedroom than when sitting in a noisy office. As a result, tinnitus patients should expect that their tinnitus will appear much louder in quiet situations, and this is one of the reasons for patients to avoid silence.

Limitation of attention

The brain is not capable of performing more than one task requiring full attention at the same time.

Our brain is capable of performing very complex tasks, which the most advanced computers available are unable to emulate. However, the brain has serious limitations as well. It is not capable of performing more than one task requiring full attention at the same time. A classical example would be to try to read a book and write a letter at the same time.

In everyday life, all our sensory systems, including the auditory system, are continuously flooded with information. We are exposed to a wide variety of different sounds and are aware of only a very small percentage of them. All sounds reach the cochlea and subconscious subcortical centers. These centers are able to process and discriminate between a number of different sounds at the same time. The brain adopts several strategies when faced with the need to deal with a large amount of information arriving simultaneously, while only one task can be placed in the focus of conscious attention at any one time.

Most repetitive activity is automated by a large number of subconscious conditioned reflexes.

The first strategy is to automate certain responses that require a standard and predictable reaction to the same stimulus, by creating a series of conditioned reflexes working at a subconscious level. A typical example of this is driving a car when we are receiving stimulation through many sensory modalities. Without conscious attention, we are able to arrive at our destination while at the same time carrying out a conversation with our passenger. The speed of reaction required to execute many different fast responses actually forces the need for automating this task. Another good example of this is playing a musical instrument while reading the notes.

Another strategy to deal with sensory overload involves classification of stimuli into important, requiring some action, and secondary or not important at all. Once this classification is performed, no significant stimuli will undergo a process of habituation, or blocking. However, when the same neutral stimulus is repeated many times over and over without reinforcement (reward or punishment), it ceases to evoke any reaction, and additionally we stop perceiving its presence. The stimulus still evokes activity at the periphery of the sensory system, and within the subconscious centers; however there are no reactions and furthermore no conscious perception. The signal is blocked or filtered out at a subconscious level in the auditory pathway and prevented from reaching the highest level, where it would be perceived. This process occurs naturally and continuously for all neutral stimuli.

Stimuli are classified by their importance; those indicating danger are dealt with first.

The next mechanism involved in solving the problem "one task at a time" is to organize all the tasks to be done according to their relative importance, and to perform these tasks in order, one at a time, starting from the most important onwards. All stimuli that indicate danger, induce fear or require immediate action in order to preserve life or insure safety are given the highest priority. It is clearly more important to detect the sound of the approaching tiger who may eat you for lunch than to detect the noise made by the turkey you are hoping to eat for your own lunch. In particular, we do not have control over the mechanism by which our attention is drawn to stimuli indicating danger, inducing fear or having general negative associations.

Consequently, it is unthinkable that a patient would be able to sit through a session of TRT counseling, paying good attention, while a tiger sits in a corner of the room, even with the assurance that the tiger has not attacked anybody, for at least a week. Once tinnitus begins to suggest potential danger, it forces our brain, at a conscious and subconscious level, to monitor its status.

Plasticity of the brain

Plasticity of the brain allows learning and creation of conditioned reflexes.

The most fundamental characteristic of the brain is its ability to undergo modification and plastic changes. These changes occur by modification of the strength of connection between neurons. This feature is the physiological basis for memory, learning at the conscious level and developing new reflexes. Because of it, we are able both to learn a new language and to perfect a golf swing. The golf swing may be relearned after initial acquisition of inappropriate body position or swing, but this generally takes longer than learning the right way from the start. It is a frequent observation that relearning takes a longer time than initial training from a naive state.

Retraining of conditioned reflexes is possible but takes time.

Furthermore, relearning of conditioned reflexes can occur only by performing proper exercises, and it requires time. It is impossible to change or remove a conditioned reflex purely by cognitive processes. Therefore, tinnitus patients need to perform, over a period of time, exercises aimed at extinction of inappropriate reflexes linking the tinnitus-related neuronal activity within the auditory system with activation of the systems responsible for anxiety, annoyance, etc. Moreover, when there is strong emotional association, relearning a reflex that was acquired with negative reinforcement takes longer.

Other systems in the brain activated by tinnitus, in addition to the auditory system.

The brain consists of many different subsystems interacting with each other in a parallel fashion, each having a different purpose and function. Analysis of the behavioral problems caused by tinnitus indicate that certain areas of the brain have a special relevance in its development, the limbic and autonomic nervous systems being of particular importance.

The limbic system in the brain controls emotions and is strongly connected to the auditory system.

The limbic system is responsible for our emotions. By experimental stimulation or destruction of a small part of this system, we can induce or abolish fear, thirst, hunger, sexual drive and anger. The limbic system is strongly and directly connected to the auditory system and so, through appropriate training, sounds can induce strong positive or negative emotional responses. For example music, the sound made by an infant offspring or the voice of an army corporal who was responsible for our military training, all evoke strong emotional reactions. Activation of the limbic system is absolutely essential for the learning process, and the lack of concurrent limbic activation during auditory stimulation results in habituation of the sound.

The autonomic nervous system controls automatic body functions and its sympathetic part controls the "fight or flight" responses.

Another important part of the brain is the autonomic nervous system. This system controls the basic functions of the body such as the heartbeat, sweating, hormonal levels, bowel functions, respiration and temperature.[1] We do not have direct control of the autonomic nervous system but we can modify its activity by fairly simple interventions such as exercising or relaxing. Only with special training is it possible to achieve some control over the basic level of activation of the autonomic nervous system. Certain disciplines such as yoga, biofeedback, special relaxation techniques and classical hypnosis make this possible to some extent.

The sympathetic part of the autonomic nervous system will be activated when there is a need for any action, physical or mental. Its prolonged activation, however, would result in feelings of exhaustion, stress and discomfort.

This system becomes highly active in situations of danger or where fear is produced, preparing us for fight or flight. During the fight or flight response, there are a number of profound changes in the body induced by the sympathetic part of the autonomic nervous system, such as increased epinephrine levels, muscle tension,

---

[1] The autonomic nervous system has two parts: a sympathetic and a parasympathetic part. The sympathetic nervous system prepares us for mental and physical activity. In extreme activation, it gets us ready for fight or flight. The parasympathetic nervous system acts in a reverse manner, preparing us for relaxation, digestion, rest and sleep. The two systems are connected in a reciprocal manner; the activation of one suppresses the other. In this book the term "autonomic activity" refers principally to stimulation of the sympathetic nervous system.

increased heart and respiration rates and reduced blood flow to the stomach and bowel. There is also an increase in the general level of alertness, which, among other things, prevents sleep. These reactions are not usually intended to be sustained for prolonged periods; if for any reason this happens, then they induce extreme exhaustion, causing profound effects on the function of the brain and body.

Note that the sympathetic part of the autonomic nervous system will be activated when there is a need for any action, physical or mental. The point to consider is how high this activation is and for how long a time it is sustained. If even relatively low levels of activation are evoked, but for prolonged periods of time, this results in the feeling of exhaustion, with high level of stress and discomfort. The increased activation can be induced by any stimulus once it is linked with the need for action, and particularly if the action is aimed at protecting us from danger or discomfort. For example, it may be induced by the sound of a police siren, the red lights from a car braking, or the voice of the boss with whom we have had problems in the past.

Tinnitus signals act as a continuous sensory input constantly activating the sympathetic part of the autonomic nervous system and maintain excitation of this system at a higher than normal level.

Tinnitus signals, once they have become associated with negative feelings or potential negative consequences, act as a continuous sensory input activating the sympathetic part of the autonomic nervous system and keeping the excitation of this system at a higher than normal level. Note that the level of activity of the autonomic nervous system relates closely to the severity of tinnitus as perceived by the individual.

The neurophysiological model of tinnitus

Tinnitus becomes a problem only when reflex activation of the limbic and autonomic nervous system take place.

Once the general features and principles of the working of the auditory, limbic and autonomic nervous systems have been presented, it is important to discuss the interaction between all these various components, and the part that they play in tinnitus and decreased sound tolerance, as described in Ch. 2. It is of particular importance to convey the message that perception of tinnitus is in itself benign, and that tinnitus only becomes a problem when inappropriate conditioned reflexes are created that link the tinnitus-related neuronal activity in the auditory system with activity in the limbic and autonomic nervous systems. Finally, the level of activity of the autonomic nervous system relates closely to the severity of tinnitus as *perceived by* the individual.

For over 80% of people who are experiencing tinnitus for the first time, the sound is not associated with any negative meaning and, therefore, it undergoes the process of spontaneous habituation.

For over 80% of people who are experiencing tinnitus for the first time, the sound is not associated with any negative meaning, and it undergoes the process of spontaneous habituation, identical to that of other meaningless external sounds, such as the sound of a new refrigerator. If, however, the first experience of tinnitus induces a high level of annoyance or anxiety, by being associated with something unpleasant or by occurring during a period of stress and anxiety, then a different scenario emerges. People experience a higher level of annoyance or anxiety linked to the meaning of the new tinnitus sound, and this results in an enhancement of activity in the autonomic and/or limbic systems; tinnitus then becomes a clinically significant problem. These patients start to monitor the tinnitus signal extensively, which further enhances its importance.

Tinnitus becomes a clinically significant problem when the tinnitus-related neuronal activity starts activating the limbic and autonomic nervous systems, resulting in annoyance and anxiety.

An early common concern is that tinnitus is inescapable and cannot be modified or altered. This results in a build-up of increasing alarm and anxiety, with further stimulation of the limbic system (Fig. 2. 11c). Since all auditory signals that indicate threat or danger are assigned a high level of priority and are closely monitored, the neuronal networks involved in their detection become highly tuned to these sounds, further enhancing their detection. The tinnitus signal is treated in precisely the same manner. Enhanced detection of the tinnitus results in a further increase of activation of the limbic and autonomic systems, which, in turn, enhances detection of tinnitus. This feedback loop creates a vicious circle of increasing annoyance and tinnitus perception. The final level of annoyance will depend on the highest level of activity in the autonomic nervous system that the subject can sustain for a prolonged period of time.

Changes in body function result from strong activation of sympathetic autonomic nervous system by tinnitus signal.

Activation of the sympathetic part of the autonomic nervous system results in a number of specific changes in body functions that are reflected in behaviors. Particularly relevant are increased levels of alertness, making sleeping difficult or impossible, alteration of heart rate and palpitations, problems with digestion and bowel activity, nausea and diarrhoea. In some patients, generally enhanced perception affecting all sensory modalities (global hypersensitivity) occurs. The quiet environment associated with sleeping also results in enhanced tinnitus perception, further interfering with the ability to go to sleep. However, patients more frequently have a problem in sustaining sleep, rather than with falling asleep.

Tinnitus-enhanced autonomic nervous system activity interferes with sleep. Sedatives and tranquilizers are not a long-term solution.

While tinnitus can indeed contribute to sleep disruption, some of the behavioral problems blamed on tinnitus result from sleep deprivation itself, as it causes problems similar to those evoked by tinnitus. There is exhaustion, lost of clear logical thinking and increased irritability; sufferers are more susceptible to making irrational associations, which can enhance their concerns and dislike of tinnitus. The very frequent consequence of sleep disturbance is that many tinnitus patients are taking sleeping pills. This has the negative effect of interfering with normal sleep patterns: decreasing the proportion of the rapid eye movement (REM) stage of sleep that is essential for the rest. Patients might be unconscious for a longer time than without medications but will not necessarily experience more REM sleep. These drugs, commonly in the tranquilizer group, produce significant changes within the central nervous system and especially the limbic system. Although they may be helpful in the short term, when there is intense distress, they do not break the vicious cycle of tinnitus reaction. It is important to recognize the negative side effects of such drugs, the possibility of development of dependence and the fact that they will not help tinnitus in the long term (Ch. 6).

Neither the level of autonomic activity nor the severity of the tinnitus is related to the psychoacoustical characterization of tinnitus perception (e.g., its pitch, loudness). The level of autonomic nervous system activity induced by tinnitus determines its severity.

Neither the level of autonomic activity nor the severity of the tinnitus is related to the psychoacoustical characterization of tinnitus perception (e.g., its pitch, loudness, etc.). It is a common experience that people with relatively quiet, simple tinnitus sounds can experience high levels of annoyance and anxiety, while others with extremely loud, complex and persistent tinnitus can experience very little annoyance or distress. The difference between those suffering because of tinnitus and others who are simply experiencing it, without significant distress, depends on the level of activation of the autonomic nervous system and not on what is happening within the auditory pathways. Ensuring that patients understand these particular relationships is an important part of the TRT counseling process.

Tinnitus is often established during a negative emotional experience with high autonomic system activity.

The base level of activity in the autonomic nervous system, and also the highest level at which this activity can be sustained for periods of time, is of importance in determining the extent of tinnitus impact in an individual. Pre-existing levels of autonomic nervous system activity at the time of tinnitus emergence are of particular significance. If an individual has an increased level of autonomic nervous system activity as a result of a previous profoundly negative and stressful experience, tinnitus emerging at that time will further increase this level of autonomic nervous system activity to a point where it will establish a vicious circle. By comparison, the emergence of tinnitus perception at a time of low autonomic nervous system activity and a relaxed state might not result in the establishment of the vicious circle, and natural habituation could take place. This explains why clinically significantly tinnitus commonly emerges during a period associated with profound emotional stress (Hazell & McKinney, 1996).

As can be seen in Fig. 2.12, the activation of the autonomic nervous system and subsequent changes in tinnitus severity can occur through two different complementary pathways. In the first one, the limbic system and autonomic nervous system is stimulated by tinnitus-related neuronal activity via subconscious pathways in a conditioned reflex manner (Fig. 2.12b). When this subconscious loop is dominant, there is generalized annoyance induced by tinnitus, with sleep disturbance, problems with attention and attacks of anxiety and panic, not necessarily associated with any particular thoughts. The conscious loop includes cortical areas, conscious thinking, verbalizations, beliefs, etc. (Fig. 2.12a). This pathway is significant when the patient exhibits more specific fears associated with tinnitus, such as the possibility of brain tumor, deafness or psychiatric illness. In practice, patients exhibit symptoms reflecting activity of both the conscious and subconscious loops, both contributing to the final reactions in varying degrees.

A subconscious loop, or vicious circle, can progressively enhance tinnitus without the patient consciously thinking about it.

The subconscious loop can work independently, resulting in autonomic nervous system activation from tinnitus even when the patient is unaware of it, while the conscious loop requires conscious awareness of the presence of the tinnitus, and thinking about it. In each case of clinically significant tinnitus, we have at least some involvement of the subconscious loop.

Tinnitus can produce phobic reactions, which are not helped by attempts at avoidance.

A small proportion of patients experience phobic reactions to tinnitus perception: a tinnitus signal evokes fear such as fears about its outcome in terms of sinister pathology, irreversible changes, its inevitable worsening and the impossibility of successful treatment. In this respect, the response and force of autonomic reaction is similar to that evoked by spiders (in arachnophobia). In this condition, each subsequent encounter with a spider produces powerful autonomic responses that can be disabling, for example sweating, palpitations or bowel disturbance. In addition, there is significant enhancement of the ability to detect spiders so that they are invariably spotted in a room before anyone else sees them, and they also appear to be substantially larger than their real size. Repetitive exposure to the spider, but without proper counseling or removal of negative reinforcement, results in a worsening of the phobia and enhancement of reflexive reactions and defensive behavior. Removal or reversal of this phobia for spiders must involve a process of learning about their true nature, growing to like them and finally being able to touch them without distress.

As with spiders, it is important that the phobic tinnitus patient does not try to avoid tinnitus by "masking," or even by blocking or distracting techniques, but should learn to experience tinnitus with increasing equanimity. Nevertheless, an important part of the management of these tinnitophobic states is the specific counseling against the notion that tinnitus can have feared and dreaded effects, which initially are a very powerful belief for the patient.

The phobic response is not mediated simply by the conscious loop but also involves the subconscious loop, just as the presence of the spider produces an automatic, conditioned reflex aversive response, without the need for any verbalization or evaluation. This phobic reaction to tinnitus is particularly difficult to overcome since, unlike the spider, it is not possible to escape easily from the presence of tinnitus.

New sounds attract our attention but habituate easily if deemed to be unimportant or without emotional association.

The first experience of a new and previously unknown sound results in excitation of the auditory pathway up to the cortex (Fig. 2.8). As the signal is new, it attracts the attention and triggers a process of cortical evaluation. As a part of a process that may eventually lead to some action being taken, the limbic and autonomic system are mildly activated at this time. If it turns out that this auditory signal is not of any particular importance and does not require any selective reaction, the specific excitation of the autonomic and limbic systems induced by this auditory pattern will weaken and gradually disappear. Further presentations of this signal will result in it being detected, but no stimulation of the limbic or autonomic nervous system will occur (Fig. 2.9a). By this stage, some habituation of perception has begun to occur, so that even when the stimulus is detected it is not consciously perceived.

A familiar example of this phenomenon can be noted after the purchase of a new refrigerator. When the machine is turned on, a quite loud, often annoying, sound is experienced. Initially, the sound of this refrigerator induces some annoyance, reflecting a stimulation of the autonomic nervous system, and even some anxiety, as it is frequently believed that the sound might indicate malfunction. As the refrigerator continues to work without malfunction, and reassurance is obtained from the store that all is well, anxiety and annoyance about this new sound gradually recedes. With continued repeated experience of the refrigerator turning on and off, awareness decreases gradually until the refrigerator is not heard, except when we are directly focusing our attention on it. This process typically takes several days or weeks.

This is a classic example of habituation, with the sound of the refrigerator undergoing a reduction of priority in the list of sounds to which we have to pay attention until it reaches the level of neutral sounds. Ultimately, there is no reaction to this sound, and we are no longer aware of its presence. Habituation of reaction and perception of this sound happens via a filtering process occurring at a subconscious level in the auditory system, with its connections to the limbic and autonomic nervous systems.

When tinnitus sounds are detected for the first time, they are treated in exactly the same way as any other new sound. Indeed, many patients are convinced that the sound of tinnitus is coming from outside and frequently open a window or look for a source of sound elsewhere in their environment. This might be an explanation why some so-called "hummers"[2] continue to be convinced that their sound is emanating from the environment (Rice, 1994). Hummers are distressed by sounds that others (often younger and with better hearing) cannot hear. Some hummers may be exhibiting a form of hyperacusis. Most tinnitus patients realize that the perception of tinnitus does not change as they move around their environment, as opposed to the perception of all external sounds, and they identify tinnitus as a sound originating within the head.

The principle of extinction of conditioned reflexes can be applied directly to the habituation of tinnitus-evoked reactions and its perception.

It is impossible to remove the tinnitus source or to attenuate the tinnitus perception by a conscious act. However, as already stressed, it is not the perception of tinnitus that is important but the reaction to the tinnitus. Fortunately, it is possible

---

[2] "Hummers" describes a group who complain about the presence of a low-frequency humming sound that they perceive as coming from their environment. Gas pipes and electrical transformers are often blamed for this by sufferers, who carry on lengthy correspondence with the relevant authorities. In some cases, a source of low-frequency sound has been detected, but in the majority of cases, it would seem that the underlying problem is either one of low-pitched tinnitus/somatosounds or decreased sound tolerance specifically for normal low-frequency sounds in the environment.

to habituate both the reactions to tinnitus and the perception of tinnitus itself using appropriate techniques, based on the extinction of conditioned reflexes. As habituation of tinnitus occurs within the brain, above the tinnitus source, it is independent of tinnitus etiology, otological diagnosis and psychoacoustical characterization of tinnitus (e.g., pitch, loudness and suppression by sound).

The principal goal of treatment is the habituation of reaction to tinnitus (Fig. 2.15a). Once it is achieved, tinnitus will still be perceived with the same psychoacoustical characterization (loudness and pitch), and it may be perceived the same percentage of the time. However, the presence of tinnitus will no longer produce any annoyance, or any emotional or autonomic response, and at the behavioral level patients will not be bothered by tinnitus, and it will have no impact on life. To achieve this outcome, it is necessary to change functional connections between the auditory system and the limbic and autonomic nervous systems responsible for the conditioned reflex arc linking the tinnitus-related neuronal activity with activation of the sympathetic part of the autonomic nervous system.

Habituation of tinnitus-induced reactions is equivalent to passive extinction of the conditioned reflexes.

The secondary goal is to facilitate habituation of tinnitus perception. Once that is achieved, patients will be aware of tinnitus for a small proportion of the time, mainly when focusing their attention on tinnitus. It is necessary to induce the process of blocking (filtering-out) the tinnitus-related neuronal activity from reaching the higher levels of the auditory system, where it would be perceived. Habituation of reaction to a stimulus can be described as a passive extinction of conditioned reflexes, as originally proposed by Pavlov (Konorski, 1948). Understanding that habituation and passive extinction of conditioned reflexes are the same phenomenon, by different names, has shown the way for the inducing and facilitating tinnitus habituation.

Typically, passive extinction is achieved by repeating the sensory stimulus but without reinforcement. This approach cannot be applied for tinnitus, as it is impossible to eliminate all reactions of the autonomic nervous system, which acts as a negative reinforcement. Therefore, a technique is used in which both the stimulus and the reinforcement are still present but decreased.

There are no methods for direct modification of the specific links between the auditory system and the autonomic nervous system (both conscious and subconscious loops). Instead, we employ a modification of a technique of passive extinction of conditioned reflexes. The classical process of passive extinction is achieved by repeating the sensory stimulus, but without reinforcement. In other words, the stimulus is moved to a neutral category by showing by example that it is no longer associated with a reinforcement. This approach, however, cannot be applied directly for tinnitus, as it is impossible to eliminate all reactions of the autonomic nervous system, which acts as a negative reinforcement. Therefore, a technique is used in which both the stimulus and the reinforcement are still present but decreased.

The first step is to reclassify tinnitus at a cognitive level as a neutral stimulus. The reclassification of tinnitus to a category of neutral or semi-neutral stimuli is essential, as habituation cannot occur without this – or would be extremely difficult to achieve.

Decrease of tinnitus-related activation of the autonomic nervous system is achieved by two mechanisms. First of all, tinnitus is reclassified at a cognitive level as a neutral stimulus. Patients are presented with information arguing that tinnitus perception and tinnitus per se are side effects of benign compensation occurring within the auditory system, typically to irrelevant dysfunction of the OHC system (following the discordant dysfunction theory) and/or enhancement of gain within the auditory system as a consequence of decreased auditory input (conductive or sensory hearing loss imitating the experiment with soundproof chamber). As a result of this reclassification, the activation of the limbic and autonomic nervous systems by the higher cognitive loop is removed or strongly decreased, and only the subconscious loop remains (Fig. 2.12b). Note that the reclassification of tinnitus to a category of neutral or semi-neutral stimuli is essential, as habituation cannot occur, or would be extremely difficult to achieve, without this.

The second mechanism involves a psychological principle that known dangers evoke a much less-powerful autonomic response than unknown ones. An example of this phenomenon is provided by a patient sitting in a dentist's waiting room. In the first scenario, he has already been counseled by telephone to expect the need for root canal therapy and all that this entails. In the second scenario, he does not know what lies ahead of him. Even though the outcome will be the same, the patient faced with uncertainty about dangerous or unpleasant experiences is much more distressed and agitated than one who knows what is coming.

In the case of tinnitus, we provide a clear explanation of the mechanisms resulting in tinnitus perception, and those involved in creating annoyance and negative emotional responses. Basically, the patient is taught crucial elements of the neurophysiological model of tinnitus. This produces a decrease in the autonomic nervous system activity resulting from tinnitus, since patients now understand what is happening and why.

Patients are taught why tinnitus is not linked to any danger.

Another way of influencing the limbic and autonomic nervous systems is to create new, positive associations with tinnitus. Generating hopefulness about the possibility of successful treatment and involving the patient actively in this process creates a strong change in emotional attitude and response. As TRT has better results than any other tinnitus treatment, the published results can be shared with the patient, a powerful tool in producing this change of outlook. It is important to avoid negative images of tinnitus. Descriptions like screeching, tearing, steam jets should be replaced by benign, more peaceful descriptions, such as "music of the brain." This reduces the negative emotions produced by the limbic system and consequently reduces autonomic nervous system activity.

The next aspect of treatment is aimed in a non-specific way at the patient's general level of arousal and stress. A high proportion of tinnitus patients have busy and demanding life-styles; they are constantly under pressure to increase performance and cope with all sorts of difficult and different problems, both at work and in domestic situations. At home, they are frequently engaged in many activities, have problems related to their busy family or have significant life challenges. All these stresses add to the overall level of activity in the limbic and autonomic systems, already enhanced by tinnitus.

Therefore, patients are advised to try to decrease the general level of stress. Different stress management strategies, biofeedback, relaxation training – sometimes hypnosis or simply proper time management – and getting involved in other pleasant activities may result in decreasing stress and annoyance levels. This reduces the general level of arousal and activation of the limbic and autonomic nervous systems and consequently weakens the feedback loop that plays a dominant role in creating a high level of tinnitus-induced annoyance. It should be realized that stress management, although extremely important for some patients, cannot on its own bring about permanent relief from tinnitus symptoms.

Distraction techniques will not affect the function of the subconscious loop, or the underlying specific neuronal activity, which will persist as before. They can only be used when the patient is thinking consciously about the tinnitus. Although distraction strategies might be useful in the initial stages of tinnitus distress, for instance to help in getting to sleep, in the long term they are counterproductive. Retraining of the reaction cannot take place in the absence of tinnitus. Furthermore, the distraction technique provides only temporary relief and may even attract the individual's attention to the presence of annoying tinnitus.

Habituation is facilitated by decreasing the strength of the signal through sound therapy.

The second part of the method used to achieve extinction of conditioned reflexes involving tinnitus is to decrease the strength of the tinnitus signal. This is achieved by sound therapy, which is the other indispensable component of TRT. It is important to explain to patients the reasons for this and to make it clear that it is sound which is important and not the method or device for producing it.

If we increase the background neuronal activity in the auditory system by adding sound, the difference between the tinnitus signal and the background neuronal activity decreases. This results in reduction of the strength of the tinnitus-related signal passing to the limbic system and the cortical areas, because all our perceptions, as well as the assessment of the strength of any neuronal activity within the brain, are based on the difference between signal and background activity (e.g., background noise). As a consequence of reducing this contrast, subcortical detection of the tinnitus-related neuronal activity becomes more difficult. This itself will increase the probability of habituation of the tinnitus signal for both tinnitus-induced reactions and perception.

When using sound therapy, it is important to realize that if suppression of tinnitus occurs, even though temporary symptom relief is experienced by some patients, this is an avoidance strategy, which by definition prevents habituation of tinnitus as the brain cannot be retrained to a signal that it cannot detect. Therefore "masking" of tinnitus is counterproductive and contraindicated in TRT, which is aimed at tinnitus habituation rather than temporary symptom relief.

Experiencing tinnitus in a state of low arousal aids habituation, whereas suppression and avoidance of tinnitus slows habituation.

In our London clinic, an exercise is used (the "ten second exercise") that encourages patients to focus on the *reaction* to their tinnitus (from time to time) and for brief periods only in order to note the strength of their dislike and body reactions to it and to try to reduce, by an act of will, these negative responses. Practicing relaxation exercises at the same time facilitates this process. The rationale for this approach is that habituation will occur to any stimulus if repeatedly experienced in a state of low arousal.

There is no drug that can be recommended for tinnitus treatment.

Use of various medications is a separate issue. While there is no drug that can be recommended for tinnitus treatment (see Ch. 6), many patients are taking some medication prescribed because of tinnitus. Typically, these drugs are aimed at affecting central nervous system function. Although there are a number of drugs that are active in reducing limbic and autonomic nervous system activity, and are commonly used in the management of anxiety, we do not recommend the use of these drugs, except in an acute emergency. However, if patients come to us who have already been taking these drugs for some time, we do not advise them to withdraw from them suddenly. Our attitude towards drugs results from the observation that none has been shown to have a positive effect on tinnitus itself without causing profound side effects. Despite the fact that these drugs may produce temporary improvement in coping with the tinnitus, they also impair plasticity of the central nervous system and, therefore, slow down the process of habituation. This is particularly relevant with the benzodiazepines (see Ch. 6).

Benzodiazepines interfere with the learning process in TRT and slow the process of habituation.

Imagine the difficulty in trying to learn a new language at night school after spending the early evening consuming several pints of beer. Many of our patients who have been taking a benzodiazepine report that even slight alteration in their perception of reality greatly interferes with their ability to think clearly and function normally, and also to undertake the mental activities involved in TRT.

Habituation to tinnitus is slow; patients must understand this and be followed carefully over time.

The processes of habituation of both reaction and perception are very gradual and take time, generally measured in months, as it is necessary to retrain conditioned reflexes while we cannot remove reinforcement totally. Some patients experience subjectively significant improvement within a month or two, but others notice a beneficial effect later in their treatment. To prevent relapse, we insist on continuing therapy for at least 12 months, and we make it clear to all patients at the beginning that they must remain under supervision for this period. In practice, we are trying to keep contact with all our patients until they do not need any additional help. For research purposes, we are following patients for several years after they ceased TRT treatment. It is usual for patients to experience partial habituation during the first six months of therapy. It is important for patients to realize that habituation may take a long time, that changes are very gradual and that they are not necessarily smooth and monotonic. It is essential to follow all TRT instructions regardless of whether or not tinnitus is less or more severe on a given day.

Patients are encouraged to choose the best treatment option based on the model.

At the end of the first consultation session, we discuss our recommendations with the patient, making clear that this is the preferred option but at the same time outlining other options and presenting the positive and negative aspects of their selection. It is very important not to put patients under any pressure to accept a particular approach, as all of those who are experiencing extreme tinnitus distress will already feel under heavy pressure. The purpose of presenting different treatment options is to have the patient agree on which is the most appropriate, rather than making a didactic enforcement of one form of therapy or another. The approach will be much more successful if it is based on the belief of the patient that it will succeed (and on understanding why), rather than accepting a forced choice imposed by the healthcare professional. The optimal option is discussed and justified on the basis of the neurophysiological model, and it is presented as the option that is most likely to succeed in the shortest time.

Patients receive all the material used in counseling for revision at home.

Finally, patients are provided with all the notes and drawings used during their counseling, as well as selected reprints of articles written in a simple and straightforward manner about tinnitus or hyperacusis. Successful study requires homework, and patients are encouraged to read this information as an important part of the reinforcement process and to contact us if they have any questions or misunderstandings that require clarification. In addition, the interview may be recorded and the patient given the tape to be reviewed later on (the practice in the London clinic but not in the USA because of legal issues). It is very helpful to allow patients to have copies of their medical reports, as such reports contain an account of the individual case and justification for the particular treatment approach that has been selected. A copy of the report of the visit is also sent to the referring physician.

In summary, tinnitus-related non-specific counseling is aimed at conveying the following ideas.

1. The perception of tinnitus does not reflect any pathological state but results from a healthy compensation of the auditory system to some disturbances of neuronal activity, typically generated in the periphery.
2. The problems and behavioral symptoms created by tinnitus do not result from the perception of the sound but from the reaction to it by the brain and body.
3. Conditioned reflexes are involved in producing tinnitus-induced reactions.
4. Conditioned reflexes can be retrained, resulting in habituation of reactions evoked by tinnitus and its perception.
5. For habituation, it is necessary to reclassify tinnitus into a neutral/semi-neutral category of stimuli.
6. Habituation can be facilitated by a decrease in the strength of the tinnitus signal, achieved by the proper use of sound therapy.
7. Habituation of tinnitus-induced reactions is the primary goal; once it is at least partially achieved, habituation of tinnitus perception will follow automatically.

3.4.2　Specific aspects of general counseling related to decreased sound tolerance

Decreased sound tolerance can accompany tinnitus or occur on its own. When present, it typically involves both hyperacusis and misophonia. The majority of tinnitus patients exhibit decreased sound tolerance to some extent, and for about 25–30%, hyperacusis is significant enough to warrant specific treatment.

General counseling for decreased sound tolerance is focused on potential mechanisms underlying its presence. For hyperacusis it is explained that the auditory system provides an automatic gain control, modifying its sensitivity at both peripheral and central levels. Consequently, when a person is exposed to a low level of the sound, this signal is amplified by OHC system by up to 60 dB (Narayan et al., 1998;

Overstreet, Temchin & Ruggero, 2002; Robles & Ruggero, 2001; Ruggero *et al.*, 2000) and still further in the central auditory pathways (Boettcher & Salvi, 1993; Gerken *et al.*, 1984; Gerken, Simhadri-Sumithra & Bhat, 1986; Salvi *et al.*, 1992).

Hyperacusis results from abnormally high gain within the auditory system.

When the average sound level increases then this gain decreases, loudest sounds potentially having the greatest effect. If mechanisms controlling this gain modification are producing higher levels of amplification when it is not needed, then overstimulation occurs within the auditory system, resulting in the perception of sounds as abnormally loud, even painful. This phenomenon is called hyperacusis. In pure hyperacusis, the limbic and autonomic nervous systems and their connections with the auditory system are normal, and their high activation is of secondary consequence to the excessively high levels of activity in the auditory pathways.

Treatment of hyperacusis is based on the desensitization principle: systematic exposure to non-annoying sound results in increased threshold of discomfort.

Treatment of hyperacusis is based on the desensitization principle: systematic exposure to non-annoying sound results in an increased threshold of discomfort. For particularly severe hyperacusis, patients start with low sound levels and gradually increase the intensity during treatment. This treatment works at a subconscious level, does not involve retraining of conditioned reflexes and does not involve cognitive processes. Consequently, the improvement of pure hyperacusis typically occurs fast, within weeks. Patients need to follow the protocol of sound therapy for hyperacusis and their understanding of the neurophysiological model can be limited.

Misophonia, the dislike of sounds, reflects enhanced connection between the auditory and limbic and autonomic nervous systems; it has the same mechanism as clinically significant tinnitus, based on conditioned reflexes.

In real-life, the situation is more complex, as the majority of patients have both hyperacusis and misophonia. Some have misophonia without hyperacusis. Misophonia, which reflects enhanced connection between the auditory and limbic and autonomic nervous systems, involves the same connections and mechanisms as tinnitus and is controlled by conditioned reflexes. Basically all principles and explanations used for tinnitus are applicable for misophonia, with the difference that the neuronal activity evoked by external sound acts in place of tinnitus-related neuronal activity. However, it is linked to the reactions of the limbic and autonomic nervous system in entirely the same fashion as clinically significant tinnitus. Therefore, the same basic approach of extinction of conditioned reflexes can be utilized for the treatment of misophonia.

To treat misophonia, a positive association with external sounds is created by systematical exposure to pleasant sounds, to which the patient is asked to pay attention. This approach is totally different from desensitization used for hyperacusis.

However, as external sounds, over which we do have control, are inducing reactions, it is possible to use more powerful methods of active extinction of the reflexes. Specifically, a positive feeling about external sounds is created by systematical exposure to pleasant sounds, to which the patient is asked to pay attention. Note that this approach is totally different from desensitization used for hyperacusis.

During counseling about decreased sound tolerance, its various components are explained, stressing the similarities and differences. When significant hyperacusis is present together with tinnitus, then counseling regarding tinnitus is abbreviated, as frequently tinnitus improves significantly after hyperacusis treatment is successful. Misophonia is discussed, stressing its similarity with tinnitus and the role of conditioned reflexes in its development.

3.4.3   General factors modifying tinnitus retraining counseling

The specifics of counseling are decided by allocation to a treatment category. However, some general factors affect the implementation. One of the factors is the strength of inappropriate beliefs. In these patients, the conscious loop plays a dominant part. It is important to address these specific beliefs and concerns in addition to the process of general "demystification." Patients need to be shown that their fears are unfounded, using the neurophysiological model and clinical and research data, as documented in peer-reviewed literature. Some patients are strongly convinced that their tinnitus indicates the presence of a brain tumor, a stroke or some other neurological disease, despite full investigations. These patients may require repeated assurance.

Culture and background affects the way people respond to tinnitus and must be taken into account during counseling.

An individual's cultural, social and educational background, profession and age can have a profound impact on thinking and the development of tinnitus. These factors have to be taken into account in the counseling process, selecting illustrations and analogies that fit the individual's profile most closely. Social acceptance of the expression of emotion shows great cultural variation and has a direct bearing on the development of tinnitus and on the methods for dealing with it. Free expression of emotion (for example in certain Mediterranean cultures) acts as a method to avoid a build-up of tension. This tends to decrease the severity of any reaction to tinnitus and hyperacusis. Conversely, the "British stiff upper lip" might be seen as an impediment to the release of these emotions, causing a build-up of greater distress and annoyance.

Independent thinking is often culturally based. It does little good to apply TRT counseling as a didactic imposition of the provider's own professional status and knowledge about tinnitus when interacting with someone who has a free and independent personality. In this situation, a much more effective approach is to work together as a team where the patient is a member. The educational background of the patient will also play a significant role in shaping the therapist's approach. While the general message is the same, the arguments and examples will vary according to the individual's educational background, and their trust or mistrust of science and research in general.

Patients need to be sure that professionals are doing their best to help them and that they have sufficient knowledge of the subject.

Different cultural backgrounds will result in a difference of the ease with which an individual will accept orders given by authority. Is there a blind belief that everything the family physician says must be absolutely true, or is there a constant questioning of all forms of advice received from any professional? This will determine the level of interaction that the patient will have with the tinnitus therapist and will decide whether the patient will treat the doctor as an authoritarian figure or as a partner with whom the problem is being solved. In each case, it is important to develop a good rapport between patient and therapist. Patients need to be sure that therapists are doing their best to help them and that they have sufficient knowledge of the subject. This is an extremely important part of TRT. A high level of trust facilitates the process of demystification of tinnitus and increases the compliance of the patient with the treatment protocol.

Partners, friends or other family members are asked to participate in counseling sessions.

When other people are influencing the patient's life and thinking, as with parents or partners, appropriate counseling must be given to them as well. Indeed it is very helpful when making an appointment to encourage patients to bring with them somebody with whom they have close everyday interaction. Partners and close friends who gain a first-hand knowledge of the neurophysiological model can be instrumental in the patient's own study, and thus help in the TRT process. This ability to provide help removes the feeling of helplessness and despair often felt by those close to a suffering patient.

The general level of the patient's scientific knowledge, particularly their ability to understand the anatomy and physiology of hearing, plays a significant role. Patients often acquire a significant knowledge of tinnitus before they come, frequently involving many misconceptions. Wide use of the Internet, combined with the total freedom to put on it any type of uncontrolled information, has a negative impact on tinnitus patients. They follow countless unsubstantiated claims about methods to achieve "miracle cures" for tinnitus; even worse, they are learning how terrible tinnitus can be, and about its presumed links with numbers of medical problems. This provides strong negative counseling, which makes·their tinnitus worse and necessitates spending time during counseling counteracting this information. However, some level of general scientific knowledge facilitates the process of counseling. The absence of a scientific background in no way precludes the ability to understand the model and follow TRT, provided that appropriate language is used to communicate the concepts and ideas.

The absence of scientific knowledge does not prevent understanding of the model.

Correctness of the model and TRT does not depend on any religious beliefs. Illustration of the model using concepts related to Darwinian evolution theory may offend some people with contrary religious beliefs; therefore such concepts are avoided during counseling.

Many people, because of religious or other beliefs, do not accept the Darwinian concept of evolution. Neither does correctness of the model depend on it. The integrity of the model is always preserved, but the delivery may vary depending on the situation. A good example is the way of describing how the brain reacts to signals indicating danger. It is irrelevant whether this ability was acquired as a result of evolution, and natural selection, or created in some other way.

Musicians are specially affected by tinnitus and hyperacusis because of their auditory training.

Patients with professional training in music, or for whom music plays an important role in life, will be sensitive to even very small modification of tinnitus perception, as detecting and evaluating sounds play a vital part in their life. They have a specially modified signal-processing and pattern-matching ability that is more acute than in the untrained individual. This is particularly applicable to professional musicians, sound engineers and other professions where the work requires identification, separation and detailed evaluation of complex sounds. As artists in general, including musicians, can have a tendency to higher emotional reactions relating to their work, they may display a more significant reaction to tinnitus or hyperacusis and, therefore, have a tendency to be more distressed by it. This is certainly confirmed by our clinical experience. Therefore, special counseling is needed, explaining to patients why certain professional training can enhance tinnitus detection.

3.4.4 Common issues for sound therapy

Sound therapy consists of enrichment of the auditory background.

Sound therapy consists of enrichment of the auditory background by several different approaches: the introduction of additional sounds, increasing the volume of existing sounds, amplification of environmental sounds by hearing aids, and finally, by wearable sound generators. Typically, more than one approach is used. Even when sound generators are used, which provide a well-controlled sound source for enrichment of the auditory background, environmental sounds are still required. Specifics of the implementation of sound therapy are determined by the treatment category for a given patient.

All patients are advised to avoid silence.

All patients are advised to avoid silence and to provide an enrichment of environmental sounds. This is not an easy or trivial matter. It is helpful to perform a detailed assessment of the sound environment in which the patient lives throughout a 24-hour period, as many people spend surprisingly long periods of time in silence. The goal of counseling about sound therapy is to convey to the patient the importance of filling every part of the day and night with background sound, which, at the same time, must not be intrusive or irritating. Listening to TV or radio, although appropriate for recreational periods, is not the proper approach. These sound sources attract attention as they contain speech, promoting the need or desire to understand what is being said.

All patients are taught sound enrichment. Sounds of nature are best.

The need for sound enrichment is heightened by the tendency to lose many natural environmental sounds in our modern society. Modern buildings tend to exclude environmental sounds. In general, the population is living longer and, with ageing, there is a tendency to become hearing impaired. Furthermore, elderly people frequently live alone, which further decreases stimulation of the auditory system. In Western culture in the past it has been the practice to impress on children the importance of keeping quiet: working and going to bed in silence. This training leaves the concept that silence is golden, when in reality it is not. In nature, there is a continuous background of natural sound – wind, rain, animals, etc. – and silence tends to occur only before an emergency (e.g., arrival of a predator). Silence, therefore, has a tendency to increase alertness, preparing for danger. The realization that the right sounds can increase relaxation has led to numerous devices that create nature sounds, both naturally and electronically. These devices are used too for increasing background sounds in office environments to avoid distraction by unexpected noise, and the detrimental effects of silence.

There are many ways to enrich the sound background, for example using table-top sound machines, CDs and ear-level instruments (called sound generators).

Introducing extra sounds is an effective and convenient method of changing the strength of the tinnitus signal and, therefore, facilitating habituation.

There are many ways to enrich the sound background. It is relatively easy to introduce nature sounds by using table-top sound machines, CDs, and ear-level instruments: called sound generators. Introducing extra sounds is an effective and convenient method of changing the strength of the tinnitus signal and, therefore, facilitating habituation.

Sounds of nature are preferred for effective sound enrichment. For most patients we recommend the sounds of nature generated by specialized electronic devices, so-called table-top sound machines. Our patients also prefer this method. It works better than recordings on tape or CD, as it provides a very constant sound, the level of which can be adjusted as needed. Sound enrichment does not need to be loud; it should be easily perceived when attention is directed toward it, without straining to hear it.

The sound used for enrichment during day and night should be neutral, non-intrusive and not annoying.

The sound used for enrichment during day and night should be, on the one hand, neutral, non-intrusive and not annoying. On the other hand, it should not be pleasant or arousing to the extent that it attracts attention. The sound should be easy to ignore. The type of sound depends strongly on the personal preference of the patient, but most patients choose first the sounds of flowing water. Nature sounds, or wide-band noise, are always better than the radio or television as they do not contain meaning. Music is not recommended for continuous background sound as it tends to induce emotion and attract attention. Meaningful sounds can attract attention and evoke emotions, consequently increasing autonomic activity. An interesting illustration of this is one of our patients who was comforted by the sound of speech of foreign language broadcasts, which he was unable to understand.

Whatever sound is used, habituation to it should occur rapidly and patients should soon become unaware of its presence. Sound enrichment should be used continuously (24-hours a day, seven days a week) because the auditory system and its connections, apart from the cortical awareness centers, are active normally during sleep. They can be stimulated at this time to promote habituation of tinnitus, as well as to decrease gain within the auditory pathways. It is common that some patients like the sound produced by a large domestic or ceiling fan; however, the level of sound produced by a fan cannot be changed, which limits its effectiveness. When the climate permits, windows may be left open or air conditioning turned on, although, again, these sources cannot be adjusted for intensity.

It is notable that many tinnitus patients, and most patients with hyperacusis and misophonia, spend much of their time seeking silence. Feeling threatened by a barrage of internal or external sounds, for which they may have developed a profound dislike, they try hard to avoid them. Patients develop a pattern of behavior that excludes all external environmental sounds on the basis that any sound is intrusive, unpleasant, can be dangerous or may make tinnitus worse. It is not a simple task to persuade such patients of the therapeutic benefits of sound! Instruction about the concept and use of sound enrichment has to be specific to the patient and must be monitored and altered according to the individual needs of each patient. It is often not a trivial task to find sounds that patients will tolerate or to which they have not already developed an aversion.

Approximately 50% of tinnitus patients have a problem with sleeping.

Sound therapy is very effective in improving sleeping by providing a neutral auditory background, which decreases the apparent strength of tinnitus and helps with falling asleep during short periods of wakefulness.

As mentioned above, approximately 50% of tinnitus patients have a problem with sleeping (McKenna, 2000). The possible mechanisms of this problem were discussed in Ch. 2. At a behavioral level, patients judge that they may be unable to fall asleep because their tinnitus is very loud, or they may wake up in the middle of the night and be unable to fall asleep again. Most people sleep in a quiet, often silent, room; in this situation, the tinnitus signal is enhanced, increasing its perceived loudness and intrusiveness significantly. Sound therapy is very effective in improving sleeping by providing a neutral auditory background, which decreases the apparent strength of tinnitus and helps with falling asleep during the short periods of wakefulness that are an integral part of a normal sleeping pattern.

Subcortical auditory pathways are very active and so are capable of being influenced by sound therapy during waking hours as well as during sleep. This is even the case under full surgical anesthesia (Wang, Ryan & Woolf, 1987). Neuronal activity measured during sleep and anesthesia was found to be the same or even higher than when fully awake. We can easily be awakened by an important signal (e.g., the sound of a baby crying), while we can sleep through loud but unimportant signals (e.g., a thunderstorm). In other words, the auditory system is continuously monitoring the sound environment, and subcortical centers are performing the vital task of selecting, categorizing and filtering signals, as described above, even during sleep. In the case of the patient with sleeping problems, night-time sound enrichment is particularly important not only to help to induce tinnitus habituation but also to help with sleeping. Sound enrichment has a beneficial effect on sleeping in everyone, regardless of the presence or absence of tinnitus.

Introducing the sounds of nature are a very effective way of enriching background sound.

For many patients, introducing sound during the night produces the first beneficial effect seen with TRT, and in many cases it provides very significant relief in a short period of time. The elderly have a shorter sleep cycle, and therefore the beneficial effects of night-time sound enrichment are more pronounced.

3.4.5 Sound enrichment in hearing loss

The same approach of background sound enrichment is used in those with impaired hearing except the sound is further amplified by hearing aids.

The approach to enriching the background sound for people whose hearing loss causes significant problems is exactly the same as for those with normal hearing. Such sound enrichment is further enhanced by appropriate amplification through hearing aids. There is one point that needs to be taken into account. Many hearing-impaired patients have normal or near-normal hearing at low frequencies. Typical environment sound contains a significant amount of energy in the frequency range below 200 Hz, which provides constant sound stimulation and thus helps to prevent an increased gain in the auditory system. These frequencies, however, cannot be amplified by hearing aids. Therefore, it is crucial to fit hearing aids with open molds to avoid blocking these low frequencies; hearing aids fitted with closed molds act as ear plugs for frequencies below 200 Hz.

Deep canal hearing aids (well-vented) in tinnitus patients are on trial in our London clinic and are suitable in selected patients. Many patients experience significant enhancement of tinnitus if the ear canals are totally or partially blocked by any means, including hearing aids.

Habituation of tinnitus is facilitated by sound stimulation and hindered by silence.

Decrease of the natural sound level increases the chance of emergence or re-emergence of tinnitus, as demonstrated by the soundproof room experiment (Heller & Bergman, 1953). As loudness of any sound depends on the contrast between this sound and background, anything that reduces environmental sound will increase perceived tinnitus loudness. In silence, tinnitus is the only sound present and will have no chance of escaping the attentional focus of the auditory system. Pattern recognition and auditory gain are enhanced during silence, increasing

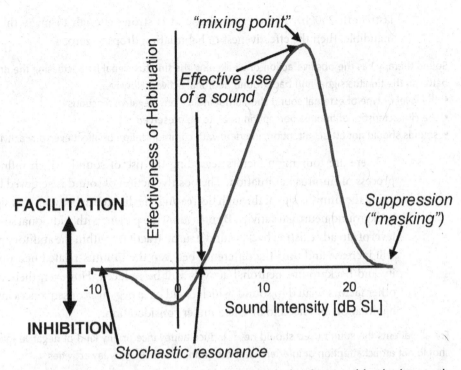

Figure 3.1   Dependence of habituation on sound intensity. Note that for sound levels close to the threshold of detection, inhibition of habituation may occur through stochastic resonance. The probability of habituation decreases to zero when the sound is suppressing tinnitus. The optimal level for tinnitus treatment corresponds to the beginning of partial suppression of tinnitus, typically described by the patient as the "mixing" or "blending" point.

the chances that tinnitus-related neuronal activity will be detected. Habituation of both tinnitus reaction and perception depend on plasticity in the auditory system and its connections with the limbic and autonomic nervous systems. Habituation of tinnitus is facilitated by sound stimulation and hindered by silence.

3.5 Sound therapy: common features

3.5.1 Selecting optimal sound

The intensity of the sound in sound therapy affects the process of habituation.

The process of habituation is affected by the levels of sound selected for use in sound therapy. The crucial elements of this dependence are shown in Fig. 3.1. When the sound level is close to the threshold of hearing, this signal can actually enhance tinnitus through stochastic resonance: the enhancement of the tinnitus signal by addition of low-level random noise (Jastreboff, 1999c; Jastreboff &

Jastreboff, 2000b). If the external sound is strong enough to make the tinnitus inaudible, then the effectiveness of habituation drops to zero.

Sound therapy has the positive action of weakening the tinnitus signal by decreasing the difference between the tinnitus signal and background neuronal activity. However,
• the level or type of external sound should not induce any negative reactions
• the characteristics of tinnitus perception need to be preserved
• sounds should not attract attention, interfere with communication or affect everyday activities.

There are four main factors regarding the use of sound, which influence the process of tinnitus habituation. The positive action of sound is achieved by weakening the tinnitus signal through decreasing the difference between this signal and background neuronal activity. By providing the patient with additional sounds, the level of already existing background neuronal activity within the auditory pathways will increase and thus the difference between the tinnitus-related neuronal activity and background neuronal activity will be reduced. However, there are three other factors related to sound, which could have negative consequences in tinnitus habituation and need to be taken under consideration.

For all patients the sound used should never induce annoyance or any kind of negative reaction. It should not attract attention or interfere with communications or everyday activities.

First, external sounds should not induce any negative reactions (e.g., annoyance) because of their loudness or quality, as this would enhance activation of the limbic and autonomic nervous systems and consequently hinder habituation. When hyperacusis is present, keeping sound below the annoyance level is the dominant limiting factor.

Habituation is a process of retraining existing conditioned reflexes, and this retraining cannot occur if the auditory system is unable to detect the tinnitus signal. Therefore, by definition, if we suppress tinnitus, we will never achieve habituation.[3] It is a basic behavioral and psychological rule that it is impossible to train, or retrain, a subject with a stimulus which is not detectable. Consequently, it is impossible to achieve habituation of tinnitus if the tinnitus-related neuronal activity is not detected by the brain because the tinnitus signal is suppressed by an external sound.

If tinnitus is suppressed ("masked") habituation will never occur.

Second, it is important to preserve the original tinnitus signal. When the tinnitus signal is modified, even if it is habituated, once the external sound source is removed, the tinnitus will return to its original unhabituated state. Consequently, there will be

---

[3] Clinical data from 20 patients who were using masking for symptomatic relief, for 15 years or more without experiencing any change in tinnitus perception or its annoyance, achieved full habituation of tinnitus after being treated with TRT for a short period.

only a partial decrease of reaction to tinnitus, based on the generalization principle. In the extreme case when the tinnitus signal is totally suppressed, by definition habituation cannot occur. When the sound level does not totally suppress the tinnitus but partly alters it, so-called "partial masking" (Moore, 1995), habituation may occur, but its effectiveness is decreased and less predictable, as the signal to be habituated will be different from the original one (Fig. 3.1).[4] To be effective, the intensity of sound enrichment should lie between the threshold for hearing it and the level at which partial suppression ("partial masking") begins to occur. This level is typically described by patients as the "mixing" or "blending" point (Fig. 3.1) and tinnitus patients perceive that the external sound and tinnitus start to interfere with each other. The use of sound above the blending or mixing point results in decreased effectiveness of sound therapy.

Therefore, the sound level used in sound therapy should be close to but below the level of partial suppression, the so-called "mixing" or "blending point." At this sound level, patients can still perceive separately tinnitus and the external sound, but the perception is that these sounds nevertheless start to interfere, blend or mix together. Further increase of sound level results in perception of tinnitus of even more different sound quality.

Note that the level at which partial suppression occurs is not simplistically related to the perceived tinnitus loudness. The loudness of tinnitus, as assessed by a loudness match, is typically stable. The perception of tinnitus, however, is influenced by its behavioral evaluation and the status of the limbic system, and this last factor influences the patient's perception of loudness. The level when partial suppression starts is related to the type and strength of the tinnitus-related neural activity and not to its perceived loudness. It should be made clear to patients that they should adjust sound levels according to the perception of "blending" or "mixing" without paying attention to how loud their tinnitus is.

Since the sound levels causing partial suppression may, nevertheless, change from day to day, patients are instructed to readjust wearable sound generators each time they are placed on the ears. However, it is not advisable to change the setting during the day, even when the levels of environmental sounds mask perception of the sound generated by the devices.

Finally, sounds used in sound therapy should not attract undue attention, interfere with communication or affect everyday activities. Treatment is aimed to be as

---

[4] This is a reflection of the so-called generalization principle (Brennan & Jastreboff, 1991). If we train a subject to respond to a certain stimulus, for example a 5 kHz tone, and after this if we test the subject on different frequencies between 1 and 10 kHz, the strongest response would be obtained using the original 5 kHz signal. As we move away from 5 kHz (for example 4, 3, 2, 1 kHz) the response will gradually diminish. If we achieve habituation of a tinnitus signal changed by "partial masking", then once the external suppressing sound is turned off, and the original tinnitus reappears, there will be less habituation since the brain was trained to habituate to a different signal: the partially changed tinnitus.

unintrusive as possible to avoid further enhancing any negative aspects of tinnitus. For instance, interference with speech discrimination would result in a straining-to-hear phenomenon, which increases tinnitus.

It is impossible to assure constant sound levels when only table-top sound machines are used to provide sound enrichment, as every movement will result in a change of the perception of the sound. This is one of the reasons for the use of ear-level, wearable sound generators. Note, however, that it is the sound that is of overwhelming importance and not the specific source or the means of its delivery. Wearable sound generators are a convenient way of delivering stable, well-controlled sound and serve as a "safety net" by not allowing outside sound levels to drop below a preset level, which could enhance tinnitus by stochastic resonance.

3.5.2 Wearable sound generators

For the majority of patients, sound therapy also involves the use of instruments (wearable sound generators or hearing aids).

For the majority of patients, sound therapy also involves the use of instruments (wearable sound generators or hearing aids). The method that provides the highest level of control of sound delivery, and seems to be the most effective mode of sound therapy, is to fit patients bilaterally with behind-the-ear or in-the-ear sound generators. These devices emit low levels of sound that, from the point of view of habituation, have several important advantages. First, the amplitude of sound generators is very stable. It is easier to habituate to external sounds that are continuous and stable, rather than changing or intermittent. In practice, after a short period of time, patients become unaware of the presence of their wearable sound generators and can very easily ignore them. Second, the level of sound can be controlled and adjusted easily by the patient to the optimal level for promoting habituation. This element of control also helps to make the sound neutral and non-threatening. In patients with hyperacusis, the ability to alter the volume of the instruments during treatment is essential.

Wearable sound generators have several advantages over environmental sound.

While a variety of sound sources could be used to stimulate background neuronal activity, wearable behind-the-ear broadband sound generators offer certain advantages. These generators share with tinnitus a physical frame of reference related to the head; therefore, their sound does not change with head and body movements. The perception of all sounds from the environment changes with even the slightest movement of the head. The brain will gradually habituate to wearable sound generators, and this ability to habituate to perception of a sound that is not changing while the individual is moving around is transferred to tinnitus. The situation is similar to learning how to ride a bicycle before learning how to ride a motorcycle.

The instruments produce a broadband noise that stimulates a reasonably wide range of neurons within the auditory pathways. These small devices do not block the ear canal and so there is no interference with environmental sound entering the ear. In addition, as a low level of sound (around 10 dB SL) is used, it does not interfere with normal hearing.

Instrument fitting must be bilateral to avoid asymmetrical stimulation of the auditory system.

Another important issue is that devices are fitted to both ears, even when the tinnitus is perceive as being localized to one ear. For all categories of patient needing sound generators or hearing aids, binaural instruments are used whenever physically possible. The reason for this is that we are attempting to achieve symmetrical stimulation of both sides of the auditory system. Asymmetrical stimulation results in reorganization of the receptive field within the auditory system, consequently impairing its ability to process sound. Unilateral fitting of hearing aids to bilateral hearing loss results in decreasing speech discrimination ability in the un-aided ear. Attempts to stimulate only one side in unilateral tinnitus frequently results in a shift of the perceived location of the tinnitus to the opposite side because of the strong interaction within the auditory pathways, and the asymmetry of sound stimulation.

For both sound generators and hearing aids, as open as possible ear-mold fittings are needed to minimize the occlusion effect and the reduction of normal access for environmental sounds.

For both sound generators and hearing aids, as open as possible ear-mold fittings are needed to minimize the occlusion effect and the reduction of normal access of environmental sounds to the ear. Making really good open ear-molds is not a trivial task. Cosmetic concerns should be recognized, as with hearing aid fitting. Until recently, only relatively large, behind-the-ear sound generators were dominant on the market and all our results in the past were obtained using these instruments. Now a variety of behind-the-ear and in-the-ear instruments are available. It is important to be aware of what the patient considers acceptable and not try to force an instrument choice, as it will not be used by an unwilling individual.

The type or make of the instrument is irrelevant as long as it provides relatively broadband stable sound with a volume that can be regulated smoothly from the threshold of hearing. The spectral characteristics of sound reaching the tympanic membrane are not crucial. In particular, we do not attempt to relate them in any way to the perceived pitch of tinnitus. It is important to realize that habituation can be achieved solely by enrichment of the auditory background; however the use of sound generators, when indicated, appears to have a higher probability of success and is likely to achieve habituation in a shorter time.

Wearable sound generators, or combination instruments, are essential in hyperacusis.

For hyperacusic patients, wearable sound generators, or combination instruments where there is also a hearing loss, are always indicated.

Optimally, instruments should be worn throughout waking hours.

Sound generators should be put on as soon as possible after patients wake up, and worn throughout the waking hours without changing the initial settings, except in hyperacusis. The general instructions are that they be put on and forgotten about. If for any reason it proves impossible to wear devices throughout the whole day, a minimum of 8 hours should be attempted, which may be divided into several shorter blocks of time. Patients should be aware that this is less effective than wearing them on a continuous basis.

The instruments should be worn particularly whenever there is a low level of background noise.

It is important that the instruments are worn whenever there is a low level of background noise, for instance in the evening. If patients have a problem wearing the devices because of discomfort (tactile hypersensitivity), they should be advised to gradually introduce the devices. This may include wearing the devices without switching them on, and building up gradually to the optimal daily usage time and appropriate volume of sound. If this approach is used, it needs to be stressed that the real treatment starts at the point where they have built up to the appropriate daily use, to avoid generating an unrealistic expectation of the time course of the treatment. We do not recommend wearing the devices during sleep as they are not comfortable and could interfere with sleep; however, some patients do this. It is preferred that free-field sound enrichment devices should be used during the night.

Without proper counseling, sound therapy alone will be ineffective.

We realize that, in the past, many professionals have advised the use of environmental sounds such as radios and ticking clocks to help patients to cope better with their tinnitus. However, it is crucial to remember that sound therapy without appropriate discussion and counseling based on the neurophysiological processes does not work. Therefore, simply giving a patient wearable sound generators will not be effective without a program involving TRT counseling, even with appropriate advice about their setting and use. The same applies to advice about sound enrichment and "avoiding silence."

3.6 Specific modifications for individual treatment categories

The previous sections have outlined a non-specific TRT approach designed to cover all categories of TRT treatment. Misophonia might be presented in all categories and requires proper counseling and a specific protocol for its effective treatment. This is also true for sleep problems.

The type of counseling and use of instruments varies with treatment category.

Counseling and sound therapies vary with the individual patient and the treatment category to which they are assigned. The modifications of both non-specific counseling and sound therapy required for each of the treatment categories are presented below.

3.6.1 Category 0: mild or recent symptoms

Treatment of patients in category 0 consists of one session of simplified counseling, including advice about sound enrichment. Follow-up appointments are still needed, but they are mainly focused on checking the patient's status.

Category 0 treatment is used for patients whose tinnitus is mild or of recent onset. Tinnitus in these patients is often already partially habituated. These patients are frequently coming to the clinic because they have very little understanding of the mechanisms of tinnitus and have a natural curiosity about what might be responsible for it.

All that is required for category 0 is simplified counseling, with information about the neurophysiological model, together with instructions about avoidance of silence and non-specific advice on the use of background sound enrichment.

All that is required in this category is simplified counseling, with information about the neurophysiological model, together with instructions about avoidance of silence and non-specific advice on the use of background sound enrichment. Typically, these patients require one session of counseling only, with a few subsequent follow-up visits to confirm that their progress is as expected. All patients are followed up in case their condition ceases to improve and then the implementation of more extensive treatment is needed to ensure a positive outcome. Counseling in this case is still thoughtful, but not as extensive as in other categories. It is particularly important to avoid presenting these patients with information describing any effect of tinnitus that is worse than they already experience. This strategy is adopted to prevent a negative counseling effect by indirectly suggesting that their tinnitus could be worse than it is at the moment.

There is no recommendation to use sound generators in category 0. Nevertheless, there will be some patients who strongly believe that it is necessary to use sound generators to achieve control of tinnitus! If a patient cannot be convinced that a sound generator is not needed, and that this is a costly unnecessary approach, then sound generators could be used. There is no fundamental problem in using sound generators for category 0 problems; the only potential negative aspect, which needs to be explained properly to patients, is that by using and manipulating sound generators some additional attention will be brought to the tinnitus.

If subjectively significant hearing loss is present (category C0/2) then proper amplification is recommended to prevent potential enhancement of tinnitus through the strain-to-hear phenomenon and a general decrease of auditory stimulation.

3.6.2   Category 1: tinnitus alone (high impact)

Patients in category 1 have tinnitus with a high impact on their life but do not exhibit hyperacusis, subjectively important hearing loss or prolonged worsening of their symptoms following noise exposure. They receive detailed counseling about the neurophysiological model and sound enrichment, and additional information related to the need for wearable sound generators, which are recommended to all of them. These patients, as those from subsequent categories, receive a full sequence of follow-up visits.

Counseling in category 1 follows non-specific counseling, which is always tailored to the individual patient, with several modifications. All issues relating to tinnitus are discussed in detail, including thoughtful presentation of the neurophysiological model of tinnitus and discussion of conditioned reflexes and the basis for habituation. The role of OHC in hearing and in the generation of tinnitus is typically included; DPOAEs, when performed, help with this explanation. If the patient exhibits misophonia, its mechanisms are discussed, pointing out that the same structures and principles are involved in both tinnitus and misophonia. The protocol for misophonia is then presented in detail. There is no need to address the issues related to hearing loss and hyperacusis; these are omitted or presented in an abbreviated form.

Category 1 patients receive detailed counseling about the neurophysiological model and sound enrichment, and additional information about wearable sound generators which are recommended to all of them.

The last part of counseling is devoted to sound therapy and to the positive aspects of using sound generators. The dependence of the effectiveness of habituation on the intensity of used sound is presented with the help of Figure 3.1. While exposing a tinnitus patient to external sound, it is possible to distinguish four specific levels of the sound: (i) the threshold of detection of this particular external sound; (ii) the level at which perception of external sound and that of tinnitus starts to interfere with each other, referred to as the "mixing point;" (iii) the level at which suppression of tinnitus occurs; and (iv) the level that would induce annoyance if the sound was presented for a prolonged period of time. The effect on the tinnitus signal, perceived tinnitus and habituation to tinnitus when sound is presented at each of these four levels is discussed with the patient. The understanding of these levels is important, since they will be used by the patient on an everyday basis to adjust the level of therapeutical sound.

Wearable sound generators should be set to just below the "mixing" point, providing that it is still below the level inducing annoyance.

The proper setting of the sound level of wearable sound generators for this category of treatment is at, or just below, the "mixing point," providing that it is still below the level inducing annoyance. Patients need to understand that it is not crucial to be exactly at or very close to the "mixing point", and that there is a range of sound levels not exceeding the "mixing point," which will be effective.

During instrument fitting, the main elements of counseling are repeated, together with instructions on how the instruments should be used. In addition to these general instructions, practical exercises are described. Patients are advised to set their instruments starting with the ear where tinnitus seems to be dominant. They should gradually increase the sound level from a switched off position to the point where they just perceive the sound from the instrument. Next, the volume is increased to the point where the sound of the device begins to mix and blend with the sound of tinnitus. Both the unaltered sound of tinnitus and that of the devices must be perceived separately. This is the maximal level of the instrument's sound that is allowed. Patients are instructed to keep the device just below this level.

The level of sound must at all times be below the threshold for causing annoyance, or producing suppression of the tinnitus.

In no circumstances should the level of sound be above that of comfortable listening, and it must at all times be below the threshold for causing annoyance or producing suppression of the tinnitus. Once the instrument has been fitted to the first ear, the second instrument is attached and its sound adjusted to create a perception of equal loudness on both sides (i.e., the same sensation level). Warnings are given about using sound generators at very low just audible levels because of the possibility of stochastic resonance increasing tinnitus (see Ch. 2).

Patients in this category may have normal hearing, according to audiologic standards, or may have some hearing loss, typically in the high frequencies. If this hearing loss is not interfering with the quality of their everyday life (i.e., subjectively it is not affecting the patient's life), we do not offer these patients the option of hearing aids.

3.6.3 Category 2: tinnitus and subjectively significant hearing loss without hyperacusis

Counseling for patients in category 2 is similar to that for category 1 but modified to address the issue of their hearing loss. More emphasis is placed on the function of the peripheral auditory system, the relevance of OHC loss to hearing loss, stressing the analogy between OHC and hearing aids. The fact that a patient with hearing loss is effectively deprived of sound for a certain frequency range is related to the phenomenon of tinnitus occurring naturally in silence. We discuss the phenomenon of increased neuronal gain in central auditory pathways following hearing loss caused by cochlear damage and its contribution to creation and/or enhancement of the tinnitus signal.

Patients in category 2 receive similar counseling to those with category 1 but modified to address the issue of their hearing loss.

The criterion for introducing hearing aids is whether or not the hearing loss interferes with the patient's quality of life, not the results of their audiogram.

The criterion for introducing hearing aids is whether or not the hearing loss interferes with the patient's quality of life, not the results of their audiogram. Therefore, patients with quite mild losses of hearing may be fitted with hearing aids and receive auditory rehabilitation, while patients with more advanced hearing loss, but who are not affected by it, might not be recommended to use aids. For instance, musicians with small degrees of high-frequency hearing loss may benefit from hearing aids even though there is no interference with communication.

Bilateral hearing aids, or combination instruments, are fitted to all category 2 patients.

Counseling needs to be detailed, including all elements covered in category 1 but enhanced by elements related to a hearing loss. Of particular importance is discussion devoted to the role and function of the OHC system. It is pointed out that OHC, while very helpful, are not absolutely essential for hearing, and even without them it is still possible to hear and understand; simply louder sounds are needed. Pointing out that OHC work as a mechanical amplifier and can be considered as "bionic hearing aids" leads to a more acceptable proposition of using external, human-made hearing aids as their substitute. The experiment is discussed which shows that practically everybody experiences tinnitus when spending a few minutes in a soundproof chamber, demonstrating that similar compensatory mechanisms are responsible for tinnitus in hearing loss.

Counseling in category 2 focuses on hearing loss and its role in triggering and enhancing tinnitus.

The fact that the perceived strength of a signal depends on how much it is above background is discussed in detail. As patients with hearing loss will have decreased average auditory input, this will enhance the difference of the tinnitus signal from background neural activity, resulting in enhanced tinnitus perception and consequent annoyance. Last, but not least, is the problem of tinnitus enhancement while trying to listen and understand despite a hearing loss: the "straining-to-hear" phenomenon. Understanding of all the above issues leads patients gradually to recognize that increasing the auditory input by amplification of incoming sounds using hearing aids, and decreasing straining to hear, will weaken the tinnitus signal and facilitate the process of tinnitus habituation.

Patients must realize that sound therapy involving hearing aids depends on the proper enrichment of background sounds, with the hearing aid acting as an amplifier. It is the patient's responsibility to provide sufficient and appropriate environmental sound enrichment to make the therapy work. When hearing aids are used, the approach is hindered by the lack of a constant level of broadband sound from wearable sound generators; consequently, it may take slightly longer to achieve tinnitus habituation. Benefits are that the straining-to-hear effect is removed and two problems (tinnitus and the hearing loss) are targeted at the same time. Recent advances in combination instruments opened up an alternative approach to sound therapy in hearing impairment.

The majority of patients with hearing loss have reasonably well preserved or even normal hearing in the low-frequency range. As it is important to enhance, or at least preserve, the level of sound enrichment at all frequencies wherever possible, the external ear is not occluded. This means that when postaural instruments are used, the mold must be an open one. In-the-ear instruments should be open or well ventilated.

Hearing aids should be used during all waking hours and not simply for communication.

In order to optimize treatment of the tinnitus, it is essential that hearing aids should be used throughout the waking hours and not simply when they are required for communication or specific activities. As one of the goals is to remove the straining-to-hear phenomenon, instrumentation needs to facilitate speech understanding while preserving hearing of low-level background sounds. This leads to the obvious conclusion that the noise cancellation programs provided in some digital hearing aids are not recommended for patients during tinnitus treatment. Careful attention is paid to assure the selection of an appropriate hearing aid and in its fitting. Counseling is directed towards auditory rehabilitation. Binaural amplification is always recommended whenever physically possible.

Hearing aids should be "open ear" or very well vented.

There is a specific problem arising in treatment in category 2. Some tinnitus patients when fitted with hearing aids find that their tinnitus is easily suppressed by sound. While this may be welcomed as a symptomatic relief, it interferes with the process of habituation (habituation cannot occur to a signal that is not detected). These patients are advised that every day they should spend a few hours without using hearing aids but exposed to environmental sound at a level adjusted so that it is clearly perceived while not masking tinnitus.

In unilateral deafness CROS or BICROS hearing aids are recommended.

A subcategory of category 2 includes patients with unilateral, total or profound deafness in one ear, and with normal or aidable hearing loss in the other ear. Where there is some residual hearing but no speech discrimination in the worse-affected ear, we might consider fitting binaural sound generators in the first instance. Otherwise we use CROS (contralateral routing of signal) hearing aids, in which a microphone on the deaf ear conveys sound to the hearing ear. Where the better ear also has a hearing loss, a BICROS system amplifies sound to this ear in addition to taking sound from the microphone on the profoundly deaf side. Simple fitting of a CROS or BICROS system, even without TRT, can produce improvement in tinnitus in the profoundly deaf ear in 35% of those affected (Hazell *et al.*, 1992).

This approach is based on the observation that within the auditory system a spatial map of the environment is created, with specific neurons responding to sound coming from a particular direction. Loss of hearing in one ear generates an environment on one side that, from the point of view of the auditory system, is devoid of sound. Transmitting sound to the hearing side from a microphone on the deaf side provides sound from this "silent" area and restores partial activity in the affected area in the auditory pathways where previously there was a strong asymmetry of function. As a result, most patients wearing a CROS aid are able to localize sound in space. This effect occurs at a higher level in the auditory pathways and so requires substantial time for reorganization and reprogramming of neural connections. Presumably, the restoration of auditory activity and awareness of a complete auditory environment, which was previously missing, decreases the contrast between the tinnitus-related signal and the background activity and promotes habituation, as described above. Good results can be obtained by TRT counseling supported either by CROS or BICROS hearing aids, with background sound enrichment. Many of these patients experience an improved quality of life through a significant improvement in their ability to localize sound in space. Consequently, a previous approach of using low-frequency sinusoidal electrical stimulation through a single-channel cochlear implant in the profoundly deaf ear (Hazell *et al.*, 1993) has been suspended at present.

Combination instruments consist of a sound generator with a hearing aid. Results with their use are very positive.

The early version of the combination instrument (known in the USA as the Tinnitus Instrument) was promoted and used quite extensively. The device combines a hearing aid and a sound generator and was useful in the past for "masking" tinnitus. Because of its technical limitations, it was not appropriate for TRT and we were not using it. There were several disadvantages with these instruments for our purposes. The main disadvantage was that they did not comply with the need for a high-quality modern hearing aid, as the hearing aid part of the combination instrument was generally of poor quality. Second, patients found the multiple controls hard to manipulate, particularly in the small in-the-ear instruments. Third, there is no longer any need for instruments producing a high level of noise as we are no longer attempting to suppress tinnitus. Fourth, the sound level from the sound generator part was above the threshold of hearing when the device was switched on. New combination instruments that do not have these limitations were introduced in the USA in 2001. Results with their use are very positive.

Electrical stimulation via a cochlear implant could be used as a substitute for auditory stimulation and as a part of tinnitus retraining in profoundly deaf patients.

Patients with profound bilateral deafness present a special challenge, as it is impossible to conduct normal sound therapy, which requires at least some level of hearing. At the same time, these patients frequently experience distressing tinnitus, which may be more of a problem than their inability to communicate. Understanding the physiological mechanism of sound therapy (i.e., to decrease the strength of the tinnitus signal by increasing background neuronal activity) provides guidance to the best approach. It is secondary if the increase of background neuronal activity is evoked by sound or by direct electrical stimulation of the auditory periphery. Therefore, electrical stimulation via a cochlear implant could be used as a substitute for auditory stimulation in deaf patients.

Cochlear implants are indicated in totally deaf patients with tinnitus.

We recommend cochlear implantation for profound deafness in the presence of distressing tinnitus and to begin TRT with counseling before surgery is contemplated. In those patients where persistent tinnitus distress might even result in the abandonment of their implant following surgery, it has been possible to produce very significant changes in tinnitus reaction and perception by TRT counseling alone.

In the past, some cochlear implant centers have used the presence of distressing tinnitus as a contraindication to cochlear implantation. However, the evidence from several studies shows a high proportion of patients with tinnitus improved after cochlear implantation, and only a few (less than 5%) experienced a worsening of their tinnitus as a result of such surgery (see Ch. 6 for details).

3.6.4   Category 3: hyperacusis without prolonged enhancement from sound exposure

Because of the need for a different approach to hyperacusis from that for tinnitus, it is essential to establish the presence and extent of hyperacusis in each patient. This is achieved by measuring LDLs and making a detailed assessment of the patient's experience with environmental sounds to identify the potential contribution of misophonia to decreased sound tolerance. Approximately 40% of our patients have decreased sound tolerance. It is important to realize that the application of a protocol for management of tinnitus that disregards the presence of hyperacusis will not only fail to help the patient but may make the symptoms worse. Treatment for hyperacusis is required in about 25–30% of all patients.

Patients in category 3 receive counseling focused on hyperacusis-related issues at the expense of information about tinnitus and they have sound therapy aimed at desensitization. It is essential to establish the extent of the hyperacusis component in decreased sound tolerance, since sound therapy will be determined by the extent of hyperacusis, disregarding misophonia, which is treated separately. The extent of hyperacusis is assessed by measuring LDLs and examining the patient's experience with environmental sounds. There is a continuum of distribution of average LDL values from equipment and legal limits (i.e., 120 dB hearing level) down to 20–30 dB hearing level in patients with severe hyperacusis and misophonia. Using an average LDL of 100 dB hearing level as the borderline for normality, about 40% of our patients exhibit decreased sound tolerance. As in the majority of patients, hyperacusis is accompanied by misophonia, all patients will receive counseling about both phenomena. This counseling is in addition to the non-specific counseling given to tinnitus patients. In those with dominant hyperacusis, and tinnitus being a secondary symptom, counseling focuses on hyperacusis-related issues at the expense of information about tinnitus, particularly the mechanisms involved in controlling the gain within the auditory pathways (control of the OHC system and modification of the sensitivity of neurons in the central auditory pathways; see Ch. 2 for details).

Hyperacusis is treated primarily by wearable sound generators, while misophonia requires special counseling and a separate treatment protocol.

These patients are taught that the auditory system, like all sensory systems, regulates its sensitivity on the basis of the average intensity of stimuli it receives. This means that in a very quiet environment we may become strongly aware of sounds that previously were inaudible, such as our heartbeat or sound produced by the movement of clothes over our body.

In the auditory system, this increased gain is achieved at two different levels. First, in the periphery, the sensitivity of the cochlea may be modified through the efferent system and the OHC, altering amplification within the cochlea. Second, in the central auditory system, the sensitivity of auditory neurons can be modified to produce a high level of enhancement (amplification) of signals. There is a gradual transition from maximal activity of the cochlear amplifier (OHC) to passive transduction of the sound. In certain circumstances, the activities of this amplifier may be altered so that amplification is provided unnecessarily for higher levels of sound coming into the cochlea. In the central auditory system, a similar scenario might exist with inappropriate amplification of neural patterns of activity induced by moderate to high levels of sound.

Many patients with hyperacusis also experience the perception of sound distortion. This might result from neurons experiencing premature saturation of activity, resulting in "peak clipping" of the signal and perceived distortion of external sounds. Once a sufficient number of neurons reach this state of saturation, defense mechanisms are triggered and sounds are perceived as being uncomfortably loud, often with pain in the ear. As a part of this defense mechanism, the limbic and autonomic nervous systems will be activated in an effort to remove the person from the presence of the perceived excessive sound, or in an attempt to suppress its source. Reports of subjects who spent even a few minutes in a soundproof chamber clearly show that the perception of external sounds loudness is enhanced, presumably as a manifestation of increased gain within the auditory pathways.

Accordingly, mechanisms evoking abnormally high auditory gain might result in the emergence of tinnitus, as well as hyperacusis. Indeed, it is a common clinical experience that tinnitus and hyperacusis emerge around the same time. The two phenomena can, therefore, be viewed in some patients as two manifestations of the same internal mechanism.

In category 3, temporary worsening of symptoms can occur after sound exposure, but never beyond a good night's sleep.

In categories 0–2, the symptoms of tinnitus are frequently worsened by exposure to sound for periods not exceeding a few hours. The same situation may happen for patients in category 3, and both tinnitus and hyperacusis might, therefore, exhibit worsening after sound exposure. While this has no effect on the proposed treatment or its outcome, this enhancement of symptoms may result in a worsening of misophonia, requiring specific counseling concerning the mechanisms of misophonia and the transient nature of the tinnitus increase. It is stressed that, even when the symptoms become worse as a result of sound exposure, this does not indicate new damage to the cochlea, as some patients believe. However, when enhanced hyperacusis or tinnitus in response to sound exposure persists after a good night's sleep, other mechanisms are implicated, and a different treatment approach is needed, as described in the next section.

In the treatment of Category 3 patients, sound therapy is aimed primarily at desensitization of the auditory system to achieve attenuation or even removal of hyperacusis. The desensitization principle is explained to the patient as making the system more resistant to louder sounds by gradually introducing sound of increasing loudness. An analogy of desensitization may be explained in terms of sunburn. Immediate exposure to tropical sunshine when the skin is very pale will result in burnt skin, and possibly serious illness. However, sunburn can be avoided by gradually increased periods of exposure to the sun. Similarly, in hyperacusis, by gradually introducing carefully controlled sound, it is possible to desensitize the auditory system and achieve the same level of sound tolerance as present in the general population.

For this category of treatment, sound generators (or combination instruments where subjectively significant hearing loss is also present) are recommended. They are fitted binaurally using open ear-molds as described above. However, the initial sound levels are determined by the patient's annoyance level, which would depend on the extent of hyperacusis. Patients are advised to increase the sound level gradually, while keeping it always below that which could evoke annoyance. For pure hyperacusis, the sound is increased to the highest level that does not induce any annoyance or discomfort, or interfere with hearing. Many patients will experience an immediate symptomatic improvement in their sound tolerance when wearing the instruments. This should not be confused with the ultimate aim, which is to use desensitization to achieve normal tolerance to sound without the need for instruments. In this category, it is particularly important to use continuous not intermittent exposure to the sound, even at the expense of using lower sound levels. It is also important to keep close and frequent contact with the patient.

Some patients experience only hyperacusis and misophonia without tinnitus. Others may experience some tinnitus, which for them is not a significant problem, while suffering severely from hyperacusis. In this group, we can omit all the counseling relating to explanations of tinnitus and focus on the hyperacusis and misophonia. Furthermore, in these patients, it does not matter if the tinnitus is suppressed by the sound therapy. The comfortable listening level for sound from the instrument is the maximal sound level to be used.

If both tinnitus and hyperacusis are present, the hyperacusis is treated first.

When significant tinnitus is present, hyperacusis is still treated first and the sound level is determined by potential annoyance; additionally, patients are instructed to avoid suppression of tinnitus if possible. Being close to the "mixing point" is a secondary goal, attempted only after substantial improvement is noted in hyperacusis.

3.6.5   Category 4: prolonged worsening of symptoms by sound exposure

The characteristic feature of patients in category 4 is that the tinnitus and/or hyperacusis are exacerbated for periods of days or even weeks by exposure to external environmental sounds. The exacerbating sound might be considered to be quite low. Although this prolonged exacerbation is relatively uncommon, it is extremely important to recognize its presence, because inappropriate treatment can have devastating results. The most important criterium is whether the tinnitus and hyperacusis are still enhanced the following morning after a good night's sleep, following exacerbation by sound. This group has the lowest probability of success, and recovery takes a long and unpredictable time. Hyperacusis is almost always the dominant problem in category 4. Consequently patients need very detailed counseling focused on hyperacusis.

The mechanism of enhancement of tinnitus and/or hyperacusis by sound exposure may be either peripheral or central. One hypothesis is that there is a mechanical dysfunction of the cochlea, principally the OHC and the basilar membrane, resulting in enhanced function of the cochlear amplifier. The overamplification may be caused by a shift in the working position of the cochlear amplifier into a higher amplification setting, where it "gets stuck."

In category 4, the mechanism of prolonged symptom exacerbation can be explained by a "kindling" or "winding-up" effect.

Undoubtably some of these cases have an explanation in central auditory dysfunction. One explanation is that a phenomenon similar to "kindling" or "winding-up" occurs. The term kindling is used in epilepsy to describe the process whereby a weak electrical stimulus initially has no effect but repetitive presentation induces a full epileptic attack. In the case of tinnitus, the term is used to describe the prolonged worsening of tinnitus and/or hyperacusis as a result of exposure to a relatively short period of moderate or loud sound. In "winding-up," the worsening of a symptom occurs from exposure to a continuous stimulus over a prolonged period of time. This phenomenon is well recognized in pain; in tinnitus and hyperacusis it describes the significant worsening to even very low levels of sound when the sound is presented for a longer period of time. The same sound presented for a shorter time has no effect. A potential mechanism might involve continued overstimulation of the auditory system when in a sensitized state, leading to a permanent resetting of central auditory filters. These then overreact to very low levels of external sound (Jastreboff, 1990; Moller, 1997).

Some patients who are severely misophonic or phonophobic may also experience the sensation of decreased sound tolerance that persists beyond a night's sleep after sound exposure. It is clearly of great importance to take a detailed history (without prompting the patient too strongly) to establish whether there are strong concerns about the possible ill effects of normal levels of environmental sound on the ears or on hearing.

The strategy in this treatment category is to avoid overstimulation and to apply levels of sound as much above the threshold of hearing as the patient can tolerate, without evoking the "winding-up" effect. Being above the point of stochastic resonance is of secondary importance in this category; however, patients need to be counseled about stochastic resonance to avoid the enhancement of symptoms. The treatment is aimed at desensitization of auditory pathways, similarly to category 3. In patients with strong misophonia or phonophobia, this approach will also avoid the possibility of causing extreme distress through overstimulation with sound therapy aimed exclusively at hyperacusis.

For category 4, binaural wearable sound generators are used, typically starting from very low sound levels and increasing with very gradual increments.

Therapy begins with the fitting of binaural wearable sound generators as for category 3, but with instructions to keep the sound level close to threshold for a period of a few weeks. The patient's status is then reviewed. Patients are frequently advised to wear their instruments initially for a week without switching them on, as a part of the problem with intolerance of the instruments may result from general sensory oversensitivity, including touch. Sequential treatment blocks of six to eight weeks follow, with small increments in sound level from the instruments on each occasion. At any time that the tinnitus or hyperacusis is exacerbated, the level of sound is reduced by one step. The need for continuous exposure to sound from the instruments is crucial. It is much better to continue for prolonged periods of time with instrument levels set just above the threshold rather than to use the alternative strategy (adopted by some centers) of brief episodes of exposure to a much higher level, which are gradually increased in duration. It must be stressed that this alternative approach has made a number of patients very much worse. This is evident from evaluation of patients coming to us for TRT who had undergone "pink-noise therapy". It is recognized that there is a risk of stochastic resonance with such low initial levels of sound, which might enhance tinnitus, but this risk is outweighed by the problems created by too rapid increases in instrument sound level, as this might itself cause prolonged worsening of symptoms. Patients should be advised that there could be some temporary increase in tinnitus through this effect.

Use of the wrong sound therapy can make category 4 patients much worse.

Some hyperacusis patients have been recommended to use so-called pink-noise therapy. This does not actually involve the use of pink noise, which is defined as noise where the acoustic energy decreases inversely with frequency, but uses a spectrum of sound with the hyperacusis frequencies filtered out. Typically, the levels recommended are quite high. While this approach is not optimal for patients with hyperacusis who fit our category 3, it can be absolutely devastating when used in the treatment of category 4 patients. When these patients are exposed to continuous high levels during pink-noise therapy, cumulative effects occur and tinnitus and hyperacusis are set permanently to a much higher level than before treatment began. Using low levels of broadband noise just above threshold avoids this exacerbation effect; over prolonged periods of time, this approach produces compensatory changes that result in a reduction of hyperacusis and tinnitus.

3.7   Follow-up and closure of treatment

Follow-up contacts are essential for maximal therapeutic effect.

Follow-up contacts are necessary to assure that TRT has its maximum impact and effect. During these contacts, continuous counseling is performed, including reinforcement of the goals we aim to achieve. The compliance of patients is checked with regard to the protocol for recommended sound therapy, the use of enrichment of background sounds, instrument settings, and the gradual withdrawal from the use of ear overprotection. Treatment progress is monitored, and patients' questions and concerns are addressed. Finally, recommendations are made regarding the next phase of the treatment.

3.7.1   Methodology of follow-up contacts

In tinnitus retraining, the follow-up sessions constitute an important part of the overall treatment, including re-presentation of the model.

It is essential to establish a structured and well-organized system of follow-up. Wherever possible, the patient should return to the treatment center. If, because of constraints of distance or finance, normal visits are prevented, then at least a telephone/fax/e-mail interaction with the patient must be maintained as long as necessary. The intervals between visits will vary according to the logistics of the center and the individual needs of the patient, but contacts will be more frequent in the initial stages of therapy. Follow-up appointments, counting from the instrument-fitting session, are scheduled monthly for the first three months, then at 6, 9, 12, 18 and 24 months. These intervals will depend on what is practical at each center, and when the final stage of treatment is reached for each patient.

Each renewed contact with the patient involves elements of tinnitus retraining counseling, the specifics of which depend on the individual patient and stage of treatment.

Each renewed contact with the patient involves elements of TRT counseling, the specifics of which depend on the individual patient and stage of treatment. This is in contrast to some traditional views about follow-up, where there is fairly simple checking with a few measurements to see "how the patient is getting on." In TRT, the follow-up sessions constitute an important part of the overall treatment. During follow-up, specific aspects of each patient's problems and the status of their tinnitus and hyperacusis at the time form the central theme of the counseling approach. Patients are encouraged throughout the program to ask any questions which come to mind, particularly based on their own experience of tinnitus and hyperacusis. Follow-up visits enable these questions, fears and anxieties about what might be happening to be vocalized, discussed and disposed of.

> Follow-up also checks the patient's compliance with the prescribed protocol; if necessary the sound therapy approach is modified.

Another part of the follow-up process is checking the patient's compliance with the prescribed protocol and, if necessary, modifying the sound therapy approach. Problems that are a natural part of auditory rehabilitation (in the hearing aid group) and those associated with instrument fitting or function are dealt with at the same time. It must be stressed that the major role of these follow-up visits is to provide repeated episodes of TRT counseling and checking that the patient really understands the concept of the mechanisms involved to a point where they become second nature.

The second major role of the follow-up process is to assess changes in patient status, as part of the outcome measures. The first part of this process involves a follow-up structured interview guided by a specific form (Appendix 1). This form mirrors the form for the initial interview. The goal of therapy is to decrease and finally eliminate the effect of tinnitus and hyperacusis from the patient's life. Questions are tailored to examine these parameters. In particular, questions are asked about activities that are interfered with, or prevented, with reference to concentration, quiet recreational activity and sleep. Since we are expecting to see a partly independent development of habituation of tinnitus reaction and tinnitus perception, questions are developed to differentiate between these two entities.

> Separate questionnaires used during follow-up assess the degree to which habituation of tinnitus reaction and habituation of tinnitus perception has occurred.

Questions relating to habituation of perception include the average percentage of time when the patient is aware of tinnitus over the last four weeks. These data are surprisingly coherent. Questions about habituation of tinnitus reaction deal with the annoyance experienced when tinnitus is present. Patients are asked the percentage time when tinnitus is annoying them. Another useful measurement is the change in frequency of "bad days" and perceived change of annoyance during the bad days. Since the perceived severity of tinnitus tends to fluctuate, this provides us with a measure of the maximal level of annoyance produced by tinnitus. Observation that the frequency of bad days is unchanged but the level of annoyance on those days is reduced indicates a habituation of reaction, while a reduction in the actual frequency of bad days indicates habituation of perception. For all parameters studied, we ask if change has occurred, and in which direction (i.e, same, better, worse).

It is crucial not to ask leading or biased questions during these interviews. The questions must be formed in a way that is neutral and leaves the patient with the option to answer one way or the other. In each case, when applicable, we ask patients the same question separately about tinnitus and about decreased sound tolerance. These evaluations are done initially and repeated on all follow-up visits. This enables statistical analysis of the changes of all these parameters over the treatment period.

The final questions are aimed at assessing commitment. First, patients are asked what their reaction would be if, because of any reason, they had to return the devices they are wearing. The majority of patients have a very strong response, indicating their unwillingness to part with them. A much smaller group has a neutral attitude towards the idea of returning them (mostly people at the end of the treatment).

LDLs are assessed at each visit for patients with hyperacusis, to guide treatment and assess improvement.

Audiometric measurements are repeated for the first time at the six month follow-up, except for patients with decreased sound tolerance (category 3 and 4) when LDL are evaluated at every appointment. Repeated LDL measurements are helpful in deciding the proper sound levels that can be used at a given stage of treating hyperacusic patients. It also provides us with a means of assessment of improvement in these patients. During the final follow-up appointment, all patients repeat the audiometric evaluations that were performed at their first session. This is primarily to ensure that there are no new developments in the auditory system unrelated to tinnitus.

The use of extensive questionnaires aimed at the evaluation of multiple parameters of tinnitus, hyperacusis and the psychological status of the patient could be extremely useful as part of a research protocol, but they have no place in TRT as they do not provide information relevant to treatment and require extra time. As the goal of our program is to improve the life quality of the individual impaired by tinnitus and hyperacusis, specific questions are aimed at measuring changes in these parameters. Improvements in psychoacoustical measurements of tinnitus will not indicate that the patient has been helped unless there has also been an improvement in the patient's life quality. This approach is in contrast to most of the published research on tinnitus, where success of a treatment is measured in terms of changes in audiometric tests. In reality, these bear no relationship to the distress experienced by the patient.

3.7.2 Potential factors related to a failure

A frequent question concerns the patients who fail in a TRT program. It is possible to identify certain classes of patient who show a lower probability of improvement. However, even these patients typically make some progress, and some of these will eventually do really well.

In general, if TRT fails to produce the expected outcome, it is important to have a plan for modified treatment and not to abandon the patient. Modification may involve changes in protocol and require additional time. Over time, a number of these patients eventually reach the level of significant improvement and do not require further help. They should not be considered as a TRT success, as the mechanism involved in their improvement may contain elements of spontaneous habituation or other non-specific effects not related to TRT. They are classified as "no-better" for the purpose of reporting results. Many professionals who practice TRT may feel unwilling ever to give up on a patient, however slow their progress. There is always the issue of allocation of resources, which means that the benefit available to the large majority of tinnitus sufferers may be compromised if too much time is spent on a single very difficult individual.

Temporary worsening of symptoms

Some patients exhibit temporary worsening of their symptoms around four to eight weeks into the treatment. It is important to be aware of paradoxical worsening, which in reality is not failure at all. Often it is related to a fast positive response to the first session and rapid habituation, resulting in initial enthusiasm about the program and a belief that symptoms are likely to continue to get rapidly better. However, on returning home and experiencing exacerbation of symptoms related to the natural variations of tinnitus, patients become despondent and begin to become anxious that the treatment might not work. Furthermore, despite counseling, many patients have an expectation of a monotonic smooth, continual improvement, whereas changes can occur in an unpredictable fashion with any complex neurophysiological process. While habituation occurs rapidly but is not strong enough to assure stable control of tinnitus, all patients will experience fluctuations of tinnitus effects and its perception. It actually reflects a positive development and results from the following processes. If the brain is able to control tinnitus only for a period of time by a process of temporary habituation, then when release of this control occurs, the original symptoms re-emerge. Compared with the time when tinnitus was under control, this is perceived as a worsening of tinnitus and a potential failure of treatment; in fact, it is just another manifestation of the contrast phenomenon. These experiences are actually an indication of fast habituation and a good prognostic sign, provided that the patient is properly and speedily counseled about the real nature of these effects. Otherwise habituation can be blocked and reversed by the patient's perception that treatment has not only failed but may have made tinnitus worse. This is a good reason for early follow-up (at four to eight weeks) and also to include a discussion of these effects in the initial counseling, stressing that it is always temporary. These patients require reinforcement of the message presented in the first session and a detailed explanation of the processes outlined above. This approach is always effective in getting patients back into the standard treatment and to proceed as expected to permanent habituation of their tinnitus. It is useful to point out to patients the positive aspect of this experience, as it demonstrates that the brain is indeed capable of achieving at least short-term habituation. Warning patients of this common experience at the initial consultation can avoid this particular problem.

Inadequate initial counseling or lack of sufficient follow-up visits

Some patients find it very difficult to follow the protocol: they fail to make the effort of following sound therapy; they think they know better or simply misunderstand instructions. Sometimes, it appears that a patient is doing the right things, but careful questioning reveals problems that need to be addressed. Repetition of the elements of the initial counseling, presented in a different perhaps simplified manner, with checking for comprehension, and increasing the frequency of follow-up visits is usually helpful. Remember that for initiating habituation of tinnitus it is essential to reclassify tinnitus to a category of neutral stimuli. It might not be achieved during initial counseling, so that repeating the description of the neurophysiological model is necessary to assure reclassification of tinnitus.

Lack of follow-up and not teaching the model properly are the commonest causes of failure.

Lack of follow-up is a common reason for failure. Sometimes, it reflects lack of full appreciation by patients or therapists that follow-up is as an essential part of the treatment, rather than visits which simply check progress. In an extreme situation, patients are being fitted with sound generators, given limited counseling and asked to report results in half a year or so, without any subsequent visit. In fact this is not TRT at all, as for TRT the counseling is the indispensable part of the treatment. Habituation of stimuli that have strong negative connotations is very difficult; consequently habituation is hindered as long as tinnitus is perceived as indicating potential problems or even danger. One intense session of counseling is frequently insufficient to convey all the information needed for reclassification of tinnitus. Therefore, all follow-up sessions must contain elements of counseling and reinforcement of the concepts of TRT.

The effects of litigation

The presence of litigation makes habituation difficult.

Patients involved in litigation, or whose income depends on the continued experience of tinnitus/hyperacusis (i.e., disability payments), typically show very slow progress or no progress at all. Putting aside the possibility of inventing or exaggerating their symptoms because of potential financial gain, these patients are constantly being interviewed by different doctors and lawyers, which brings tinnitus/hyperacusis constantly to their attention, reinforcing its negative aspects, especially feelings of anger and grievance. This works directly against the approach and principles of TRT.

Subconsciously, the awareness that tinnitus distress may enhance any payments or income (disability) received through the legal process can also militate against habituation of tinnitus. It is essential to ask patients about impending litigation and to warn them about the possibility of a negative impact on treatment. Where appropriate, it is advisable to counsel patients about the benefits of avoidance or speedy conclusion of legal activity, after which TRT can proceed as in other patients.

Severe psychological problems

Some of our patients experience depression or high levels of anxiety before the emergence of tinnitus. Others have long-standing psychiatric illness that has resisted effective treatment. These patients are frequently on medications for anxiety or depression or others that might enhance tinnitus or hyperacusis and impair the plasticity of the brain necessary for habituation to occur. Such medications can also impair their ability to understand new concepts (Beckers *et al.*, 2001a; Busto, 1999; Gerak *et al.*, 2001; Kilic *et al.*, 1999; Lader, 1999; Longo & Johnson, 2000; Munte *et al.*, 1996; Verwey *et al.*, 2000; Ziemann, Hallett & Cohen, 1998).

Patients who experience depression purely as a result of tinnitus/decreased sound tolerance do well, particularly if they are not on psychotropic medications.

Patients who experience a depressive illness purely as a result of tinnitus/decreased sound tolerance do well, and their depression tends to improve with the improvement of their tinnitus, particularly if they are not on psychotropic medications. In this group, it is important that patients realize that, even if tinnitus/decreased sound tolerance is effectively treated, they may still experience anxiety and depression caused by other factors. Patients whose depression or anxiety hinders effective TRT may need separate treatment by a psychiatrist or psychologist simultaneously with TRT before progress can be made. Patients who have previously been resistant to such treatment, or who frequently relapse, may occasionally prove impossible to be helped by TRT.

Effects of medications

Psychotropic drugs slow habituation but should only be withdrawn slowly, under the direction of a physician, and after tinnitus retraining has begun.

It is common for many patients, especially the elderly, to be taking various drugs. Furthermore, since significant tinnitus frequently produces or enhances depression and anxiety, patients are often being treated with psychotropic drugs. Some centers are using these drugs for the treatment of tinnitus in spite of a lack of clinical results showing their effectiveness. Unfortunately, many of these medications reduce the ability and speed of learning and plasticity of the brain, thus hindering the process of habituation. Finally, some drugs have the properties of enhancing tinnitus or hyperacusis by direct effect or as a result of withdrawal (e.g., Alprazolam, Fluoxetine; for details see Ch. 6). When patients are on medications, it is essential to have a close interaction with all physicians who are prescribing for the patient, in an attempt to minimize the number of drugs and their dosage. In particular, drugs prescribed in the false belief that they are helping tinnitus should be gradually withdrawn.

As patients get older, they get more sensitive to many drugs. As they tend to develop more medical problems, they are prescribed still more drugs or have their dosage increased because of lack of therapeutic effect, with profound and unpredictable effects on the central nervous system, tinnitus and/or decreased sound tolerance.

Category 4 patients

Category 4 patients typically show a slower response to tinnitus retraining and should be tested for Lyme disease.

Patients in category 4 typically show a slower response, with a lower probability of success. The most complex situations in this category are patients with Lyme disease (borreliosis), who have a number of profound neurological problems in addition to having very significant hyperacusis, all correlated with the extent and the stage of the disease. A confounding problem in all category 4 patients is the inability to use higher sound levels for sound therapy. There is also a tendency for a greater degree of fluctuation of symptoms, which makes setbacks more common. In this category, it is important to check the possibility of predisposing, underlying medical conditions requiring specific treatment, or medication that might be implicated.

This category challenges the proficiency of the TRT practitioner more than any other. The application of sound therapy in a very slow and careful way, without aggravating the symptoms, has to be combined with skilled counseling of a patient who may be profoundly misophonia. It is necessary to be prepared, and to make the patient prepared, for slow and irregular progress.

Suppression of tinnitus evoked by hearing aids

Tinnitus suppression induced by the use of hearing aids can slow the habituation process.

Paradoxically, patients are more complex to treat if it is very easy to suppress tinnitus with hearing aids. Here tinnitus can be totally suppressed by environmental sounds amplified by hearing aids. While it is always possible to adjust the sound level of sound generators to prevent suppression of tinnitus, it may not be achievable with hearing aids without losing the benefits of improved communication. Some patients will be in a program of "tinnitus masking" and strongly attached to the relief of symptoms this method brings to a few people. With hearing aids, it is important to spend some time each day, perhaps when there is nothing much to listen to, with hearing aids turned down or even switched off so that tinnitus is audible, and to apply standard methods of sound therapy. With patients, who, in some cases, have been fully "masking" their tinnitus for up to 20 years, we have been successful in gradually converting them to a TRT program and achieving habituation of their tinnitus. This has been achieved by gradual reduction in sound generator level, together with the implementation of appropriate counseling.

Focusing on a cure

Any patient who is deeply convinced that a certain approach is effective (e.g., masking, allergy, homeopathy) may have difficulty in accepting the principles of TRT and, therefore, may not benefit from this approach. An additional group includes those who are so focused on the need for total eradication of tinnitus that they will not settle for anything less, even though they may improve substantially. These patients generally conduct a fruitless search from place to place to achieve a goal of not hearing their tinnitus at all. The secret is in teaching a correct understanding of the neurophysiological model, which can refute and contradict the wrong beliefs about the mechanism of their tinnitus and its effective treatment. Some patients seem to make a career out of being unhelpable and may have rather specific personality defects that will prevent TRT from succeeding.

3.7.3   Closing the treatment

With any treatment that continues over a long period of time, it may be difficult to decide when to stop treating the patient. With TRT, there is no precise way to identify the end-point of treatment, or to decide when a significant therapeutic effect has been achieved. During treatment, the improvement occurs very slowly, with the rate of change gradually decreasing, making it even more difficult to determine when the treatment can be considered to be finished. Moreover, group data show that there is a smooth continuum of the extent of improvement and, therefore, it is impossible to identify any specific value as a "significant" or "sufficient" change.

Closing the treatment depends on patient expectation. Avoid sudden changes.

Each patient has a different expectation and goal of what they hope to achieve during the TRT program. The same level or habituation or extent of improvement can be considered highly satisfactory by one patient and inadequate by the other. Some patients will be delighted with a small reduction in their tinnitus annoyance, while others will continue in treatment until they reached a point where they can hardly perceive their tinnitus at all (Jastreboff, 1999a; Sheldrake *et al.*, 1996).

When to stop

Most patients at the beginning of treatment will have significant scores on our analogue scales relating to most symptoms; apart from those in category 0, patients will typically have values between 5 and 10. We expect scores on these scales to reach 1 or 2 before deciding to stop the treatment. Values for tinnitus awareness should be around 10% or less, and annoyance as close to zero as possible, indicating that habituation of reaction, the goal of TRT, has occurred. In every case, the time to stop treatment must be agreed upon with the patient, when the conclusion is that no formal further appointment is needed, although the door is always left open.

How to stop

Throughout TRT, it is important to avoid rapid changes, and this principle applies to the termination of the treatment as well. Rapid changes may result in alterations in neuronal activity, with increases of reaction and perception of tinnitus. This may make patients feel that they still have problems. Do not do anything that will unnecessarily attract attention to the patient's symptoms. For instance, in stopping the use of wearable devices, it is important not to do this by reducing the wearing period to part of a day, resulting in the patient putting on and taking off the devices and drawing attention to their symptoms. Rather, they should stop wearing devices for certain days during the week. Gradually they stop the use of sound enrichment. The use of sound during the night should be the last thing to be withdrawn, but it may be that the patient prefers to continue with this strategy as sound enrichment during the night often improves sleep quality regardless of the presence of tinnitus or decreased sound tolerance.

3.7.4 What to do in case of relapse

If tinnitus re-emergence is experienced after successful therapy, subsequent retraining is usually fast and effective.

Although re-emergence of troublesome tinnitus is uncommon following a full TRT program, it does happen occasionally. New and different sounds may be noticed following some unconnected events, either emotional or ear related, and tinnitus emerges again as a problem, usually after a long period when no tinnitus was experienced at all. Though this is often what patients fear most, they should be strongly reassured that the subsequent emergence of tinnitus is easy to treat, because they have already acquired the skills inherent in the retraining program. They should be advised to start at once with the information review and sound enrichment, and to make renewed contact with their professional support. In our limited experience of this quite uncommon problem of recurrent tinnitus, we have had universally good results and a fast return to a state of habituation. It is worth telling patients about this possibility before closing the treatment, so that if it should occur, any concern will be minimized. Paradoxically, the complete disappearance of tinnitus for long periods of time followed by subsequent emergence of quite trivial tinnitus can evoke great alarm. The lessons of the neurophysiological model may have been forgotten rather than rehearsed from time to time, and the patient can feel that all is lost. The situation is preferred where tinnitus is experienced from time to time, without any feelings of threat, danger, or any negative reaction, as this will ensure a process of continued habituation.

It is often desirable to be able to make contact with patients after they have ceased formal contact with your center. One reason for this is the important collection of long-term data for research. Another is that patients who have gone through a successful program and habituated to the tinnitus can be very useful in helping with present or prospective patients, and also with providing positive publicity for the media. In our experience, many grateful patients are only too happy to oblige, but usually after a period of time ask to be left alone. It is essential not to endanger your patient's well-being by risking a recurrence of the problem through re-awakening memories of tinnitus distress.

3.8 Minimal requirements necessary to perform TRT

The procedures outlined in this chapter present the optimal implementation of TRT. This version is effective for all types of patient but requires commitment of sufficient time; therefore, it may be difficult to implement in centers that do not specialize in tinnitus and decreased sound tolerance and do not have a physician as a part of the team. Nevertheless such centers may wish to provide TRT. Consequently, the frequent question is what are the minimal requirements necessary to conduct TRT.

3.8.1 Evaluation

The essential information is contained in the forms for initial and follow-up interviews (Appendix 1) and all these questions must be asked and responses recorded. Although it does not take long to acquire answers to these questions by interviewing the patient, in the traditional management of tinnitus patients the majority of these questions are not asked. The most important audiometric measurement is of LDLs, which should be measured across the full audiometric range (125 Hz to 8 kHz; P. J. Jastreboff measures them up to 12 kHz), together with the pure-tone audiometric threshold to establish the dynamic range of the ear. Secondary, but frequently useful, is speech discrimination. Specific "tinnitus measurements" are unnecessary for treatment but can be useful for counseling.

The other important component of the initial evaluation involves the exclusion of other pathologies involving the auditory system. This can be achieved by investigations already performed by another specialist, the patient bringing proper documentation to show that this has been done and that they have a clean bill of health with respect to vestibular schwannoma etc. Alternatively, these investigations may be organized as part of the initial evaluation according to accepted otological and audiological practice. This information is needed for two reasons: first to be used in the process of counseling the patient against the presence of sinister pathology, which may be a part of their anxiety, and second, of course, to avoid overlooking serious pathology.

3.8.2 Treatment

The essential part of treatment is a process of TRT counseling of the patient, which requires a deep understanding of the neurophysiological model and its clinical implications. Some degree of ability to counsel patients in the prescribed manner must be acquired, and the therapist must fully understand and believe the model himself/herself. It is essential that each patient is treated as an individual, and that there is a completely flexible approach to each individual, involving sensitivity and awareness of the patient's problems. Giving the same lecture to everybody will not provide TRT counseling and will not be effective. Therefore, providing patients with lectures/counseling on videotapes, or counseling in groups, cannot be regarded as TRT.

The next essential need is a good understanding of the principles of sound therapy, and that it is not a particular device, but sound, which is important in TRT. The ability to fit wearable sound generators or hearing aids properly is very helpful, as these instruments are needed for the majority of patients. While fitting hearing aids by a third party under appropriate instruction is possible, in our experience this has typically caused problems and failure when these professionals are not trained in TRT. Therefore, we recommend that fitting of all instrumentation should be performed in the center that provides TRT. This is even more important for combination instruments, as their fitting and protocol of use is more complex than for sound generators or hearing aids alone. It is important to stress that the fitting appointment includes rigorous counseling related to sound therapy.

While the majority of patients do receive some kind of device as they are a very convenient way of applying sound therapy, they are not always necessary for TRT.

While the majority of patients do receive some kind of device, and while they are a very convenient way of applying sound therapy, these devices are not absolutely necessary for TRT. A majority of the patients can be helped without any instrumentation whatsoever. Additionally, category 0 does not involve instrumentation by definition. The sound, which is provided by environmental sound enrichment, has no requirements for a specific method of delivery.

Proper use of instrumentation facilitates progress in TRT.

However, proper use of instrumentation facilitates progress in TRT, and centers providing TRT should master the art and science of instrumentation as described here.

3.8.3   Follow-up

Follow-up contacts are necessary to achieve a high rate of success.

Follow-up contacts are necessary to achieve a high rate of success; without such contacts, some patients may develop problems, in particular poor compliance with TRT principles. Furthermore, without follow-up, the therapist has no means of knowing whether his/her technique is effective or not and loses the opportunity to improve skills as a TRT practitioner. For this reason, we strongly discourage embarking on TRT programs without the ability for following patients.

During follow-up visits, the essential component is continued TRT counseling, and modification of the protocol when needed. Repeated audiological measurements are not essential to the follow-up procedure, except in hyperacusic patients. Some follow-up contacts can be performed by telephone conversations. However, face-to-face contact remains a much more powerful and effective way of applying TRT, and it has more predictable results.

4

Evaluation of treatment outcome and results

The initial results of Tinnitus Retraining Therapy (TRT) from treatment centers in Baltimore, Atlanta and London are presented, together with more recent results from other centers. The methods of patient assessment and data collection are described, together with a justification for these approaches. Approximately 80% of patients exhibited a significant improvement following the protocol within a period of about 1 year. While these results were obtained with rigorous protocols for patient treatment, they were generated in everyday clinical practice and not in specifically designed research studies.

4.1 Introduction

Our goal is the habituation of tinnitus with the ultimate outcome of abolishing the impact of tinnitus on the patient's life.

When severely distressed tinnitus sufferers first arrive seeking help in one of our clinics, they generally have one requirement; the permanent eradication of their ability to hear tinnitus so that they will never hear it again. They also want to achieve this very rapidly. The need relates to the severe effects tinnitus has had on their lives, and the patients' perception that this can only be improved by entirely removing tinnitus. Achieving this would represent a cure for tinnitus in the traditional sense. To our knowledge, it is at present impossible, although it remains a goal for on-going research. From the previous chapters, it is clear that our goal is the habituation of tinnitus, and that this process requires some time. The ultimate outcome is abolishing the impact of tinnitus on the patients' lives. As such, our goal is identical to that of the patients, but the specifics of achieving it are often different. Initially, patients believe that relief from tinnitus can be achieved only by totally removing tinnitus perception.

Before progress can be made, we may need to change patients' expectations: first about the speed at which improvement may occur, second, about final goals and, finally, about the means by which we are trying to achieve these goals.

Therefore, before progress can be made, we may need to change patients' expectations: about the speed at which improvement may occur, about final goals, and about the means by which we are trying to achieve these common goals. The demand for never hearing tinnitus again decreases as the patient achieves deeper understandings of the neurophysiological model of tinnitus and the mechanisms of tinnitus distress. Moreover, as the feelings of distress and alarm are the first symptoms to improve during the initial stages of habituation induced by TRT, there is a gradual realization that it is the distress caused by the tinnitus rather than the perception of the tinnitus sound itself that is the problem to be solved.

Where there is a discrepancy between patient expectations and the realistic goals, even if there is improvement in tinnitus-induced symptoms, the patient will be dissatisfied, and the treatment will fail.

Where there is a discrepancy between patient expectations and the realistic goals that we are proposing, even if there is improvement in tinnitus-induced symptoms, the patient will be dissatisfied, and the treatment will fail. This underlines the importance of getting patients' expectations correct from the beginning. In the overwhelming majority of our patients, this is achieved by appropriate counseling during the initial consultation. In some patients, it takes some time to accept the model and expected outcome, and a few, who cannot accept our approach, remain dissatisfied even when it has been shown that the quality of their life has improved substantially.

4.2 Methods of data collection

Data are initially presented from our own centers in Baltimore USA and London UK, where TRT was first implemented. More recent results from these centers, and from the other centers around the world, are presented later.

The lack of objective methods for detecting tinnitus and evaluating its severity makes the selection of proper methods and criteria for assessing the effectiveness of a treatment extremely important.

The lack of objective methods for detecting of tinnitus and evaluating its severity makes the selection of proper methods and criteria for assessing the effectiveness of a treatment extremely important. A variety of questionnaires to evaluate tinnitus as a problem have been developed and used over time. Questionnaires can be completed by individual patients, saving the time of healthcare professionals and removing the personal bias of an interviewer. However, patients can misunderstand some questions or focus attention on unimportant issues and so our preference is towards performing structured interviews in patient assessment.

To evaluate the extent of habituation and changes in the patient's status during treatment, we used forms that guide a structured interview during initial and follow-up visits.

The extent of habituation and changes in the patient's status during treatment was evaluated by structured interview forms, which were used during initial and follow-up visits. To reduce the possibility of contaminating our results with a placebo effect, the criterion for inclusion was that a patient had undergone at least six months of treatment; in the London study, the period was at least one year. Since we wanted to reach all patients fulfilling this criterion, the telephone interview was used as well. The forms are given in Appendix 1 and the instructions for their use have been published (Henry *et al.*, 2003).

On the basis of the combined responses and the criteria presented below, a patient was classified as (i) showing significant improvement (referred to as "better"), (ii) with tinnitus that was the same or slightly improved ("same") and (iii) "worse".

The data were entered into a Microsoft Access database. All descriptive statistics were obtained using Access queries. Statistical calculations were performed following standard methods (Keppel, 1991; Ridgman, 1975).

4.3 Criteria for improvement with respect to the neurophysiological model

Because there are no objective measures for tinnitus, the assessment and evaluation was based on standard forms for structured interviews (see Appendix 1). The final goal of removing the impact of tinnitus on the patient's life is achieved in TRT by tinnitus habituation. Tinnitus habituation consists of two components, habituation of reaction induced by tinnitus, and habituation of its perception. Consequently, evaluation of patients included scales for assessing the changes in annoyance induced by tinnitus (reflecting habituation of reaction) and percentage of time when patients were aware of tinnitus (habituation of perception). For assessing the final outcome, global measures were used, such as impact of tinnitus on the patient's life, number of activities affected by tinnitus and ranking tinnitus as a problem in life. A number of other measures reflecting specific aspects of tinnitus were helpful in monitoring and modifying treatment were used as well and are listed below.

4.4 Technical aspects of measurement

The same questions were asked on initial and all follow-up visits.

The same questions were asked on initial and all follow-up visits. The impact of tinnitus on life quality was estimated in two ways. First, a statement is made about the way in which tinnitus and (separately) decreased sound tolerance interfere with a standard list of activities. The patient was also requested to include other affected activities that are not on the list and that are important for their everyday life. Patients were asked as well to indicate any change in their activity list during each follow-up visit. This provided a double checking of the validity of the subjective report of the patient. Second, the patient was asked to rate on a scale of 0 to 10 the effect of tinnitus on their life on average, during the last month. The extent of annoyance induced by tinnitus was estimated by asking patients to rate on a 0 to 10 scale their subjective perception of annoyance, on average, during the last month. Assessment of habituation of perception of tinnitus was estimated by asking patients the percentage of time they were aware of tinnitus during their waking hours over the last month. On each visit, they were also asked if this percentage changed, and in which direction.

Because of the importance of category 4 patients (prolonged enhancement of symptoms following sound exposure), there was a separate question asking patients if sound exposure caused symptoms to become better/stay the same/get worse, for minutes/hours/days. In those indicating prolonged worsening, there was an additional specific question to discover if the worsening effect persisted after a night's sleep.

To help in differentiating between the categories further, patients were asked to rank on a scale from 0 to 10 the importance of tinnitus, hyperacusis and hearing loss. This is useful as well in assessing progress and judging the relative importance of these three problems. For instance, in many patients who reported all three problems initially present, hearing loss may subsequently emerge as the dominant factor when other symptoms diminished.

Other questions were helpful in the general assessment of the progress of treatment, but they were not essential for judging the significance of a patient's improvement. All questions were asked during an interview, with the forms serving as a means to record results and maintain consistency. All questions were asked in a neutral and similar manner to avoid bias. The concept of misophonia was introduced in 2001 (Jastreboff & Jastreboff, 2001a, b). Moreover a Tinnitus Handicap Inventory (THI) evaluation was incorporated into tools for patient evaluation starting in 1999 (data from Atlanta). Consequently, initial evaluations did not involve misophonia and THI.

4.5 Specific criteria for scoring the significance of individual improvement

The standard approach to assessing effectiveness of any treatment is to run a statistical comparison between control and treated groups, or with a treated group using before and after treatment data.

The standard approach to assessing effectiveness of any treatment is to run a statistical comparison between control and treated groups, or with a treated group using before and after treatment data. While this approach tells about the validity of the average response, it provides no information about how many patients improve and by how much. In addition, in a sufficiently large group of patients, even a slight improvement that is not noticeable for an individual subject can become significant if the majority of patients are experiencing it. For example, a statistically significant change in minimal suppression level (MSL), while supporting the validity of the model, has no practical value in assessing individual patient progress nor is it noticed by the individual patient (Jastreboff *et al.*, 1994). By comparison, a very large improvement, clearly perceived by individuals, might be judged as non-significant if it exists in only a small proportion of patients (i.e., 50% of improvement but experienced only by 10% of patients will change the mean only by 0.5% and most probably will not be detected). Furthermore, the group data are of little help in guiding the treatment of individual patients. Unfortunately, an approach utilizing any criteria of improvement in an individual patient has a weakness in the total subjectivity of the criterium selected.

The crucial issue is what should be accepted as a criterium of significant improvement for any individual patient.

The crucial issue is what should be accepted as a criterium of significant improvement for any individual patient, which can be applied to all patients. The commonly used condition of simply recording whether individual patients consider they have improved is inadequate as it varies greatly from patient to patient, with patient mood, attitude to therapist, etc. and is extremely subjective. By analyzing various components of habituation, without the patient realizing the full significance of the questions asked, and by obtaining objective evidence of activities no longer inhibited by tinnitus or hyperacusis, a more impartial assessment can be made. As the goal is to reduce the effect of tinnitus/hyperacusis on life, a prerequisite for classifying a patient as significantly improving is that at least one activity previously prevented or strongly affected by the symptoms is enabled.

The second issue is to separate some slight improvement from changes that are having a real impact on the patient's life.

The second issue is to separate some slight improvement from changes that are having a real impact on the patient's life. Comparing results from our scales with verbal interviews with the patients over years, it was initially decided to require at least 20% change of the initial value. Finally, we required that more than one of the measured variables was improved by this much. The criterium that fulfills the above conditions identifies those patients who readily report a subjective improvement and are, with time, seen to make steady and continuous progress through the habituation process.

In the group of patients who are classified as "same," there are a number of patients who are perceiving and reporting some improvement. In this group, there is often a large fluctuation of severity of problems, or progress is very slow and if TRT is discontinued it is likely they will relapse. In our experience, those patients satisfying the criterium for significant improvement do not relapse after finishing the treatment, even when assessed several years later.

It is important to impose a clear time limit for assessing tinnitus outcome and to repeat evaluation several times.

It is important to impose a clear time limit for assessing tinnitus outcome, and to repeat the evaluation several times. Too short a time for assessment of outcome will result in influencing results by the placebo effect, which in the case of tinnitus can be approximately 40% (Duckert & Rees, 1984). However, accepting unlimited time for showing improvement, without following all the patients, will result in an artificial increase of success rate, as patients who are not showing improvement will have left the study and only those doing well will return. Therefore, although we have data from as short a period as a few weeks after starting treatment and for several years, for the purpose of evaluation we used data obtained between 6 months and two years.

4.6   Placebo effect and spontaneous recovery

The placebo effect is the temporary improvement of symptoms, not related to the effect of the treatment only its presence.

The placebo effect is the temporary (two to three months) improvement of symptoms not related to the effect of the treatment, only its presence; with tinnitus, the placebo effect ranges around 40%. Therefore, the potential impact of a placebo effect on results should be examined very carefully. With our protocol, the placebo effect should be limited because patients are assessed not only soon after the start of treatment, when the placebo effect can be quite strong, but again, typically more than once and after a long time delay. Sustained results over 6–24 months cannot be a placebo effect.

Our long-term results do not show any evidence of a relapse.

Importantly, long-term results do not show any evidence of a relapse. Although we should expect relapse to occur in some patients, its incidence is so low that we observed only single cases, usually associated with other medical and surgical problems. It is also possible that patients can have a subsequent emergence of completely different tinnitus and triggered by some event unrelated to the first episode. In such cases, it is common for habituation to start automatically and progress rapidly. Patients alarmed that this might be a relapse or regression of their condition and seeking help for a second time can be reassured that, as they have already learned to habituate to one specific tinnitus signal, the habituation of the new signal is achieved by the same mechanism more rapidly than before by following the basic principles of TRT.

Neither placebo effect, nor spontaneous recovery can explain the results obtained in TRT.

The effect of spontaneous recovery should be taken into account when assessing TRT results. In London, a study was performed on a group of 113 tinnitus sufferers who were not receiving any specific treatment for tinnitus and who belonged to the British Tinnitus Association. They completed the same questionnaires at the start and finish of a 12-month period in which they were asked to estimate the percentage of awareness of tinnitus, its annoyance and the effect of tinnitus on life. Only 6% showed significant changes in their tinnitus according to these measurements. A separate study, comparing tinnitus when it first emerged with just before treatment started, showed that spontaneous recovery is unlikely in patients requiring treatment (Sheldrake et al., 1996). Accordingly, neither placebo effect nor spontaneous recovery can explain the results obtained in TRT.

4.7 Effectiveness of tinnitus retraining therapy

To assess the effectiveness and validity of the treatment, the results of our centers are presented here.

4.7.1 Baltimore

In Baltimore (late 1990s), 223 more recent sequential cases from over 1000 patients, without any initial preselection, were evaluated on the basis of initial interview, follow-up visits or telephone interviews if patients were not contacting the center. These patients were treated according to our TRT protocol and were not a part of a specific trial.

The criteria for significant improvement included at least one activity initially prevented by tinnitus/decreased sound tolerance restored to normal, and at least 20% improvement of the initial value in at least two of the following factors: annoyance, awareness or effect of tinnitus on life.

The criteria for significant improvement were as described above, with at least one activity initially prevented by tinnitus/decreased sound tolerance restored to normal, and at least 20% improvement of the initial value in at least two of the following factors: annoyance, awareness or effect of tinnitus on life. The data were gathered with the help of forms for structured initial and follow-up interviews

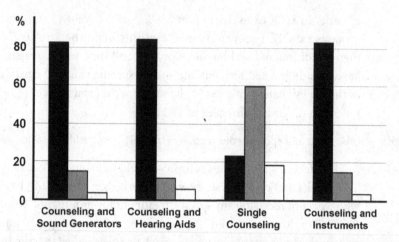

Figure 4.1   Treatment outcome for Baltimore patients. The percentages of patients fulfilling criteria of significant improvement (black bars), not improving significantly (gray bars) and reporting worsening (open bars) are presented for various treatment approaches: multiple counseling and sound generators, counseling and hearing aids, one session of tinnitus retraining counseling only, and combined first two groups.

(see Appendix 1). Patients reporting improvement but not fulfilling these criteria were classified as showing no change. Those who reported worsening of their symptoms were counted as such.

All patients received intensive initial counseling, which included explanation of the model, advice about avoiding silence and using sound enrichment (sounds of nature, radio, television). Two main approaches were implemented for instrumentation: 79% of patients received behind-the-ear sound generators (Viennatone Am/Ti) and 9% were fitted with various kinds of hearing aid according to their needs, with specific, proper counseling following TRT protocol for patients with hearing loss (category 2). The remaining 11% received an initial session of counseling but decided not to continue with the protocol. They were followed mainly by telephone interviews.

The group with sound generators and hearing aids had a similar proportion of patients showing significant average improvement of 82.0%. Notably, in the group which received only one session of counseling, only 22.7% of patients showed significant improvement.

The group with sound generators and hearing aids had a similar proportion of patients showing significant improvement, 81.8% and 83.3%, respectively, with an average of 82.0% (Fig. 4.1). No change was reported by 14.5% and 3.5% reported worsening of their problem. Notably, in the group that received only one session of counseling, only 22.7% of patients showed significant improvement, with 59.1% without significant change and 18.2% reporting worsening of their problems. Comparison of the effectiveness of the full treatment versus

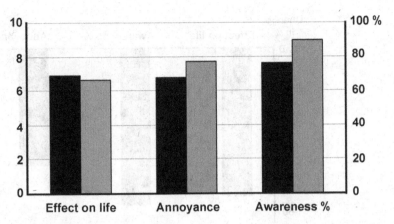

Figure 4.2   Initial characterization of tinnitus in Baltimore patients. Average initial scores recorded during the first visit for patients who subsequently showed significant improvement (black bars) and for remaining patients who did not fulfill the criteria of significant improvement (gray bars). Effect on life and annoyance were measured on 0 to 10 scale; Awareness % shows the average percentage of time patients were aware of their tinnitus.

the single counseling session was statistically significant ($p < 0.001$; $\chi^{-2} = 37.04$, degrees of freedom (df) $= 2$ using "better", the "same", "worse" classification and $p < 0.001$; $\chi^{-2} = 36.77$, df $= 1$ using significant improvement versus lack of significant improvement classification).

The values of measures used in assessing the treatment outcome were basically the same at the beginning of the treatment for the "better" and "same" categories of patients (Fig. 4.2). To focus on the change occurring in individual patients, the effect of the treatment for each variable, the difference was expressed as a percentage of the initial value, and those values were averaged separately for improvement and no-improvement categories. As expected, individual measures relating to treatment outcome (annoyance, awareness, effect on life) showed changes consistent with both elements of the habituation of tinnitus (habituation of reaction and perception) occurring concurrently. In the combined groups with sound generators and hearing aids, patients classified as showing significant improvement had an average decrease of awareness by 42.6%, annoyance by 57.7% and effect on life by 54.9% (Fig. 4.3). The changes were clearly smaller in groups classified as "same" (10.7% effect on life, 12.2% awareness and 11.5% annoyance). Nevertheless even in that category, there was a shift in the direction of this improvement for all the measures.

The question of whether the presence of hyperacusis has an impact on treatment outcome was addressed in a study of 163 patients. The patients were grouped into category 1 and 2 (no hyperacusis) and category 3 and 4 (with hyperacusis). The results show that 27% of patients needed to be treated for hyperacusis, and that the success rate is actually higher for patients with hyperacusis (95%) than for those

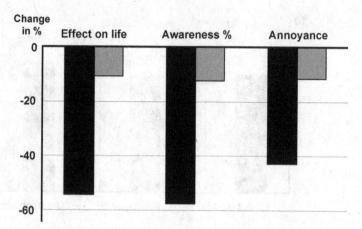

Figure 4.3   Changes in tinnitus following treatment in Baltimore patients. The averages of percentage changes calculated for individual patients. All other descriptions as in the previous figure. Note decrease of presented parameters to about half of initial values, and that some improvement was observed even in patients who did not meet criteria of significant improvement.

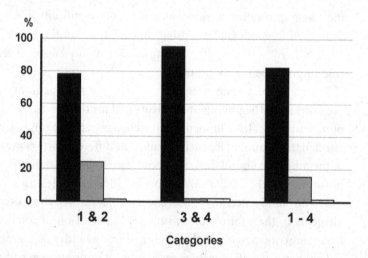

Figure 4.4   Comparison of treatment effectiveness for tinnitus only (categories 1 & 2), tinnitus and hyperacusis (categories 3 & 4), and for all (categories 1 to 4) patients. Note higher effectiveness of the treatment for patients with hyperacusis. Bars as in Fig. 4.1.

with only tinnitus (78%) (Fig. 4.4). The overall effectiveness for all these patients was 82%.

In a subpopulation of 223 patients where full data were available, cumulative distributions for each of the parameters recorded before treatment revealed some interesting findings (Jastreboff, 1999a). There were no significant differences between the distributions of these parameters for different categories, suggesting that the effects of tinnitus on patients do not depend on our categorization. The median values for severity, annoyance and impact on life were in the range 5–7 (on 0 to 10 scale). These distributions were uniform, after exceeding values of about 3–4, with approximately 10% below these values. This finding indicates homogeneity and continuity of these data, suggesting a value of approximately 3 for the threshold for clinically relevant tinnitus. In the case of awareness, the threshold value is approximately 20–30% (of the total time), with a rapid increase in the number of patients for values greater than 90%. Perhaps patients severely affected by tinnitus believe that they are perceiving tinnitus all, or nearly all, of the time.

To assess the effect of the treatment, the initial value for each parameter was subtracted from the value recorded during the following-up visit and presented as a percentage of the initial value. Analysis of cumulative distributions of these values showed that the median change was approximately 50%, with the exception of severity, which showed a smaller change. This is not a surprise, as patients were using the term severity to describe perceived tinnitus loudness. Audiological loudness match does not change with treatment, and reported changes reflect modification in perceived significance of tinnitus.

Patients with hyperacusis show greater improvement than those with only tinnitus.

Patients with hyperacusis show greater improvement, despite the groups being statistically similar in other respects. This finding supports the theoretical prediction of the neurophysiological model of tinnitus; hyperacusis should be easier to decrease/remove as the desensitization method used for its treatment in TRT does not involve retraining of conditioned reflexes and consequently is easier to achieve. Improvement in hyperacusis results in a decrease of general anxiety level and thus facilitates the habituation of tinnitus. Clinical data fully confirm this prediction and, as shown in Fig. 4.4, patients with hyperacusis tend to have a higher probability of improvement. Moreover, they recover faster.

To gain a deeper insight into the effects of TRT, a cumulative distribution is used to show the percentage of patients improving in a given variable by a relative extent (from 0 to 100%) (Fig. 4.5). The horizontal axis shows the percentage change for the parameter that is showing maximal change. Each patient was assigned a number that represents the maximal change observed among those parameters (the largest relative improvement). The reasoning for this way of data representation is that it would be most closely related to the subjective perception of improvement by the patient. Consequently, zero indicates no improvement in any of the parameters and minus 100% indicates that at least one of the parameters totally disappeared. The y axis gives the percentage of patients for whom this value of maximum change is equal or larger than the value shown on the x axis.

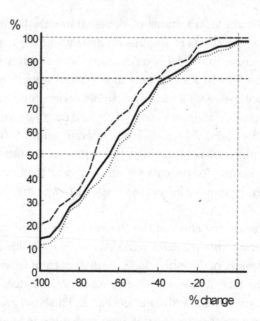

Figure 4.5   Cumulative distribution of patients experiencing a given level of improvement for at least one parameter. Solid line presents the average for all the subjects. Horizontal dashed lines show the median and the proportion of self-reported improvement. Note the smooth functional dependence, and that patients with hyperacusis (dashed line) exhibit a tendency to larger improvement than patients with tinnitus only (dotted line).

Only about 1% of all patients reported no improvement or worsening for all parameters. At the same time, 14% of all patients reported a decrease of at least one parameter to zero (−100% change; Fig. 4.5, continuous line). Half of the patients reported the change of at least one parameter by 65%. There is a tendency close to the level of significance (Smirnov test) for larger improvement in patients with hyperacusis (Fig. 4.5, dashed line) compared with tinnitus only (Fig. 4.5, dotted line). Additionally, twice as many hyperacusic patients (22%) experienced decrease of one of the parameters to zero compared with category 1 patients (no hyperacusis; 11%). Finally, the change of approximately 40% can be seen for 82% of patients.

These results further support the data presented in Figs. 4.1–4.4, which show that TRT, when implemented in an optimal manner according to the neurophysiological model, provided significant relief for approximately 80% of the patients receiving full treatment.

4.7.2 Atlanta

In 1999 P. J. Jastreboff moved to Emory University School of Medicine, Atlanta, Georgia and created a new Tinnitus and Hyperacusis Center. Treatment of patients started in 1999 utilizing a modified TRT protocol (e.g., improved counseling with stress on conditioned reflexes, modified setting of sound generators with more emphasis on avoiding annoyance and avoiding close-to-threshold sound levels), which is presented in this book. At the moment, results from the work at Emory are being analysed, but some preliminary data have been reported (Jastreboff *et al.*, 2001; 2003b; Jastreboff & Jastreboff, 2002).

The method of data analysis presented in the previous section was based on a specific criterion of treatment outcome, and success was defined as the proportion of patients who fulfilled this predetermined criterion. While this approach allowed identification of improvement in a given patient, its main weakness is that the validity of the chosen criterium may be questioned, and that the results of the evaluation may be biased by the choice of the specific criterion. Analysis of the results in these earlier sections, using a multifactorial criterion of success, yielded success rate of over 80%. This criterium was, however, purely subjective.

The other approach is to analyze statistically the changes of multiple parameters recorded before and during treatment in a group of patients. This approach does not allow analysis of individual patients but does provide information about the effectiveness of a treatment in a group of patients. The results from Atlanta are reported using a statistical assessment of the significance of changes in a population of patients treated with TRT, without making any assumptions about what constitutes the criterium for success.

The results of 120 consecutive patients with tinnitus, hyperacusis, misophonia and hearing loss treated at the Emory Tinnitus and Hyperacusis Center are presented. All patients underwent identical initial and follow-up interviews (see Appendix 1) and were asked to complete the THI questionnaire (Newman, Jacobson & Spitzer, 1996). Patients were evaluated and assigned to the proper category and treated with the variant of TRT appropriate for this category. Attempts were made to perform the follow-up visits at 1, 2, 3, 6 and 12 months from the initial visit. Since many patients came from distant locations, some of the early follow-up visits were omitted or substituted with telephone consultations. In follow-up interviews, patients were asked to evaluate an average for a given variable for the last month. Only the most relevant variables from structured interviews (i.e., percentage of time when the patient was aware of tinnitus; the percentage of time when the patient was annoyed by tinnitus; tinnitus severity, how strong/loud it was, how annoying it was; how much was tinnitus affecting life; and how big a problem was the tinnitus) are presented together with the THI results.

The collected data are not normally distributed (as they are percentages or ranks from 0 to 10); consequently, non-parametric statistics had to be used. The Wilcoxon test was used to calculate statistical significance of the differences between beginning of the treatment and a given point of time (two-tailed test). Means and standard

Table 4.1 Distribution of patients into categories and acceptance of recommended instrumentation

Patient category	Number of patients (% of population)	Number following recommended instrumentation (% of those recommended)
0	13(11.8)	13(100)
1	47(42.7)	44(93.6)
2	19(17.2)	16(84.2)
3	31(28.2)	27(87.1)
4	10(9.1)	9(90.0)
All	120(100)	109(91.8)

Note that for category 0, there is no instrument recommendation.

errors of means (SEM) presented on some figures are for an illustrative purpose only and should not be used to judge statistical significance of differences among means.

There were 77 men (64.2%) and 43 women (35.8%) in this group. The mean age was 48.9 years (SD $= 14.57$). The youngest patient was 10.5 years and the oldest was 75.5 years. Table 4.1 presents the distribution of the patients into categories and how many followed a recommendation regarding instrumentation. Sound generators or hearing aids were recommended for 89% of the patients and 92% of these patients followed this recommendation.

Evaluation of subjective self-assessment of the treatment by the patients showed high levels of satisfaction: 81.8% patients stated that they were clearly better.

Evaluation of subjective self-assessment of the treatment by the patients showed high levels of satisfaction: 81.8% patients stated that they were clearly better ($p < 0.0001$; Sign test); 98.5% stated that they were satisfied with the treatment, with 1.5% not sure ($p < 0.0001$; Sign test); and 100% continued the use of instruments after 8 months ($p < 0.0001$; Sign test).

The changes in the percentage of time when patients were aware of their tinnitus, and when they were annoyed by it, during the treatment are presented in Fig. 4.6. It is possible to observe rapid improvement, followed by further more gradual change for the better. Notably, after only three months of treatment, both variables showed highly statistically significant improvement (Wilcoxon test). As tinnitus awareness reflects habituation of tinnitus perception, while percentage of time when patients are annoyed by tinnitus reflects the combined effect of habituation of perception and reaction induced by tinnitus, these data indicate that significant habituation

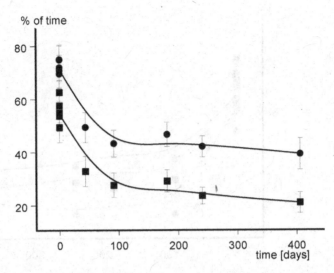

Figure 4.6   Changes of percentage of time when patients were aware of their tinnitus (circles), and when they were annoyed (squares) by it during the treatment. Results on this graph and subsequent similar figures are divided into initial visit and four time blocks: 0–59, 60–119, 120–269 and longer than 270 days (e.g., 0–2, 2–4, 4–7 and longer than 9 months). Multiple values for time 0 represent means for subgroups corresponding to given time of follow-up. Values on the time axis represent average time between initial and follow-up visits for a given group. Line (on this and subsequent graphs) shows spline approximation of the data. The statistical significance of changes were as follows: for percentage of time awareness $p < 0.01$ for first interval, and $p < 0.001$ for all remaining intervals (Wilcoxon test); percentage of time annoyed for $p < 0.05$ for first interval, $p < 0.01$ for second and $p < 0.001$ for remaining intervals. Note that both variables improved significantly during the treatment, with high levels of significance reached after 3 months.

of tinnitus occurred within the first three months of the treatment and that this reached an even higher level of significance later on.

This postulate is further supported by data showing the changes of tinnitus severity, annoyance and effect on life during treatment (Fig. 4.7). All variables showed statistically significant improvement for times longer than two months. These data strongly support the postulate that TRT results in statistically significant habituation of tinnitus and in a significant decrease of the impact of tinnitus on patients' life.

The THI has now gained some recognition and is used in various centers involved in tinnitus treatment. It consists of 25 questions divided into functional, emotional and catastrophic subscales. Initially we assessed the specificity and usefulness of individual subscales. If these subscales represent independent assessment of various aspects of tinnitus-induced problems then their normalized values should be

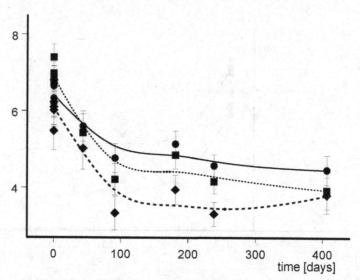

Figure 4.7   Changes of tinnitus severity (circles and solid line), annoyance (squares and dotted line), and effect on life (diamonds and dashed line) during treatment. Changes in severity were non-significant for first interval and $p < 0.01$ for remaining intervals; changes in annoyance were $p < 0.05$ for first interval and $p < 0.001$ for remaining intervals; effect on life was non-significant for first interval, $p < 0.01$ for second and $p < 0.001$ for remaining. Note that all variables showed statistically significant improvement for times longer than 2 months.

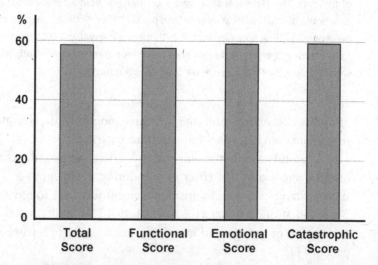

Figure 4.8   Normalized initial values of Tinnitus Handicap Inventory (THI) for the total score and for the functional, emotional and catastrophic subscales. Maximal value for total THI is 100; the subscales have been normalized to 100 to allow direct comparison of results for subscales. Note that average values for the total and all subscales are practically identical.

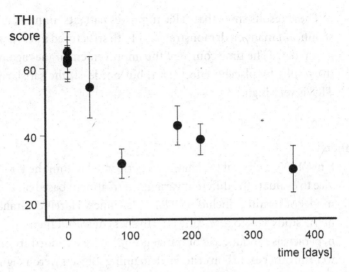

Figure 4.9   Change of the Tinnitus Handicap Inventory total scores during TRT treatment. The results for one month are not significant, while for all subsequent intervals a highly significant improvement is present ($p < 0.01$).

different. If, however, they reflect a random selection of questions, then their values should be close to each other. Our results (Jastreboff, Jastreboff & Mattox, 2001b) strongly suggest that the latter is true as the averages of normalized values, and the variability for the total and for all subscales, are practically identical (Fig. 4.8). Therefore, division into subscales is not providing any benefit and only the total score should be used. This postulate was confirmed in an independent study by other investigators (Baguley & Andersson, 2003). Therefore, there does not seem to be any advantage in using subscales, and the total score should be sufficient for the evaluation of patients.

The changes of the Tinnitus Handicap Inventory total scores during tinnitus retraining treatment are completely consistent with other results and fully support the postulate of significant improvement occurring during TRT treatment.

The changes of THI total scores during TRT treatment are completely consistent with other results (Fig. 4.9), and fully support the postulate of significant improvement occurring during TRT treatment. While the change observed after one month of treatment is not significant, for all subsequent time intervals there is a highly significant improvement ($p < 0.01$). The failure to detect any significant change at one month but significant changes at longer intervals suggests that the observed improvement is not a placebo effect, which would most likely manifest at the shortest time interval, decreasing gradually over time.

These results show that TRT improves patients' tinnitus in a highly statistically significant manner, demonstrated by both structured interviews and the THI using group data. The time course of the improvement argues against contamination of the results by placebo effect. Last, but not least, the satisfaction of patients with TRT is very high.

4.7.3 London

Since 1995, a clinical trial has been performed within the UK National Health Service to evaluate the different variants of treatment based on the neurophysiological model of tinnitus, including TRT (McKinney, Hazell & Graham, 1999). One aim of the study was to assess the effectiveness of sound therapy in TRT. Subjects with hyperacusis (about 25% of initial group) were excluded from the study but there were no other exclusion criteria. Remaining subjects were assigned to different treatment groups. All groups received the same counseling, including the instruction to avoid silence. Two groups, 36 patients each, received broadband sound generators set at two different levels of sound: just at the threshold of hearing, and at the "mixing" point. The final group (54 patients) received only counseling, with limited information about sound therapy and no instruments. Additional groups were fitted with hearing aids and are not reported here. Consequently, using TRT categorization, reported results involved only category 1 patients, and only one group (with sound generators set at the mixing point) directly followed TRT. Selection for the groups was sequential and random except those with a significant hearing loss, who were aided appropriately. Furthermore, 113 subjects from the British Tinnitus Association underwent an identical initial and follow-up evaluation (at 12 months). They were not receiving any treatment, or even seen by the London team, and they constitute a comparison group.

All patients received intensive counseling at the initial session and at each of the follow-up sessions over a period of one year, with further follow-up after two years. Data collection was very close, though not identical with the Baltimore study. Specifically, activities affected by symptoms were not recorded, but this difference still allows for comparison of the results.

At the initial session, patients went through the initial interview (Appendix 1), received intensive TRT counseling, teaching of the neurophysiological model, (by J. W. P. Hazell), and audiometric investigations. The treatment program was outlined, and ear-mold impressions were made for subsequent instrument fitting.

Patients were then seen at 1, 3, 6, 12 and 24 months. Each session consisted of the follow-up interview, repetition of the audiometrical evaluation and appropriate counseling. Patients who did not return for follow-up visits were contacted by telephone but not interviewed, and they contribute towards missing data. All

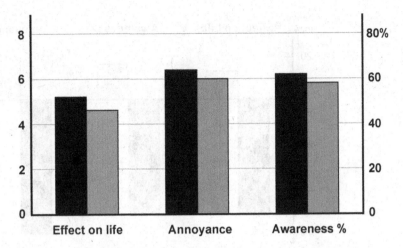

Figure 4.10 Initial characterization of tinnitus in the London study. See Fig. 4.2 for details.

patients, except those who defaulted and represent missing data, received full TRT treatment.

Individual activities affected by tinnitus were not analyzed; however, the patient was required to show at least 40% improvement in at least two categories; the effect on life, awareness or annoyance, to qualify as showing significant improvement. The main results were presented during the *Sixth International Tinnitus Seminar*, Cambridge, UK in 1999 (McKinney *et al.*, 1999).

The data were presented in a similar manner to the Baltimore results. The values for all patients before treatment were divided into "better" and "no-better" categories. The values of measures for annoyance, the effect on life and awareness were very similar between the two categories before treatment (Fig. 4.10) and are similar to those observed in Baltimore (Fig. 4.2). They differ in having generally lower values for all parameters, showing that these patients were not affected as much by tinnitus as those in the Baltimore study. Values recorded at the beginning and during the treatment were used to calculate the change occurring in each individual as a result of treatment; these are displayed by dividing them into populations of patients showing and not showing improvement.

Awareness, annoyance caused by tinnitus and its effect on life decreased by about 50%.

As with the Baltimore patients, there is a decrease of awareness, of annoyance caused by tinnitus and in its effect on life by about 50% (Fig. 4.11). Comparison of initial values with those two years later showed a highly significant improvement for all patients combined. Using the Friedman test (annoyance F: $\chi^{-2} = 180.336$, df = 5, p = <0.001; life quality: F: $\chi^{-2} = 194.868$, df = 5,

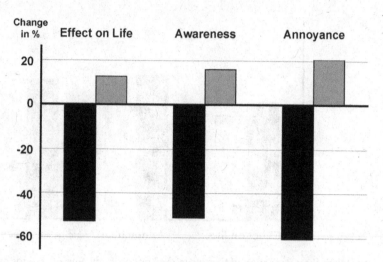

Figure 4.11 Changes of main parameters of tinnitus in London study. See Fig. 4.3 for details.

$p = {<}0.001$; loudness: F: $\chi^{-2} = 109.363$, df $= 5$, p $= {<}0.001$; awareness (percentage of time): F: $\chi^{-2} = 197.998$, df $= 5$, p $= {<}0.001$).

When patients were treated with sound generators set at the mixing point, as needed for TRT, 83.3% showed significant improvement. The group that received sound generators set just above the threshold of hearing, potentially affected by stochastic resonance, showed significant improvement only in 66.7%.

The most interesting result, however, came from a comparison of groups using sound therapy in different ways. When patients were treated with sound generators set at the mixing point, as needed for TRT, 83.3% showed significant improvement. The group without instrumentation and without full counseling about sound therapy showed success in only 72.2%. Finally the worst results (only 66.7% success) were seen in the group that received sound generators set just above the threshold of hearing and, therefore, had sound within the range of stochastic resonance (Fig. 4.12).

Previously we have shown that change of the average MSL can be linked to a treatment outcome (Jastreboff *et al.*, 1994). This observation supports one of TRT's postulates: TRT induces plastic changes within the auditory pathways, detuning neuronal networks from tinnitus detection. Consequently, a lower level of external sound is required to suppress the tinnitus-related neuronal activity and tinnitus perception.

The finding of statistically significant correlation of minimal suppression level and the treatment outcome strongly supported the neurophysiological model of tinnitus.

This finding was strongly supported by results of the study by McKinney *et al.* (1999). Analysis of the raw data, kindly provided by McKinney, revealed that MSL

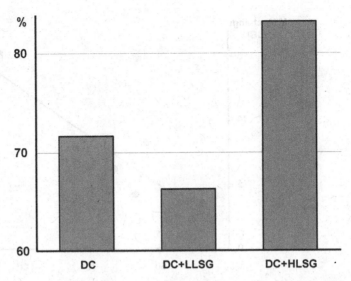

Figure 4.12 Dependence of treatment outcome on variant of sound therapy used. Note the highest effectiveness when sound generators were set at the mixing point (DC + HLSG), as needed for TRT, and lowest effectiveness when sound generators were set at the threshold of hearing (DC + LLSG), which can be explained by an effect of stochastic resonance. DC, directive counseling alone.

for the treatment groups showed changes (calculated for each individual patient and averaged for a given group) that were significantly correlated ($r = 0.8864$, $F_{1,4} = 14.66$, $p < 0.02$) with the effectiveness of treatment for each of the groups (Fig. 4.13). This finding strongly supports the neurophysiological model of tinnitus.

Treatment was continued for one year, and patients followed for a further year, when tinnitus was reassessed. Despite the absence of formal treatment, all scores were maintained or improved, showing that the results of TRT are maintained or improved well after treatment is finished.

In the comparison group of 113 tinnitus subjects from the British Tinnitus Association, who were not treated, only 6% improved. Consequently, the effectiveness of TRT could be expressed as 83.3% compared with 6%. (Note that the use of the term "comparison group" in this context is acceptable according to the literature (Rosenfeld, 2001; Jastreboff, 1999b).)

A subsequent retrospective study was performed in London on a separate clinic population (Sheldrake *et al.*, 1999). The data came from a separate group of private patients of J. W. P. Hazell, whose 311 patients were followed for one year and 124 for up to three years. The distribution of the initial 483 patients was 49 (10.1%), 145 (29.8%), 152 (31.7%), 118 (24.4%) and 19 (3.9%) in categories 0–4, respectively (Fig. 4.14). The effectiveness of treatment using a 40% criterion was 70.1% after 1 year and 83.9% at the last visit.

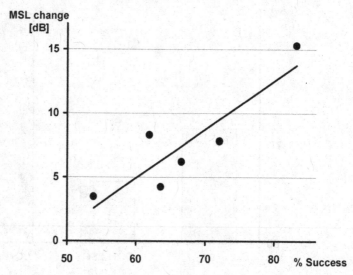

Figure 4.13 The relationship between changes in minimum suppression level (MSL) and treatment outcome measured as the percentage of the group fulfilling the criteria of improvement. The change of MSL was calculated for each individual patient and averaged for a given group. Note significant correlation between variables ($t = 0.8864$, $F_{1,4} = 14.66$, $p < 0.02$). This result strongly supports the postulate that TRT induced plastic changes in neural centers processing the tinnitus signal.

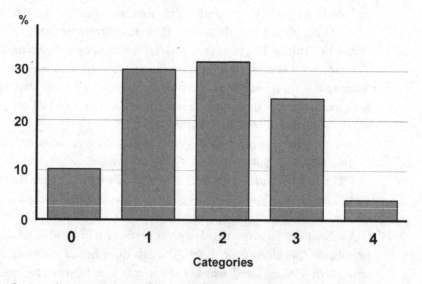

Figure 4.14 Distribution of patients by treatment category in the London clinical practice.

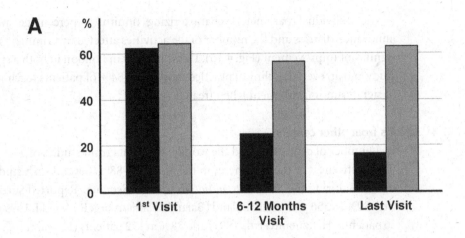

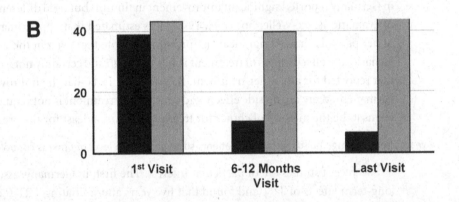

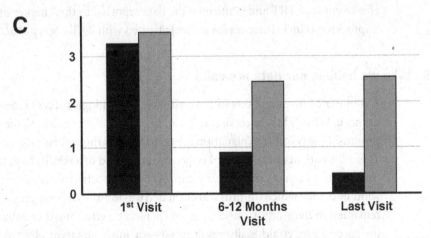

Figure 4.15 Changes in awareness (A), annoyance/distress (B) and number of activities affected (C) in patients treated in the London clinical practice. Better (■); no better (□).

The individual parameters characterizing tinnitus – percentage awareness, annoyance/distress and the number of life activities affected by tinnitus – showed a significant improvement (Fig. 4.15). Data obtained in London in both a systematic study and an everyday clinical practice showed 83–84% of patients reaching a level of significant improvement when treated with TRT.

4.7.4 Results from other centers

In a number of centers around the world, initial data from studies of TRT indicate the effectiveness of the treatment, in the range 70–88%. Several such studies were reported during the *Sixth International Tinnitus Seminar.* Reported success rates were 80% in 556 patients in Poland (Bartnik, Fabijanska & Rogowski, 1999), 84% in 56 patients (Heitzmann *et al.*, 1999) and 88% in 172 patients (Herraiz *et al.*, 1999) in Spain and 82% in 223 patients in the USA (Jastreboff, 1999a). A study of 122 patients in Germany reported significant improvement in tinnitus but used different criteria of evaluation(Lux-Wellenhof *et al.*, 1999); it is estimated that approximately 80% of her patients showed significant improvement. Note that even in the worst case scenario, the effectiveness of treatment is still very high and certainly not worse than that reported for any other treatment. Based on the facts that the improvement is permanent, there are no side effects and continuing treatment is not required, TRT seems to be the method of choice for treating tinnitus, at least for the present.

Five years after initiating tinnitus retraining, patients sustained a high level of tinnitus control.

Two recent studies are of particular interest. The first, in Germany, assessed the long-term effects of TRT and found that five years after initiating TRT (i.e., about four years after finalizing the treatment) patients sustained high levels of tinnitus control (Lux-Wellenhof & Hellweg, 2002). The second study used THI for assessing effectiveness of TRT and confirmed the data reported in this chapter of significant improvement in THI scores for patients treated with TRT (Berry *et al.*, 2002).

4.8 Why we believe our data are valid

A number of investigations in the past have shown high success rates of 60–70% or more. Why did these reports not lead to a successful solution to the problem of tinnitus? One possible explanation relates to the way the success rate was estimated. Typically, patients were assessed only once at the end of a relatively short period of treatment, using as a criterium any improvement reported by the patient. If the time window during which tinnitus was evaluated was infinite, only successful candidates remained in the study. Considering a 40% placebo effect, further enhancement of the success rate could easily result in 60% or more apparent effectiveness of the treatment.

Another approach has been adopted for assessing the effectiveness of tinnitus "masking" (tinnitus suppression by sound). In this case, if patients were still using maskers 6 months after starting treatment it was considered to be a success (Johnson, 1998), without measuring if patients had indeed experienced any improvement.

A large number of clinical trials of drug therapies have been performed, with initial results of 60–80%. Again a high level of placebo effect, combined with the short-coming of assessment methodology, may explain why, in spite of all these efforts, there is no drug that is in regular use with tinnitus patients (see Ch. 6).

In the past, the focus was on the psychoacoustical measurement of tinnitus, but studies using these methods were unable to show relationship with treatment outcome. Psychoacoustical characterization of tinnitus has very little relationship to the symptoms, which are important to the patient, shows a wide intra- and intersubject variability and (with the exception of MSL) does not measure changes in neurophysiological mechanisms involved in tinnitus. Currently, investigators are still using different methods for assessing patients, and only recently have there been some efforts to create criteria that can be generally accepted.

4.9   Conclusions

The results presented in this chapter show that a large proportion of patients experience a significant improvement in their tinnitus and in their sound tolerance as a result of TRT. The results are sustained, without the need for further treatment and do not seem to be contaminated by a placebo or spontaneous recovery effects.

The crucial difference between our approach and those that have been tried previously is that TRT has been based on a neurophysiological model of tinnitus. This mechanism has a good scientific basis and involves a number of systems in the brain, with the auditory system being one such system but not the dominant one (Jastreboff, 1990). Treatment is aimed at changing processing of tinnitus-related neuronal activity and not on improving coping strategies or on eradicating the source of tinnitus, which at the moment is not realistic. Treatment that is symptom based and does not relate to the mechanisms of the underlying complaint is unlikely to succeed, except by chance. This is the reason for poor results in treatments based on the concept that tinnitus is a purely cochlear phenomenon.

The underlying mechanisms for tinnitus and decreased sound tolerance (particularly misophonia) do overlap. There is often a need for the concurrent or sequential treatment for both problems. Similar strategies can be used for treating tinnitus and decreased sound tolerance. Patients can be classified by their specific combination of tinnitus, hyperacusis and hearing loss and this forms the basis for specific variations in the treatment protocol. However, in each case the goal is to achieve habituation of tinnitus and to remove or attenuate decreased sound tolerance.

The negative aspects of TRT are the time taken to achieve effect, the need for intensive one-to-one interaction with patient and that TRT has to be performed by personnel who need additional specialist training.

The positive aspects of TRT are its harmlessness and absence of side effects, its effectiveness regardless of the etiology, the ability also to treat somatosounds and decreased sound tolerance, the fact that results are independent of psychoacoustical characterization of tinnitus, the restricted duration of treatment period, the rarity of relapse and, finally, the potential ability of TRT to incorporate additional supplementary treatments that have a synergistic effect, such as medication, hypnosis, etc. At the moment, we are not aware of any other treatment for tinnitus and hyperacusis offering these advantages.

5

Prevention

> Tinnitus prevention is an area that has largely been ignored. A knowledge of the neurophysio-logical model makes it clear that avoidance of silence and the routine use of sound enrichment will reduce the incidence of tinnitus and hyperacusis. General education of both public and professionals about the dangers of negative counseling will reduce the development of aversive reactions, resulting in tinnitus persistence. Damaging loud noise increases the risk of hearing loss, in which tinnitus prevalence increases, but it is important not to overplay this issue, as the majority of hearing-impaired people do not suffer from tinnitus.

The maxim that prevention is better than a cure should be applied to the problem of tinnitus too. The prevalence of clinically significant tinnitus is very high, estimated to be up to 4% of the population, and any efforts that can be made to reduce this onset of distressing and disabling problem should be made. Based on an understanding of the neurophysiological model, there are a number of areas that can now be effectively applied to reduce tinnitus prevalence and potentially prevent its emergence in many individuals.

5.1 Avoidance of silence

The vast majority of our patients describe the initial emergence of their tinnitus during a period of silence. This is often while lying awake at night or while sitting in a quiet room in their home during the day. Many such environments are excessively quiet because of the widespread use of double glazing and the dislike for any external noise intruding into periods of sleep or quiet recreational activities. We have identified an at-risk population who before the emergence of tinnitus had a significant dislike for external sounds (misophonia). These patients, in addition to avoiding sound and, thus surround themselves with silence, may have abnormalities of central auditory processing involving increased gain, manifesting as hyperacusis.

Both sound avoidance and increased gain within the auditory pathways makes some people more liable to detect the tinnitus signal.

Both avoiding sound, and increased gain within the auditory pathways makes it more liable to detect the tinnitus signal. In some patients, decreased sound tolerance is so severe that it leads to the installation of special sound-proof rooms in their homes. Such individuals are unwittingly performing the experiment in which 94% of all normal hearing individuals developed tinnitus after being placed in a sound-proof room for more than five minutes (Heller & Bergman, 1953). In the original experiment, tinnitus did not persist because the subjects returned to normally noise-filled environments, did not become unduly attentive to the tinnitus and did not try to repeat the experiment. In particular, they did not develop any anxieties over the meaning of the sounds that they heard in the sound-proof room, because of their understanding that this was a completely normal and natural phenomenon. The importance of avoiding silence and enriching the auditory background is poorly appreciated, while the negative aspects of exposure to sound are often overemphasized. Excessive campaigning about the dangers of noise exposure can lead individuals to overprotect themselves with plugs and muffs; this, in turn, can result in the development of tinnitus and decreased sound tolerance.

5.2 Provision of sound enrichment

The presence of background sound decreases the strength of potentially emerging tinnitus and reduces auditory gain, from which hyperacusis might also develop.

As avoidance of silence is an essential feature in tinnitus and hyperacusis prevention, we are also recommending the general and continuous use of sound enrichment by natural means or electronic devices. For thousands of years, the Japanese have promoted the concept of sound enrichment, through sounds of wind and water, as a relaxing and beneficial adjunct to any environment in which a person lives. The presence of background sound decreases the strength of any emerging tinnitus and will reduce auditory gain, from which hyperacusis might also develop. Any increase in auditory gain would also enhance pre-existing tinnitus. Consequently, sound enrichment decreases the chance of tinnitus perception emerging.

Another well-known effect of the sounds of nature is that they have a calming effect on the individual by lowering activity of the autonomic nervous system. Therefore, the presence of continuous background sounds from water features, wind chimes and the like will also create an environment in which clinically significant tinnitus is much less likely to emerge. We recommend the use of sound-generating devices (e.g., table-top sound machines, CD players, water fountains) that make sounds chosen by individuals for their pleasant characteristics, which will be easily habituated and will not cause aversion.

5.3   Avoidance of excessive noise

> While hearing conservation is a very important issue when considering exposure to excessive sound levels, people should not seek out noise-free environments at other times.

Another group of individuals who are particularly at risk of developing persistent tinnitus includes those who have been exposed to high levels of noise, particularly following a visit to a disco or working in a very noisy environment (e.g., while using power tools, heavy machinery, etc.). Everyone should use ear plugs when exposed to excessive sound levels, to protect against potential hearing loss. Short breaks (10 minutes per hour) from loud sound are beneficial. While hearing conservation is a very important issue, we believe it is particularly important that such individuals should not seek out noise-free environments at other times. They should make sure that there is always a reasonable background level of noise, particularly in the place where they sleep. This is because there is an increased prevalence of abnormal signals coming from the cochlea following noise exposure and these may result in a perception of tinnitus that may then become persistent if an aversive reaction develops.

Excessive noise eventually causes damage of the outer hair cells (OHC), with an increased prevalence of tinnitus. Even small temporary changes in the OHC system following noise exposure can act as a trigger for tinnitus emergence. Impulsive or explosive types of noise seem to be particularly dangerous in this respect. Many people are exposed to sound levels that cause hearing damage only gradually over a prolonged period of time. While there may be a slow but steady reduction in the OHC population, tinnitus is frequently not experienced as there is enough time for natural compensation to occur. Habituation of the tinnitus signal is the mechanism of this natural compensation.

5.4   Avoidance of negative counseling

> Negative counseling, frequently from healthcare professionals, patient support groups and the Internet, is a potent trigger mechanism for making tinnitus worse.

Negative counseling, frequently from healthcare professionals, patient support groups and the Internet, is a potent trigger mechanism for worsening tinnitus. In many cases tinnitus that initially excited only a mild interest or curiosity becomes loud, intrusive and anxiety provoking in the face of information that it is permanent, untreatable and must simply be accepted. In many cases, such counseling comes from family physicians and otolaryngologists, who honestly believe that there is nothing that can be done about tinnitus and do not wish to waste time with something that they cannot cure. The effects of such counseling, however, can be devastating, and we have documented this time and time again in our patients (Jastreboff, 1999d).

A nationwide program is needed in each country to alert healthcare professionals to the dangers of negative counseling of tinnitus patients.

A nationwide program is needed in each country to alert healthcare professionals to the dangers of negative counseling of tinnitus patients. This has already been undertaken in several countries, including the UK. The approach that is needed is one that is more upbeat and optimistic, and truly reflects the statistics: approximately 80% of those who develop tinnitus will habituate to it without any treatment at all; the most likely outcome is that initial distress, insomnia and interference at work and with quiet recreational activity will gradually disappear, even though the tinnitus will still occasionally be perceived. TRT allows counseling of an even more optimistic nature; that with TRT the unpleasant emotional associations will disappear or strongly decrease (habituation of reaction), and that the proportion of time that tinnitus will be perceived will reduce substantially (habituation of perception).

5.5 Emergency help line

Much can be done to improve the situation of tinnitus patients simply by talking to them over the telephone.

The efforts of organizations providing a national telephone help line have shown that much can be done to improve the situation of tinnitus patients simply by talking to them over the telephone. This is the case when the information includes the reassurance that tinnitus can be improved. National programs need to increase general awareness about the benign nature of tinnitus perception. In addition, such advice should be available as soon as possible after the emergence of tinnitus and before significant fears and anxieties have developed. This would result in a drastic reduction in the number of chronic cases of severely disturbing tinnitus. Such information needs to be available in the national press, in doctors' offices and as part of health training during school or university education.

5.6 Identification of subjects with predisposition to tinnitus

Individuals who have a combination of factors predisposing them to the onset of tinnitus should be identified by healthcare professionals and given appropriate counseling before a problem develops.

Individuals who have a combination of factors predisposing them to the onset of tinnitus (e.g., pre-existing hyperacusis combined with a very stressful environment, hearing overprotection, some hearing disability and regular noise exposure) should be identified by healthcare professionals and given appropriate counseling before a problem develops. The message needs to be widely disseminated that for most people tinnitus perception is far from indicating any medical problem and is, in fact, a perfectly natural and benign experience which can be easily habituated. In rare cases when tinnitus perception is related to a medical problem (e.g., vestibular schwannoma), it is actually a friendly warning that something needs to be checked. If nothing medically significant is detected then there is no need to worry. This information will at least partially protect people from the development of negative associations in respect to tinnitus perception and thus prevent development of clinically significant tinnitus.

The problems caused by negative counseling cannot be overstated. Very often people are exposed to negative information about tinnitus well before its onset by some inappropriate reading, a television program, a conversation with a friend, etc. People who have a predisposition to tinnitus will be particularly prone to the effects of even relatively mild negative counseling for several reasons: systematic noise exposure increases the probability of OHC damage; high stress levels make it more likely that an individual will over-react to a new stimulus (tinnitus); pre-existing hyperacusis increases the chance of hearing overprotection and the tendency to decrease the average background sound level. Hearing overprotection plays a specific role, as it promotes both tinnitus and hyperacusis, so it is particularly dangerous.

5.7   Basic principles of prevention

The provision of proper education to both the general population and professionals involved in medical and audiological care is fundamental.

Providing proper education to both the general population and the professionals involved in medical and audiological care is fundamental. It needs to be clearly understood that tinnitus perception is only weakly related to tinnitus-induced distress. That is, while it is necessary to perceive the tinnitus signal initially to induce the negative reactions of the brain and body involved in tinnitus-induced distress, the characteristics of this signal (e.g., how it sounds) are irrelevant. Just perceiving tinnitus does not mean that these negative reactions have to develop; indeed in the majority they do not. Proper information, from reputable sources, should be easily available, particularly to those who have just noticed tinnitus for the first time and are naturally curious about its meaning.

It is also advisable to provide basic TRT counseling before procedures that have a chance of inducing tinnitus (e.g., stapedectomy operation or gamma knife treatment for vestibular schwannoma) to prevent the development of clinically significant tinnitus should tinnitus perception emerge after the treatment. Such counseling would be very helpful in the standard training of professions who, by definition, are exposed to high levels of the noise while under significant stress, for example the military, police, fire-fighters, etc.

The message that both sound overexposure and overprotection are harmful needs to be strongly emphasized in both public and professional health education.

The message that both sound overexposure and overprotection are harmful needs to be strongly emphasized in both public and professional health education. An image of sound should be promoted as an integral part of our life, essential for our well-being.

6

Critical overview of selected tinnitus treatments

This chapter describes and critically evaluates recently used or historically important methods for treating tinnitus, including medications, surgical approaches for neurotological problems, treatment of medical conditions associated with tinnitus and hyperacusis, masking, hearing aids, psychological treatments, electrical stimulation and alternative therapies. Although each of the listed therapies has been helpful for some individuals, none has been proven to be effective for a significant proportion of sufferers. Because drugs are particularly attractive for both patients and physicians, medications are reviewed in a more comprehensive manner.

The high prevalence of tinnitus, and the typical fluctuation of its intensity and annoyance, has resulted in patients reporting improvement following a wide range of therapies aimed at treating tinnitus or other unrelated problems. Often this was a chance relationship or spontaneous improvement of tinnitus.

Anecdotal reports of improvement triggered attempts to validate reports of a therapy being helpful.

Anecdotal reports of improvement have triggered attempts to validate these reports, usually by uncontrolled open trials. For example, in a drug therapy, a group of patients was given a medication and told it might be helpful. Unfortunately, the initial positive results failed to be confirmed by other centers and consequently were not accepted. Positive results in open trials were enhanced by a placebo effect, which in the case of tinnitus has been shown to be as high as 40% (Duckert & Rees, 1984).

Placebo effect in tinnitus has been shown to be around 40%.

In drug therapy, the placebo effect is the report of a change while the patient is taking a substance containing no active ingredient (placebo). The appropriate method for controlling the placebo effect is a randomized, double-blind study where neither the patient nor the experimenters know whether the patient is receiving the active substance or not. The placebo is without any active ingredient but cannot be detected by the patient as being different by looks, taste or side effects from the tested drug. Moreover, patients are assigned to active or placebo group in a random manner.

The placebo effect can vary greatly for the treatment of different medical conditions. In this respect, the classic paper of Duckert and Rees (1984) is of particular importance and provides reliable information that can be used as a frame of reference for assessing the validity of tinnitus treatments. In their well-conducted study, Duckert and Rees examined 20 patients who previously were given placebo injections and were aware of this. The patients were invited to continue the study and informed that this time they would receive an active substance, lidocaine. They were told of favorable responses to lidocaine that others had experienced. They were also told that their particular response could not be predicted, they would not experience side effects and their tinnitus could be temporarily increased, decreased or unchanged. In the experiment a 5ml injection of saline (i.e., a placebo) was given intravenously over three minutes. To complete the deception, electrocardiogram and blood pressure monitoring was performed. Before and after the injection, patients had pure tone audiometry, tinnitus matching and a subjective assessment of tinnitus on a scale from a positive change of 100% to a change for the worse of 100%. Changes greater than 25% were classified as significant:

Results showed that 40% (8 out of 20) of subjects reported greater than 25% changes in their tinnitus after saline administration. Saline injections can have no direct effect on tinnitus. Consequently, these reported changes resulted exclusively from the placebo effect, which, because of the expectations of the tinnitus patients, was very high.

The best approach for any trial is to conduct a double-blind study where neither subject, nor experimenter is aware whether active or placebo treatment is being given. Unfortunately this is not always possible.

Since the design of Duckert and Rees's study (1984) was very similar to the typical design of an open study for tinnitus treatment, we might expect a placebo effect of the same order in any open study. Consequently, the best approach for any trial of tinnitus treatment is to conduct a randomized, double-blind study. While desirable, it is unfortunately not always possible.

However, if the improvement is sustained for a prolonged time after treatment finishes, it is unlikely to be a placebo effect as this typically lasts no longer than two to three months. Commonly, the benefits reported in the literature for tinnitus treatments are short term rather than long term, and they are frequently similar to the effects of a placebo, making the validity of these reports questionable. The placebo effect might explain many reports in the literature of initial good results for many tinnitus treatments that, during subsequent studies, turned out not to be effective (e.g., Carrick *et al.*, 1986; Dobie, Hoberg & Rees, 1986; Penner & Bilger, 1989; Rendell *et al.*, 1987; Shulman, 1985).

Even in some studies that were described by the authors as a double-blind trial, the anonymity of patients (who is taking the drug, and who the placebo) was often compromised by the experience of side effects in those taking the active substances (Huynh & Fields, 1995). Such studies cannot be considered double blind, as patients are aware if they are being given active substance or placebo by the presence of side effects from the active substance. Unfortunately, this possibility is rarely mentioned in the literature. For example, some of the drugs under investigation for tinnitus, such as tocainide (no longer available) and alprazolam (Xanax), have a very high incidence of side effects (major and minor), which make patients aware when they are taking the drug as opposed to placebo. This effectively converts a double-blind trial into an open study (Huynh & Fields, 1995).

Randomized, double-blind studies are relatively easy to implement for drugs, more difficult for surgery and very difficult, or impossible, for treatments having counseling as a significant component. An assessment of published clinical trials for tinnitus treatment was presented in a recent paper (Dobie, 1999). The author concluded that the validity of the vast majority of reports had been compromised by poor methodology, and that there is a real need for well-planned and properly conducted studies.

Clinical results showed that auditory nerve section does not help tinnitus in the majority of patients and in about 8% actually makes tinnitus worse. Additionally, it was shown that 50% of patients without tinnitus who had acoustic nerve section for other reasons experienced tinnitus postoperatively.

Since tinnitus is a perception of sound, it is often judged to be coming from the ear. The inner ear is responsible for the transduction of sound into neural impulses and, consequently, it was natural to assume that indeed the inner ear is the dominant, or even exclusive, factor responsible for tinnitus (see Ch. 1). As a result, many treatments were aimed at the inner ear, even to the extent of cutting the auditory nerve in an attempt to separate tinnitus generators from central auditory pathways in the brain. Clinical results showed that auditory nerve section does not help tinnitus in the majority of cases and in about 8% actually makes tinnitus worse (Harcourt, Thomsen & Tos, 1997). Additionally, in about 50% of those without preoperative tinnitus, it emerges postoperatively (Berliner *et al.*, 1992; Catalano & Post, 1996; Levo, Blomstedt & Pyykko, 2000).

Focusing on the ear as the exclusive cause of the problem resulted in tinnitus being classified as "peripheral," or "central" if no ear-related event could be found. As argued in previous chapters, in each case of clinically significant tinnitus, there is strong central component responsible for tinnitus-induced distress. At the same time, it is possible that some peripheral dysfunction acts as a trigger of the tinnitus-related neuronal activity in the majority of patients. According to the neurophysiological model of tinnitus, separating these components and focusing only on the peripheral or central element is counterproductive. Even in the case of hearing loss, when there is some relationship with the probability of emergence of tinnitus, the relationship is indirect.

Hearing loss cannot be used as a predictor of tinnitus.

Hearing loss cannot be used as a *predictor* of tinnitus, as tinnitus commonly exists in people with normal hearing (Heller & Bergman, 1953; Hazell & McKinney, 1996) and tinnitus is also frequently absent in total deafness (Hazell *et al.*, 1995).

In the absence of effective treatment, desperate patients tend to cling to unproven remedies.

In the absence of effective treatment, desperate patients tend to cling to unproven therapies. An example of this is the self-imposition of severe dietary restriction, frequently combined with unnecessary dietary supplements. Patients will restrict caffeine, alcohol, salt and various types of food, while, at the same time, taking large doses of vitamins and minerals.

While dietary restrictions do not help patients with their tinnitus, they often decrease an already depleted quality of life. In a desperate search for help, patients are willing to try any treatment, whether proven or not. This is graphically demonstrated by a patient of one of the authors, who happened to be a pharmacist and had systematically treated herself with every substance contained in her pharmacy (trial and error method).

The lack of any effective treatment for tinnitus leads to the promotion of coping strategies.

The lack of any effective treatment for tinnitus leads to the promotion of coping strategies and general therapies for reducing stress and anxiety: the problems that tinnitus patients frequently experience. Coping approaches are temporarily helpful for some patients even though they neither change the tinnitus signal itself nor its perception; they may help in tinnitus-induced problems such as anxiety, inability to sustain concentration or depression. Because of the lack of proper criteria for assessing tinnitus severity, confusion has been caused by some researchers reporting an improvement in coping with tinnitus as an improvement in the tinnitus itself (Budd & Pugh, 1996; Sullivan *et al.*, 1994). Similarly to coping strategies, some medications used to help tinnitus patients, such as antidepressant or anti-anxiety drugs, are not specific to tinnitus but offer help with the associated problems. The negative implications of such drugs are that they frequently reduce overall reactiveness and affect interaction with other people in the family and work environment. These psychotropic drugs may change the personality of the patient to the point where the drug is not tolerated by the patient, or by their family and friends. These drugs slow down the process of tinnitus habituation, by impairing the ability of the individual to learn (Beckers *et al.*, 2001b; Coull, Frith & Dolan, 1999; Fleishaker *et al.*, 1995; Munte *et al.*, 1996; Rickels *et al.*, 1999; Ziemann *et al.*, 1998).

6.1 Medications

In this chapter drugs are referred to first by the active ingredient or approved pharmacological name, followed in the first instance by the best know proprietary preparation or brand name, where this is in use. Among the brand names, those in use in the USA are given before those used elsewhere.

No drug has been proved effective against tinnitus without also having very significant side effects.

Western society tends to search for a quick and easy solution to medical problems and pharmacology seems to offer a convenient, fast and relatively inexpensive answer to many problems. It is important to recognize that practically all drugs tested on tinnitus were selected because of anecdotal reports, and without relating to the presumed underlying mechanisms. Quite frequently, they were reported as being helpful in an initial open study, but when repeated by other groups failed to confirm their effectiveness. Randomized double-blind studies, which should be performed for any drug, are unfortunately very rare in the tinnitus field (Dobie, 1999). Still, many desperate sufferers search for drugs that would offer them fast relief. It is worth stressing that practically all of the drugs that have been reported to have an effect on tinnitus have significant side effects; at the moment, the authors are unaware of any medication that will abolish tinnitus permanently.

Drug therapy may play a part in the management of conditions of which tinnitus is a symptom, or in the management of coexisting anxiety and depression.

However, this is not to say that drug therapy has no part to play in the management of certain conditions of which tinnitus is a symptom: so-called "syndromic tinnitus." There are specific diseases such as Ménière's syndrome that are amenable to medical treatment, and successful management may lead to an improvement in the tinnitus, which is one of the symptoms making up the syndrome. However these cases account for a small proportion of the patients seen in a tinnitus clinic.

Another role for drug therapy is in the management of coexisting anxiety and depression. Strong emotional responses are very common in severe tinnitus, and with careful monitoring, drugs have been helpful, for example antidepressants and, in the short term, anxiety-blocking medicaments or tranquilizers. With very few specific exceptions, we seldom recommend these drugs to our patients or find them necessary when TRT is used properly.

It is a mistake to consider that psychotropic drugs on their own are a treatment for tinnitus. They help people to cope temporarily with tinnitus, but they are not changing tinnitus itself (Sullivan *et al.*, 1994). They should be used only in very carefully preselected patients with severe anxiety or depression, and they should be prescribed by a psychiatrist, preferably a member of the tinnitus treatment team. Patients coming to a tinnitus center who are currently on psychotropic medications should continue on the current dose until initial improvement of their tinnitus is observed. Even then, these drugs should be withdrawn very gradually, under close supervision, to avoid making tinnitus worse.

As drugs have been used to treat tinnitus without any relation to presumed tinnitus mechanisms, we have grouped them according to their general physiological action: vasodilators, local anesthetics, sedatives/tranquilizers, antidepressants, anticonvulsants, anti-allergic/anti-inflammatory, calcium channel blockers, other drugs, and dietary supplements. Many drugs have multiple actions and could be included in several categories. We made a subjective choice listing them in a specific category.

In most tinnitus patients, the initial reason for recommending the drug was empirical and without scientific basis. For instance, the sudden onset of tinnitus was compared to a sudden onset of cochlear deafness. The unspoken assumption that tinnitus must result from cochlear damage in each case led to recommendation of the same treatments for sudden-onset tinnitus as for sudden deafness. While this may be appropriate for patients who have a sudden onset of both hearing loss and tinnitus, in the majority emergence of clinically relevant tinnitus is not associated with a change in cochlear function and there is no sudden hearing loss. The often radical intervention (steroids, intravenous infusions of various medications) is unjustified, expensive and might be actually harmful (Fattori *et al.*, 1996; Kau *et al.*, 1997; Pilgramm, Lamm & Schumann, 1985). Unfortunately, these treatments are also being recommended for well-established tinnitus, when an initial cochlear-based mechanism for tinnitus emergence is no longer relevant.

In the future, a better understanding of the neurotransmitters in the brain involved with emergence and persistence of tinnitus may lead us to develop compounds that will block or alter tinnitus through a modification of tinnitus-related neuronal activity (Chen & Jastreboff, 1995; Eggermont, 1990; Jastreboff, 1990, 1995; Kaltenbach, 2000; Kaltenbach & Afman, 2000; Kaltenbach, Zhang & Afman, 2000; Milbrandt *et al.*, 2000; Ochi & Eggermont, 1997). Some of these drugs could potentially be used in parallel with retraining therapy to speed up the process of tinnitus habituation. Until now, most drug therapies have been born of desperation, on the part of either the medical specialist or the patient, demanding that something should be done.

6.1.1   Drugs used for tinnitus treatment
Vasodilators

Vasodilators are presumed to enhance cochlear blood flow.

Vasodilators are agents that cause dilation (enlargement) of blood vessels and are presumed to enhance cochlear blood flow. They are widely used in the management of acute cochlear deafness, even when this is thought to be the result of viral infection of the cochlea. Some authorities believe that improving the microcirculation of the cochlea, which may be shut down following certain types of insult or trauma, can help in the recovery process (Hultcrantz, 1988). While such a postulate is disputable, as a double-blind study showed that the vasodilator effect does not alter tinnitus (Hulshof & Vermeij, 1987), nevertheless many approaches aimed at improving brain and cochlear circulation have been and still are being used. Vasodilators are also combined with steroids to combat supposed inflammation, as well as carbon dioxide with oxygen inhalations to increase cerebral blood flow. The opinion has been expressed often that it is unethical to withhold such treatment. The validity of this approach to treating sudden deafness has itself not been proven, and as some spontaneous recovery even after cochlear shutdown occurs in many cases, it is impossible to say whether these treatments are really effective. This approach aimed at enhancement of cochlear blood flow certainly has no rationale or useful effect in treating well-established tinnitus.

Betahistine (Serc, Betaserc) is widely used as a treatment for Ménière's syndrome.

Betahistine (Serc, Betaserc) is widely used outside the USA (it is not licensed in the USA) and was extensively advertised at one time as treating the "vertigo, deafness and tinnitus" of Ménière's syndrome. While the authors are convinced that betahistine is effective in treating Ménière's syndrome (Ryan & Hazell, 1995), this condition is very rare compared with tinnitus on its own. Unfortunately, the effectiveness of the drug for Ménière's syndrome resulted in a misunderstanding that it could treat any kind of tinnitus, and it was widely prescribed for tinnitus patients who did not have Ménière's syndrome, without any effect other than considerable cost (Kay, 1981; Oosterveld, 1984).

Histamine and dextran infusions have been given intravenously for sudden deafness.

At one time, histamine and dextran infusions were given intravenously for sudden deafness. Currently, they are no longer recommended because of significant and sometimes dangerous side effects (Clemis & McBrien, 1996). The treatment with intravenous drugs for the acute onset phase of tinnitus is very common in parts of Europe, particularly Germany, where there are specific directives about the management of acute conditions affecting the ear.

Local anesthetics

Intravenous lidocaine is one of the few drugs that can reliably attenuate tinnitus for a short time.

Intravenous lidocaine (a local anesthetic,[1] also called lignocaine) is perhaps the only drug that can reliably attenuate tinnitus for a short time, as has been demonstrated in a number of controlled trials (Duckert & Rees, 1983; Israel *et al.*, 1982). The relief was observed at plasma concentrations 1.5–2.5 µg/ml; however, notable side effects were observed at plasma concentrations greater than 2.0 µg/ml (den Hartigh *et al.*, 1993). To be effective, the drug needs to be given by intravenous administration and it can be administered only for a short time because of its side effects; lidocaine produces profound changes in nerve transmission throughout the central nervous system and also affects other organs such as the heart and liver. Local applications of lidocaine to the middle ear have been tried to see the effects on tinnitus by "anesthetizing the cochlea." This was largely ineffective, further suggesting that tinnitus is not solely a cochlear event (Coles, Thompson & O'Donoghue, 1992; Hazell, 1981; Podoshin, Fradis & David, 1992).

Recently, a treatment using a combination of intravenous and transtympanic injection of lidocaine was reported (Shea & Xianxi, 2000). While it was proposed that this combination has long-lasting positive effects on tinnitus, this claim has not been confirmed by others. Interpretation of the results was further complicated by the fact that all patients received alprazolam and other psychotropic drugs as a part of the treatment.

Lidocaine is inactive when taken orally, but oral analogues such as tocainide and mexilitene (Mexitil) have been tried in the past (Coles *et al.*, 1992; Duckert & Rees, 1983; Emmett & Shea, 1980; Hulshof & Vermeij, 1984; Lenarz, 1986; Vermeij & Hulshof, 1986). Results of an early double-blind study showed no significant effect on tinnitus with physiologically acceptable doses of tocainide (Hulshof & Vermeij, 1985). As this drug can cause serious bone marrow depression its use has now been withdrawn. Other related drugs such as mexilitene and flecainide have been tried without any significant effect on tinnitus (Kay, 1981).

Iontophoresis (transporting ions by a small electric current) of local anesthetics has been used extensively to desensitize the tympanic membrane for minor surgery, for example insertion of ventilation tubes. A strong solution of lidocaine is placed in the external ear canal and a direct current is used to drive the active local anesthetic through the intact membrane of the eardrum. In some patients, it is possible that absorption of lidocaine into the bloodstream may occur, and it might act in a similar way to intravenous lidocaine. As some patients with tinnitus reported an improvement while undergoing this procedure, it has been marketed extensively

---

[1] Local anesthetics are used for the interruption of the nerve transmission of pain sensations. They act at the site of application to prevent perception of pain.

in Germany as "tinnicure." The device for iontophoresis has been evaluated by sequential double-blind trial on 40 patients (Willatt *et al.*, 1987). This trial showed no effect better than a placebo. Other studies were equally negative (Hazell, 1981; Laffrëe, Vermeij & Hulshof, 1989; Welkoborsky & Bumb, 1988).

Sedatives and tranquilizers

Sedatives and tranquilizers can reduce the severe anxiety and panic that often accompany tinnitus.

Some sedatives and tranquilizers[2] can reduce severe anxiety and panic, which often accompany tinnitus. In our opinion, behavioral techniques that have been shown to be effective in helping patients with anxiety (such as relaxation therapy, thought blocking, etc.) are much preferable because tranquilizers can cause dependence and worsen tinnitus during withdrawal.

Tinnitus is one of the withdrawal side effects after use of benzodiazepines.

Tinnitus is one of the withdrawal side effects after benzodiazepine use (Busto *et al.*, 1986). In our clinics, the introduction of TRT resulted in decrease of anxiety and tendency to panic, and this enabled the gradual withdrawal of these drugs from our patients. With the exception of alprazolam (Johnson, Brummett & Schleuning, 1993), there have been no reports that these drugs have any direct action on tinnitus.

Most patients with significant tinnitus experience sleep disturbance. Patients may have difficulty falling asleep because of the intrusiveness of tinnitus. Frequently, they cannot relax because of accompanying anxiety. In addition, they might have a problem getting back to sleep during periods of wakefulness in the night. Early morning waking is another sleep issue that can result in many hours of listening to distressing tinnitus before the day begins. In some cases, sleep disturbance is something that improves spontaneously after some weeks or months following tinnitus emergence, but in over 50% of patients insomnia persists (Alster *et al.*, 1993; McKenna, 2000). Sleep disturbance is more common in those who had poor sleep patterns before the onset of tinnitus, and management here may be different and difficult. Sedatives have a calming effect; they can relax muscles and decrease anxiety. Many of them produce drowsiness. All these effects may help with sleep problems. Therefore, in the acute phase of insomnia, hypnotics (promoting sleep) may be appropriate when prescribed by the attending physician and used for a limited time, but relaxation techniques are always to be preferred. The use of sound

---

[2] A sedative quiets nervous excitement. Often has an action on a particular area, e.g., cardiac, cerebral, respiratory, spinal. A tranquilizer promotes tranquility by calming, quieting or soothing without having sedative or depressant effects.

enrichment throughout the night, as a part of TRT, is a very effective remedy for tinnitus-related sleeplessness, without the need for other treatment.

Many tinnitus patients experience anxiety and consequently are treated by benzodiazepine tranquilizers[3] which are also frequently prescribed for sleep disturbance. There are no convincing data for their effectiveness in tinnitus treatment (Dobie, 1999; Murai *et al.*, 1992) and, moreover, benzodiazepines have several features that are of particular concern and necessitate strict medical supervision during their use. Because tinnitus is one of the side effects of benzodiazepine withdrawal (Busto *et al.*, 1986) the increase in tinnitus during the withdrawal process tends to cause patients to panic and return to the original dose. Second, benzodiazepines create a physiological dependence (Busto, 1999; de Las *et al.*, 2000; Juergens, 1991; Lader, 1994 1999; Longo & Johnson, 2000; Thormodsen *et al.*, 1999), making it difficult and painful to withdraw from their use. The third problem is benzodiazepine-induced changes in personality, which are sometimes quite profound. Finally, as they decrease brain plasticity and the ability to learn (Beckers *et al.*, 2001a; Butefisch *et al.*, 2000; Kilic *et al.*, 1999; Rush *et al.*, 1994; Thiel *et al.*, 2001; Verwey *et al.*, 2000; Vidailhet *et al.*, 1999; Ziemann *et al.*, 1998, 2001, 1998), they hinder the process of TRT, which involves learning and the plastic reorganization of the connections between the auditory and the limbic and autonomic nervous systems, as well as within the auditory system. While benzodiazepines are not indicated for prolonged use for any reason, in practice many patients take them for years, and some become highly addicted to them.

Diazepam (Valium) has stood the test of time for short term treatment of anxiety and sleep problems.

The earliest member of the benzodiazepines, diazepam (Dizac, Valium) has stood the test of time for treating anxiety and sleep problems. Dependency is less of a problem than for other benzodiazepines, so it may be used on a short-term basis for drug-based anxiety management. Although it has been frequently prescribed for patients exhibiting tinnitus distress, there is no evidence that it gives significant relief from tinnitus (Kay, 1981; Longridge, 1979).

Powerful addiction to lorazepam (Ativan, Alzapam) is frequently encountered.

Lorazepam (Ativan, Alzapam) was a popular benzodiazepine in the 1970s, used for a wide variety of psychological problems. While still frequently prescribed, there are no data showing its effectiveness for tinnitus suppression. Powerful addiction is frequently encountered, with profound withdrawal symptoms that have been described by patients as equal to that of withdrawing from heroin.

---

[3] A group of chemical compounds with a common molecular structure and similar pharmacological effects, used as antianxiety agents, muscle relaxants, sedatives and hypnotics. They can give rise to dependency and addiction. Tinnitus and hyperacusis frequently emerge during withdrawal from these drugs.

Clonazepam (Klonopin, Rivotril), used in the treatment of epilepsy, is frequently prescribed for tinnitus even though it has been shown to be ineffective (Murai *et al.*, 1992).

Any use of alprazolam for tinnitus must take account of the problem of strong dependency, which has been well documented following even short-term treatment. In addition its withdrawal frequently causes the emergence or re-emergence of tinnitus, or exacerbation of pre-existing tinnitus.

Alprazolam is a very powerful benzodiazepine and has been advocated for the treatment of tinnitus. A double-blind trial indicated that it was effective in reducing tinnitus loudness (Johnson *et al.*, 1993), but in this study improvement in tinnitus severity and impact on life was not evaluated. The inevitable presence of side effects accompanying alprazolam in the doses used makes it likely that this study was in reality an open trial (Huynh & Fields, 1995). The problem of dependency, even following medium term treatment with alprazolam has been well documented (Busto, 1999; de Las *et al.*, 2000; Juergens 1991; Lader, 1994, 1999; Longo & Johnson, 2000; Thormodsen *et al.*, 1999). In no case should treatment last longer than three to four weeks; withdrawal will frequently result in the re-emergence of tinnitus (Busto *et al.*, 1986).

We have seen many patients in our tinnitus clinics who have experienced extreme difficulties during alprazolam withdrawal, including exacerbation of their tinnitus. In many cases, the enhancement of tinnitus during withdrawal pushes the patient into ever-increasing doses of the drug, without a positive effect on tinnitus. Even for anxiety alprazolam is not recommended for longer than four months because of its addictive nature and possibility of inducing personality change. Even if it was effective for tinnitus, the drug would need to be taken continuously to provide continuous relief, a trial period would be to no purpose. All of these negative characteristics are sufficient to oppose strongly its use for tinnitus.

Alprazolam, and other benzodiazepines impair plasticity in the brain and reduce learning ability, thus counteracting TRT. We strongly oppose the use of alprazolam (xanax) for tinnitus.

However, there is another reason specific to TRT why we oppose its use for tinnitus. It has been already well documented that alprazolam, as other benzodiazepines, impairs brain plasticity and reduces or even prevents the ability to learn (Beckers *et al.*, 2001a; Butefisch *et al.*, 2000; Kilic *et al.*, 1999; Rush *et al.*, 1994; Thiel *et al.*, 2001; Verwey *et al.*, 2000; Vidailhet *et al.*, 1999; Ziemann *et al.*, 1998, 2001). As brain plasticity and learning skills are absolutely crucial for TRT, or indeed any habituation-based therapy, all benzodiazepines are counterproductive. For these additional reasons we strongly oppose its use.

The responsible social use of alcohol should not be prohibited; there is no evidence in the literature of increased alcoholism among tinnitus patients.

Ethanol (alcohol) may variously make tinnitus worse, has no effect or improves it (Pugh, Budd & Stephens, 1995). Patients who find dramatic improvement of their tinnitus from alcohol have occasionally become alcohol dependent against their wishes (but this is quite rare; five patients over 20 years (J. W. P. Hazell, personal observation)). Moreover, a systematic study did not show increased alcoholism among tinnitus patients (Stephens, Pugh & Jones, 1996). Therefore, the responsible social use of alcohol should not be prohibited.

Often patients will find that particular types of alcohol (e.g., certain wines or spirits) may produce an acute exacerbation of tinnitus, and here it is clear that substances other than alcohol in the beverages being drunk are responsible for enhancing the tinnitus.

Antidepressants

Many patients with tinnitus have coexisting or pre-existing depression. In individual cases short- to medium-term antidepressant therapy can be valuable.

Many patients with tinnitus have coexisting or pre-existing depression. They are frequently prescribed antidepressants. Tricyclic antidepressants (trimipramine (Surmontil), nortriptyline (Aventyl, Allegron), imipramine) and, fluoxitine (Prozac) are most commonly used in depressed tinnitus patients. If depression is linked to tinnitus emergence, then a proper explanation of the mechanism of tinnitus and a good understanding of the neurophysiological model of tinnitus frequently provides fast relief to the patients with mood elevation, counteracting any depressive state. We have found that the advent of TRT has dramatically reduced the need for antidepressants in our patients. In individual cases, short to medium-term antidepressant drug therapy can be valuable, but still it should only be seen as an adjunct to proper tinnitus management by TRT. In patients with clinical depression and pre-existing tinnitus emergence, careful consideration must be taken for their total needs. Good liaison with the patient's psychiatrist is essential.

There are a few studies assessing the effect of antidepressants on tinnitus. Mihail et al. (1988), after a double-blind trial of 26 patients, concluded that tricyclic antidepressants did not have a positive effect on tinnitus and that there was a large placebo effect. Nortriptyline was found to be just better than placebo in improving patients' depression and well-being, but there was no effect on tinnitus itself (Dobie et al., 1993). Interestingly, imipramine was associated with a 1% emergence of tinnitus, mostly in the second or third week of treatment, which subsequently disappeared (Tandon, Grunhaus & Greden, 1987).

Fluoxetine is a relatively new antidepressant (Stanford, 1996). Reports of exceptional improvement in long-standing depressive illness and related psychological disturbance have resulted in its widespread use for depression and a variety of psychological ailments. It has also been promoted in tinnitus treatment despite a lack of supporting data. In our experience, dependency and unacceptable side effects have made it inappropriate as a tinnitus therapy. Patients report vivid dreaming, personality changes, decrease in libido and difficulty in withdrawing from the drug. Its use is not recommended, except when prescribed by a psychiatrist for reasons other than tinnitus.

Anticonvulsants

Patients taking various anticonvulsant (antiepileptic) drugs were noticed to have an improvement in tinnitus, leading to trials of some of these drugs for tinnitus treatment (Brummett, 1995). Results from animal research have supported the possibility of epileptic-like brain activity in tinnitus, with very high frequency bursts that appear to be related to tinnitus perception (Chen & Jastreboff, 1995). Furthermore, these data also suggested that disinhibition was mediated by gamma-aminobutyric acid (GABA, an important inhibitory neurotransmitter). Recent animal data with tinnitus and hearing loss induced by sound overexposure fully supported the hypothesis that tinnitus-related neuronal activity might be in the form of bursting activity, while the general increase of spontaneous activity appeared to be related to the extent of the hearing loss (Jastreboff *et al.*, 1999b; Kwon *et al.*, 1999). Unfortunately, none of the antiepileptic drugs tested proved to be effective against tinnitus.

Many other anticonvulsants have been also tried to help tinnitus patients (e.g., barbiturates, carbamazepine (Tegretol), baclofen (Lioresal)). Phenobarbital (barbiturate) was the first such drug to become available, in the latter half of the nineteenth century, and for over 60 years was used as an antiepileptic and as a general sedative. Amylobarbital (Amytal, Sodium Amytal) (Donaldson, 1978) has been used for the treatment of tinnitus without success (anon, 1981b).

Carbamazapine has been advocated since the 1980s as a tinnitus suppressant (Emmett & Shea, 1980). It is still one of the most frequently prescribed drugs for tinnitus, in spite of the fact that in a double-blind trial its effect was the same as placebo, and it frequently has significant side effects (Donaldson, 1981; Hulshof & Vermeij, 1985). Some improvement is reported in palatal myoclonus (a somatosound) (Rahko & Hakkinen, 1979).

There is growing evidence of involvement of the GABA system in tinnitus, which drew attention to the potential use of baclofen (an agonist for type B receptors for GABA) for the treatment of tinnitus. While the effect of baclofen on the evoked potentials recorded from auditory pathways in animals has been documented

(Szczepaniak & Moller, 1996) and there are anecdotal reports of benefit in some patients, a recent double-blind study failed to reveal any difference from placebo (Westerberg, Roberson & Stach, 1996). The significant side effects, presumably associated with one of the racemic[4] forms present in the commercially available baclofen, prevented use of higher doses of the drug. Presently, this drug is being tested in an animal model to assess whether other agonists at the type B GABA receptor might be useful for tinnitus treatment.

Other antiepileptics, such as primidone (Mysoline; Shea et al., 1981), valproate (Depacon, Epilim; Mansbach & Freyens, 1983) and lamotrigine (Lamictal; Simpson et al., 1999), have been tried in open trials for therapeutic effect; none has become established in tinnitus treatment, mostly because of the unacceptable side effects and the lack of clear benefit for tinnitus.

Antiallergic, anti-inflammatory drugs

Drugs that reduce or inhibit allergic reactions or that reduce inflammation by acting on the components of the inflammation (without acting against the causative factor) have long been considered of potential use. Steroids (anti-inflammatory) are indicated as part of the treatment for sudden hearing loss, and there is a consensus that they should be administered as soon as the cochlear deafness is identified. They may sometimes be indicated in the long-term therapy of hearing loss and tinnitus caused by autoimmune disorders, where the body produces antibodies against the cochlea (Haynes et al., 1981). However, they should not be used in the absence of a proven autoimmune disorder or sudden hearing loss. If they are used for a short period of time, the side effects should be minimal. There are also studies on the injection of steroids into the middle ear (Shea & Ge, 1996; Silverstein et al., 1996), but their results are confounded by the selection of participants (mostly those with Ménière's syndrome).

Cinnarizine (Stugeron; an antihistamine (antiallergy) drug), which is used principally as a vestibular sedative in balance disorders, was indicated as having an effect on tinnitus. The manufacturer claims that the drug has an effect on central cerebral function. Open trials on tinnitus have not shown it to be effective (Gananca et al., 1988; Podoshin et al., 1991).

In rare instances where somatosounds resulting from spontaneous otoacoustic emissions in the cochlea are heard by the patient, they can sometimes be suppressed by treatment with aspirin (acetylsalicylic acid) (Penner & Coles, 1992). While the presence of spontaneous otoacoustic emissions in tinnitus patients is a common finding, in the vast majority of cases these emissions have nothing to do with

---

[4] Many chemicals exist in two sterically different forms that are mirror images of each other and can be distinguished by their ability to rotate light. The two forms often have differing drug activity as the body can distinguish between them. Commercially produced preparations often contain both: they are racemic.

their tinnitus, and patients are unable to hear them (Penner & Burns, 1987). The identification of spontaneous otoacoustic emissions as being responsible for the sound heard by the patient is complex and requires careful analysis with equipment only available in a research setting (Hazell & Sheldrake, 1992; Norton, Schmidt & Stover, 1990).

Calcium channel blockers

There are a number of calcium channel blockers[5] and several have been considered for tinnitus. Nimodipine (Nimotap), one of the dihydropyrimidine class of drugs, is an antagonist of L-type calcium channels (having slow conductive properties) and has been shown to abolish tinnitus in animals (Jastreboff & Brennan, 1988), and also in about 16% of patients when tested in an open study (Davies, Knox & Donaldson, 1994). Nimodipine differs from other dihydropyrimidines in its ability to cross the blood–brain barrier. It has been shown to affect brain blood flow, act directly on neurons in the central nervous system and affect function of OHC in the cochlea (Bobbin *et al.*, 1990; Guth *et al.*, 1992; van Benthem *et al.*, 1994). A study with the animal model of tinnitus shows that this drug affects salicylate-induced tinnitus in a dose-dependent manner (Jastreboff & Brennan, 1988, 1996; Jastreboff, Brennan & Sasaki, 1991). A study comparing nimodipine effectiveness with another drug from the same family, nifedipine (Adalat, Procardia), showed that nimodipine attenuated tinnitus by directly affecting the hair cells in the cochlea, and also brain neurons, but not by changing cerebral or cochlear blood flow (Jastreboff & Brennan, 1996). We feel that this drug has some potential for tinnitus treatment.

Flunarizine (Sibelium) was recommended originally for tinnitus on the basis of its presumed ability to enhance cerebral arterial blood flow and ability to prevent narrowing of blood vessels (vasoconstriction), which was linked to tinnitus. In a double-blind study of 50 tinnitus patients (Hulshof & Vermeij, 1986) this drug failed to show any significant results.

Other drugs

The belief that tinnitus was related principally to cochlear dysfunction lead to the use of furosemide (frusemide; Lasix), which can modify cochlear properties through its diuretic action. Additionally, it was suggested that in high, but still therapeutic, doses furosemide can modify the endolymphatic potential (Guth *et al.*, 1992; Risey, Guth & Amedee, 1996). Recent research has shown that furosemide, in doses used clinically, affects the central nervous system and has anticonvulsant

---

[5] A class of drugs that have the ability to inhibit movement of calcium ions across the cell membrane. These agents are used to treat hypertension, angina pectoris and cardiac arrhythmias; examples include nifedipine, diltiazem and verapamil. They are also known as calcium antagonists or slow channel-blocking agents.

properties (Gutschmidt *et al.*, 1999; Hochman *et al.*, 1995), but does not alter the endolymphatic potential as had been proposed initially (Guth *et al.*, 1992; Risey, *et al.*, 1996). Misconceptions regarding the level of its action in the nervous system led to a proposal that furosemide could be used as a tool for distinguishing tinnitus of "cochlear origin" from "central" tinnitus: if furosemide was effective, then tinnitus was considered to be peripheral. As furosemide in a high dose can actually cause cochlear damage and has not been shown to be effective for tinnitus (Bian & Chertoff, 2001; Freeman *et al.*, 1999), we do not recommend it.

The observation that many patients could enhance tinnitus by muscle contractions of one kind or another led to trials of the muscle relaxant Eperisone (Myonal in Japan), to help tinnitus patients (Kitano *et al.*, 1987). A study performed on 164 tinnitus patients showed that 23% of treated patients and 4% on a placebo were considered to have an 80% improvement. However, the effects described were measured immediately after drug administration and no long-term benefits were recorded (Murai *et al.*, 1992).

Glutamate, an excitatory neurotransmitter in the brain, is the most likely link in the cochlea between IHC and afferent fibers of the auditory nerve. It was suggested that dysfunctions in this system might cause tinnitus (Pujol, 1992; Pujol *et al.*, 1993). Therefore glutamic acid diethylester (Acidutex, Tinnex, Lefederivin), an antagonist of glutamate, was used for treating tinnitus (Ehrenberger & Brix, 1983; McIlwain, 1987). Except in the initial open study there was no evidence of its effectiveness. Caroverine (competing with glutamate for one of its receptors (the AMPA[6] receptor) and, at higher doses, blocking a different glutamate receptor (the NMDA[7]) receptor), was also reported to be effective (Denk *et al.*, 1997; Oestreicher *et al.*, 1999). Any medication acting on glutamate should be considered with great care, since glutamate is the major excitatory neurotransmitter in the brain, and its manipulation might cause profound side effects.

Ginkgo biloba directly influences brain function, decreases stress level, and increases memory and test solving abilities.

Ginkgo biloba (EGb 761, Ginkgold, Tanakan), an extract from the Japanese maidenhair tree, has been widely promoted for the treatment of tinnitus. It contains a number of active components that are claimed to promote blood flow in the brain, thereby directly influencing brain function and, through this action, improving tinnitus. The specific extract of this tree is produced under license from the French and German governments (labeled EGb 761) and is sold as Tanakan (Europe) or Ginkgold (USA). It was variously shown to decrease spontaneous activity in several areas of the brain (Duverger, DeFeudis & Drieu, 1995; Lamour *et al.*, 1992),

---

[6] Alpha-amino-3-hydroxy-5-methyl-4-isoxazole propionate.   [7] *N*-Methyl-D-aspartate.

decrease stress levels and increase memory and test-solving abilities in both animals and humans (Bolanos-Jimenez et al., 1995; Rapin et al., 1994; Rodriguez de Turco, Droy-Lefaix & Bazan, 1993). Furthermore, it was shown to be more effective in old animals and elderly people (Barkats et al., 1994; Deberdt, 1994; Huguet, Drieu & Piriou, 1994). Specific experiments on tinnitus have shown attenuation of salicylate-induced tinnitus in animals in a dose-dependent manner (Jastreboff et al., 1997; Shengtai et al., 1996). However, control trials in humans have been controversial (Coles, 1988; Hoffmann et al., 1994; Holgers, Axelsson & Pringle, 1994; Meyer, 1986), and a recent double-blind study failed to reveal any action of the drug on tinnitus (Drew & Davies, 2001).

Some trials have attempted to show benefit by combining ginkgo extract with "soft laser" treatment (Plath & Olivier, 1995; von Wedel et al., 1995). The proven positive effects of Ginkgo (on stress, memory and problem-solving abilities) might indirectly be helpful to tinnitus patients. Indeed, patients who claim to benefit from ginkgo described an increased ability in coping with tinnitus and a general feeling of improved well-being, but no real change in their tinnitus.

It is important to recognize that there are a number of different extracts of ginkgo, which vary dramatically in their composition, and the above comments relate to a specific extract EGb761, which offers a uniquely stable composition because of government regulations. EGb 761 or other extracts derived from the Japanese maidenhair tree may play a role in a combined therapy in the future.

Dietary supplements

It has been suggested that zinc levels below normal range could be a cause of hearing loss and tinnitus (Gersdorff et al., 1987a; Shambaugh, 1986, 1989). We have measured zinc levels in serum of patients in our London tinnitus clinic for nearly 10 years and have discovered only five patients who have abnormally low levels of zinc. In two patients, there was an associated hearing loss, which improved slightly on zinc administration. We have not identified a patient whose tinnitus was improved by zinc therapy. These negative results are supported by other published data (Gersdorff et al., 1987b; Paaske et al., 1991).

There is a general tendency to take large doses of vitamins to cure any kind of a medical problem, which ignores the fact that an adequate diet contains all the vitamins necessary for health. Additional supplements are passed through the body, at best are irrelevant and at worst can cause damage. With the absence of effective tinnitus treatment, ingestion of large doses of vitamins is commonplace, sometimes under the label of "molecular orthogonal medicine." We would like to bring particular attention to nicotinic acid (Niacin, Niacinamide), part of the vitamin B complex, which has been used for tinnitus ignoring the fact that it can be dangerous in large doses and may cause cardiovascular collapse (heart attack).

A double-blind study failed to show any beneficial effect of Niacin on tinnitus (Hulshof & Vermeij, 1987).

6.1.2 Drugs and substances that might cause tinnitus

Some patients believe that their tinnitus is made worse by various drugs and food substances.

The issue of drugs that are reported to cause or aggravate tinnitus is complicated by the formal procedure used during the approval of medicines. All side effects that have been experienced while taking a drug during clinical studies have to be reported to the appropriate national bodies, even if they might just appear accidentally and are also equally present in the control group taking a placebo. Causal reading might create the impression that these drugs are frequently inducing tinnitus while, in fact, the effect is just as strong in the placebo group. In many countries, there is a system by which physicians can report any side effect perceived to result from drug ingestion. As tinnitus is such a common symptom, almost all the drugs in the *British Pharmacopeia* have been blamed unfairly for causing tinnitus.

Many unfounded fears about drugs causing tinnitus relate to the fact that tinnitus emerges, or is aggravated, as a result of the condition that is being treated rather than the treatment itself. Increased stress levels associated with the process of illness, as well as the disturbance of normal body functions, tend to enhance tinnitus. Patients, however, tend to associate the worsening of tinnitus with the medication they are taking for their illness. If there is a concern that a drug is aggravating tinnitus, it is important to have a trial period without this substance and then to reintroduce it, while checking whether tinnitus is changing. Psychotropic drugs[8] frequently act on the limbic and autonomic nervous systems (crucially involved in the emergence of clinically significant tinnitus) and have the potential for enhancing tinnitus. This is another reason why we do not recommend these drugs to be used unless they are currently being prescribed for other conditions. The majority of complaints about drugs are about those administered for the treatment of depression and anxiety.

Considerable anxiety is experienced by patients who believe that their tinnitus may be made worse by various food substances. Many tinnitus sufferers live an almost monastic existence, abstaining from a wide range of foods and drinks that previously had contributed significantly to their life quality. They also refuse simple drug therapies that had controlled other intermittent problems, such as headache, night cramp and acute infections. Two patients of J. W. P. Hazell contracted cerebral malaria after refusing antimalarial medication, which they feared would make tinnitus worse.

---

[8] Drugs capable of affecting the mind, emotions and behavior, they are used in the treatment of some mental illnesses.

At the same time, some therapeutic agents have indeed been shown to induce or enhance tinnitus. A summary of drugs that may be inducing tinnitus, and other hearing disorders, has been prepared by Seligmann *et al.* (1996). It is interesting that the majority of drugs that have been vigorously applied in attempts to cure tinnitus are also reported as causing it. This underlines the lack of understanding of tinnitus mechanisms and the typical irrelevance of drugs that are being taken coincidently during the process of tinnitus emergence. Another confounding factor is that elderly patients are often more susceptible to drugs and require smaller doses to achieve the same therapeutic response as younger subjects. This is sometimes not recognized, and tinnitus emergence occurs with doses that would not affect younger people.

Patients should not be deterred from taking small doses of aspirin prescribed to guard against heart attack and stroke or for pain relief.

Aspirin in a high dose (several grams a day) can induce tinnitus very predictably. Some doctors in rheumatology have used the emergence of tinnitus as a way of estimating the maximal dose of aspirin to be used by a patient (Mongan *et al.*, 1973). Importantly, salicylate-induced tinnitus disappears once the dose of the drug is decreased. Patients should not avoid taking small doses of aspirin and other related analgesics nor fear to use aspirin in managing pain. There is no evidence at all that small doses are responsible for tinnitus emergence nor that chronic therapeutic dosing damages the cochlea. Many older patients with tinnitus experience arthritis and other skeletal problems, and appropriate analgesia is an important part of managing pain during the day and promoting undisturbed sleep at night. Similarly small doses of aspirin are effective in the prevention of heart attack and stroke in some patients and they should not be deterred from taking it.

Quinine sulfate (Legatrim, Nicobrevin) is not presently in use except for night cramps, which are common in older people. It is known that quinine does increase tinnitus in the short term (Jastreboff *et al.*, 1991; Roche *et al.*, 1990; McFadden, 1982), but this temporary effect on tinnitus should not stop patients from using it if it is the only solution for night cramps (Man-Son-Hing, Wells & Lau, 1998). Night cramps may well keep the patient awake at night, a time when tinnitus itself can be more troublesome; therefore, avoiding quinine might actually enhance the severity of tinnitus impact on the patient's life.

Patients often worry about taking antibiotics. This is frequently because they are aware that some antibiotics are considered ototoxic. Aminoglycosides[9] (e.g., streptomycin (Agri-Strep, Agrimycin) and gentamycin (Garamycin)) actually

---

[9] A group of bacteriocidal antibiotics that are effective against aerobic Gram-negative bacilli and *Mycobacterium* tuberculosis (causing tuberculosis).

can damage the cochlea when administered in high dose by injection. Ototoxic antibiotics are either destroyed by stomach acid or are not absorbed from the gut and, therefore, must be given by injection to be effective. Antibiotics given by mouth, such as penicillin, generally will not harm the ear or cause tinnitus.

Many of the powerful drugs used in cancer therapy, particularly cisplatin (Platinol) (Moroso & Blair, 1983), can cause cochlear damage and contribute to tinnitus emergence (Alberts & Noel, 1995; Anderson *et al.*, 1988; Kopelman *et al.*, 1988). Tinnitus of this kind is fully amenable to TRT and often improves after cancer therapy, when health improves. All patients undergoing chemotherapy are exposed to high stress levels and anxiety about the disease being treated; they also often have concerns regarding potential side effects of the drugs used. This usually plays a part in the mechanism of tinnitus distress.

Some patients blame the onset of their tinnitus on taking marijuana, cocaine and other prohibited substances. There is no evidence that these drugs are responsible for tinnitus, and such experiences are probably coincidental. They may, however, be associated with metabolic changes induced by these drugs or resulting from their sudden withdrawal, where dependency has developed. In many individuals, there are complex guilt feelings associated with drug taking, which can enhance tinnitus once it has emerged.

Much distress is caused by withdrawing coffee and tea in the mistaken belief that this will help the tinnitus. There are no data linking tinnitus and caffeine in a systematic manner.

In our experience, much distress is also caused by withdrawing coffee and tea in the mistaken belief that this will help the tinnitus. These pleasant beverages are so much a part of cultural tradition that their exclusion from the diet almost always results in a reduction in life quality, with no benefits to the tinnitus. In those patients particularly sensitive to caffeine, a simple personal trial of exclusion will tell whether or not caffeine is causing a problem. There are no data linking tinnitus and caffeine with tinnitus in a systematic manner.

6.1.3   Summary for applicability of medications

Drugs should be considered only if indicated by conditions other than tinnitus.

Presently, there is no evidence that any drug is effective in treating tinnitus, without profound side effects. We believe that medications should be considered only if indicated by conditions other than the tinnitus, and on a temporary basis for a small group of patients who experience very high level of distress. Even then, psychological approaches are preferred. Benzodiazepines particularly should be avoided because of their profound negative side effects, including decrease of the brain plasticity, which is necessary for TRT. Dietary modifications are discouraged, as there are no clear data showing that diet can reduce or improve tinnitus.

6.2   Surgical approaches for neurotological problems

There is no surgical solution for patients with tinnitus.

In the search for a cure for tinnitus, it is not surprising to find that many hopes have been attached to a surgical solution. This frequently indicates the desperation of tinnitus sufferers and their surgically orientated medical advisers, some of whom are still suggesting destructive surgery as a way of "getting rid of tinnitus." Such an approach is based on an assumption that tinnitus is contained within the cochlea. The knowledge that potential mechanisms of tinnitus are not confined to the cochlea has changed the philosophy of surgical practice when tinnitus is a presenting symptom. In consequence, a strong attempt should be made to preserve cochlear and auditory nerve function, even when speech discrimination is poor. An increase of auditory input by appropriate enrichment of environmental sounds, amplified by hearing aids when needed or provided by sound generators, can be a powerful tool in helping with tinnitus. We argue very strongly against destructive surgery in terms of labyrinthectomy or acoustic nerve section, unless necessitated by medical conditions.

Unfortunately, the presence of distressing tinnitus is used by some authorities as a contraindication to rehabilitative surgery (e.g., myringoplasty (repair of damaged tympanic membrane), stapedectomy or cochlear implantation for total deafness). Our strategy is that anything that will improve peripheral input to the auditory system has a good chance of reducing tinnitus perception and its annoyance.

Only a small percentage of patients presenting at our tinnitus clinics have identifiable surgical pathology that is amenable to specific forms of treatment, either medical or surgical. This partly reflects the fact that many of these patients are referred from specialists who would have already identified such pathology and treated it.

Tinnitus can change following surgery to correct specific pathologies, for example perilymphatic fistula, otosclerosis or Ménière's syndrome.

Tinnitus can change or can be induced by procedures performed to correct a specific pathology (e.g., perilymphatic fistula, otosclerosis, Ménière's syndrome). It is very important to counsel patients *before* operation that tinnitus may temporally increase or emerge just after surgery as a consequence of blocking of the ear canal and middle ear with blood clot and/or a surgical dressing. Failure to do this may cause serious alarm that temporary postoperative tinnitus, which is common, is an indicator that something has gone wrong with the procedure. As a result of this anxiety, tinnitus may increase and become persistent.

6.2.1   Ablative surgery to eradicate tinnitus

The persistent requests from a patient deeply distressed by tinnitus to have the "offending ear" removed by ablative surgery are occasionally heeded by the equally desperate surgeon who does not have a solution for the patient's tinnitus. Destroying the ear in an attempt to eradicate tinnitus, or cutting the auditory nerve, is a naive approach that frequently fails and is based on lack of knowledge of the mechanisms of the neurophysiological processes involved in tinnitus. In fact, clinical data show that cutting the auditory nerve induces tinnitus in 50% of patients who previously did not experience it (Berliner *et al.*, 1992). As can be predicted from the neurophysiological model, patients with the highest level of distress, most likely to seek this extreme treatment, are those least likely to benefit from altering a peripheral component of tinnitus. It is possible to expect that in these patients there are the strongest connections between the auditory system and the limbic and autonomic nervous systems, and thus the relative importance of the peripheral signal is much smaller than in other tinnitus patients.

Research indicates that the tinnitus-related neuronal activity may emerge as a modification of the spontaneous activity in auditory neurons in the brainstem and may be related to decreased activity coming from the cochlea, more specifically from dysfunctional OHC and imbalance of activity arising from stimulation of IHC and OHC (Chen & Jastreboff, 1995; Jastreboff & Sasaki, 1986; Kaltenbach, 2000; Kaltenbach & Afman, 2000). Moreover, this activity undergoes further enhancement in the auditory pathways and their connections with the limbic and autonomic nervous systems (Jastreboff, 1995). Therefore, section of the auditory nerve or destruction of the cochlea, which are peripheral to the brainstem, would not be expected to have any positive effect on tinnitus and could even make it worse (Jastreboff, 1990, 1995). From this perspective, it seems highly inappropriate to use ablative surgery for treating tinnitus, even if the precise anatomical localization of the centers involved in the processing of tinnitus could be identified. Nevertheless, some authorities still strongly promote this kind of surgical treatment (Pulec, 1995).

Even in profound hearing loss and the absence of cochlear hair cells, there is a random pattern of resting discharge potentials that represents the "code for silence" (Moller, 1984). This activity is blocked by subcortical filters and, therefore, no sound is perceived. Sectioning of the auditory nerve results in scarring and sometimes in the growth of an electrically active "stump neuroma," a benign swelling on the end of the cut nerve. This can lead to increased auditory nerve discharge, together with a synchrony of firing in various auditory nerve fibers: a phenomenon which in the normal auditory system results in the perception of a sound. It is interesting that in a somewhat analogous situation where a patient is suffering from severe pain, the concept of cutting the peripheral nerve has been almost totally abandoned because of the typical lack of improvement and the frequent establishment of phantom pain after the surgical procedure (Melzack, 1992).

In the literature, there are a limited number of reports of auditory nerve section for tinnitus alone. Fisch (1970) reported that one of four patients had a positive response with respect to tinnitus. Most data on ablative surgery come from studies of the treatment of Ménière's syndrome or vestibular schwannoma (Baguley, Moffat & Hardy, 1992; Harcourt et al., 1997; Silverstein, Haberkamp & Smouha, 1986; van Leeuwen et al., 1996). In Ménière's syndrome, labyrinthectomy or vestibular nerve section often result in a rapid recovery from incapacitating vertigo, but tinnitus is typically unchanged. The elevation of a mood state may result in a dramatic improvement in general stress level, and through this mechanism alleviate tinnitus in some patients.

6.2.2 Vestibular schwannoma

Vestibular schwannoma (frequently called acoustic neuroma) is a benign swelling on the vestibular nerve, which may compress the auditory nerve and interfere with the blood supply to the cochlea. Tinnitus is the first symptom in 11% and is present in 85% of patients with vestibular schwannoma (House & Brackmann, 1981). Nevertheless, in vestibular schwannoma it is relatively uncommon for tinnitus to be particularly severe or annoying. Enormous resources are poured into vestibular schwannoma diagnosis and although current techniques using magnetic resonance imaging (MRI) with gadolinium contrast or "fast spin" are highly specific and sensitive, only an extremely small percentage of patients with clinically significant tinnitus actually have schwannomas (Baguley et al., 1997; Moffat et al., 1998). Patients with schwannoma who also have tinnitus may be diagnosed relatively early. Nevertheless, diagnostic procedures have to be undertaken very carefully for a number of reasons. Drawing a patient's attention to the fact that their tinnitus could be related to a brain tumor can greatly enhance the severity of the tinnitus. In addition, patients with hyperacusis who may also have anxiety or phobic states can find the experience of undergoing MRI quite devastating, both in terms of the high sound levels produced by the scanner and by having movement severely restricted for a period inside a small metal tube. Many tinnitus sufferers are claustrophobic. It is crucial to give patients waiting for MRI appropriate counseling so that the experience does not exacerbate their tinnitus. It is helpful to suggest that the MRI is looking at the anatomy of the auditory nerve and organ of hearing rather than mentioning the need to exclude a brain tumor, unless the patient specifically asks. Make sure that the patient understands exactly what the experience will entail, and that he or she is provided with well-fitting ear-plugs for attenuating the sound levels experienced inside the scanner.

Prevalence of tinnitus preoperatively is approximately 70% in those undergoing surgery for vestibular schwannoma. Postoperatively, approximately 30% improve, 7% worsen and 40% develop new tinnitus.

Reports from patients undergoing surgery for vestibular schwannoma, which frequently involves auditory nerve section or destruction of the inner ear, show basically similar results: prevalence of tinnitus preoperatively was around 70%, improvement was noted in approximately 30%, tinnitus worsened in approximately 7% and new tinnitus developed postoperatively in 40% (Andersson *et al.*, 1997; Catalano & Post, 1996; Harcourt *et al.*, 1997; House & Brackmann, 1981; Levo *et al.*, 2000; Matthies & Samii, 1997; Rigby *et al.*, 1997; Wiegand, Ojemann & Fickel, 1996).

Two large studies of 1579 cases (Acoustic Neuroma Registry (Wiegand *et al.*, 1996)) and from 1000 sequential patients (Matthies & Samii, 1997) showed similar findings: 55% of patients reported tinnitus before operation; 31% were unchanged postoperatively; 24%, improved; and 7% became worse (Wiegand *et al.*, 1996). Interestingly, tinnitus was more prevalent in hearing (51%) than in deaf patients (21%), and it persisted in 46% after operation (Matthies & Samii, 1997). Andersson *et al.* (1997) reported that out of 141 patients, 70% had tinnitus before and 60% after surgery. The severity of tinnitus did not change as the result of operation. In this group, there was a 35% risk for developing tinnitus when no preoperative tinnitus was present, and a 15% chance that tinnitus would disappear when presenting preoperatively. Similar data were reported by Levo *et al.* (2000) with 39.8% risk for developing tinnitus.

Preservation of hearing may be an important factor for tinnitus. In one study of surgery for vestibular schwannoma, where hearing was not preserved, tinnitus remained in 62% and new tinnitus started in 33%; if hearing was preserved, tinnitus remained in only 40% and no tinnitus-free patients developed it postoperatively.

Preservation of hearing may be an important factor for tinnitus. Catalano and Post (1996) studied a sample of 51 patients. In 25 patients in whom hearing was not preserved, tinnitus remained in 62% (8 out of 13), and new tinnitus appeared in 33% (4 out of 12) of those who did not have it before surgery. Results were quite different in patients in whom hearing was preserved (26). Tinnitus remained in 40% (4 out of 10), and none of the remaining 16 patients who did not have tinnitus before operation developed tinnitus postoperatively. Harcourt *et al.* (1997) reported that 75% of 161 patients had tinnitus preoperatively. After operation, tinnitus was absent in 45%, lessened in 17%, was unchanged in 30% and worsened in 8%.

Predictions from the neurophysiological model of the negative effects of consistently decreased auditory input were supported by data from vestibular schwannoma surgery. Therefore, the emphasis should be on preserving and improving hearing, wherever possible, in any type of otological surgery. In our clinics, this has led to the promotion of operations that are conservative with respect to preserving hearing, such as endolymphatic sac surgery and vestibular nerve section in Ménière's syndrome rather than labyrinthectomy, although the last procedure may be simpler to perform. The preservation of residual hearing, even in the absence of speech discrimination, may be desirable so that the sound therapy part of TRT, in the form of a sound generator or amplification of background sound by hearing aids, can increase peripheral input, reduce central auditory gain and consequently help to reduce tinnitus distress.

6.2.3   Tympanic membrane perforation

Tympanic membrane perforations are frequently encountered in everyday otological practice. It is usually necessary or desirable to close the perforation (myringoplasty) in order to improve conductive hearing loss and avoid infection. In the majority of patients where the perforation is successfully closed, a simultaneous improvement in preoperative tinnitus is observed. It is unusual for tinnitus to worsen, unless there are complications of surgery.

A useful preoperative technique that is a routine in our London tinnitus clinic is to perform a "patch" test prior to decisions about myringoplasty. Place a small piece of thin paper soaked in an appropriate topical ear preparation over the hole in the eardrum and repeat the pure tone audiogram and tinnitus evaluation. The most important part of this procedure is to obtain the patient's subjective impression of what has happened to the tinnitus and the hearing. The patch may be left in place for the patient to go home (it generally falls off after two or three days) so that the patient can make an assessment of what the tinnitus is like in a natural environment. The outcome of the patch test influences strongly the decisions about surgery. Even if there is no improvement in tinnitus, an ear in which there has been recurrent discharge should be grafted so that it becomes practical to fit appropriate hearing aids or sound generators and thus facilitate TRT when needed.

6.2.4   Perilymphatic fistula

Leakage of perilymph from the oval or round window can result in sensory hearing loss, tinnitus and vertigo or unsteadiness. In some cases, it may be difficult to distinguish the symptoms from those of Ménière's syndrome. Diagnosis of fistula is difficult even on careful examination of the middle ear during surgery. In the absence of a definitive test, the diagnosis has frequently been doubted, to the extent that some authorities do not acknowledge its existence. Some data indicate that effective closure of a leakage of fluid from the round window results in a long-term improvement of tinnitus in about 50% of patients, while helping the hearing and removing of vestibular problems as well (Hazell, Fraser & Robinson, 1992b). It is an important diagnosis to remember, particularly following stapes surgery and after accidents involving head injury or barotrauma (e.g., diving accidents). Positional audiometry and fistula tests using a balance platform while modifying the air pressure in the ear canal, while not providing a final answer, can be helpful in making the diagnosis (Black & Homer, 1996). Any potential improvement or maintenance of hearing is helpful in improving the implementation of the sound therapy part of TRT. Additionally, stress levels are typically improved by removing vestibular symptoms, which is helpful in achieving better results with TRT.

6.2.5 Cochlear implants

Another category of surgical procedures involves the surgical placement of a cochlear implant for the treatment of total deafness. Since a number of profoundly deaf tinnitus sufferers express relief of tinnitus during electrical stimulation provided by the implant, this approach has been considered for hearing patients as well. Unfortunately, attempts to put implants into patients with tinnitus but otherwise normal hearing did not relieve their tinnitus (Berliner & Cunningham, 1987; Leone *et al.*, 1984). Therefore, it cannot be considered a "final method" when other approaches failed. There is a theoretical potential for using electrical stimulation via a cochlear implant to stimulate auditory pathways and use it as a substitute for the sound therapy part of TRT.

6.2.6 Otosclerosis

There are far too few studies of the results of otosclerosis surgery that consider the outcome with respect to tinnitus. Typically, the surgeon is focused solely on closing the air–bone gap and restoring hearing. Preoperative complaints about tinnitus being the most severe symptom are often disregarded. Although otosclerosis surgery is successful in good hands in over 95% of patients (Gukovich, Avramenko & Moroz, 1974; Shea, 1981), it is such a common procedure that it is not difficult to encounter patients who have had failed surgery, resulting in damage to the cochlea. Many of these patients, in addition to profound deafness, have very severe tinnitus.

However, some patients with severe tinnitus and otosclerosis, perhaps with a degree of sensorineural hearing loss, have been refused surgery because of the surgeon's fears of worsening the tinnitus. Tinnitus should not be an automatic indication for refusing patients stapedectomy or stapedotomy (Causse *et al.*, 1985). Such patients can benefit from an improvement in their hearing, which could facilitate the effective use of hearing aids and restore some degree of auditory input.

Improved hearing, with or without appropriate aiding, is an important part of tinnitus management as a whole, facilitating the implementation of sound therapy.

6.2.7 Ménière's syndrome

Ménière's syndrome is a condition affecting the whole labyrinth. The symptoms comprise fluctuating low-frequency hearing loss, tinnitus (typically low frequency, roaring) and prolonged attacks of vertigo, often with nausea (Beasley & Jones, 1996; Knox & McPherson, 1997; Marchbanks, 1997; Merchant, Rauch & Nadol, 1995; Schuknecht, 1981; Watanabe et al., 1997). It is commonly believed that this syndrome results from raised pressure in the endolymphatic space, sometimes to the point where rupture of the cochlear membranes occurs; consequently, it is often referred to as endolymphatic hydrops. However, human data strongly suggest that Ménière's syndrome may occur without hydrops, and vice versa. This observation argues against the indiscriminate use of methods aimed at decreasing endolymph pressure (diuretics, surgery) to alleviate tinnitus. Furthermore, it is likely that a mild increase of endolymphatic pressure might result in fluctuating hearing loss, or vertigo, alone and some other conditions might cause identical symptoms (e.g., perilymphatic fistula). Consequently, Ménière's syndrome is one of the most frequently misdiagnosed conditions, leading to inappropriate treatment. In fact it is rare, with estimated prevalence from 10 to 150 per 100 000 (Johnson & Lalwani, 2003).

Tinnitus associated with Ménière's syndrome can sometimes be helped by the medical or surgical cochlear-orientated approaches used in Ménière's treatment. A combination of medical and surgical treatments produces an improvement in Ménière's syndrome-related tinnitus in roughly half of the patients (Bertran & Alvarez, 1999; Fucci, Sataloff & Myers, 1994; Moffat, 1997; Hazell & Ryan, 1995; Soderman et al., 2001; Tewary, Riley & Kerr, 1998; Thomsen et al., 1998). It is important not to presume that these approaches will have any effect in non-Ménière related tinnitus, which accounts for the vast majority of tinnitus.

In the early stages of Ménière's syndrome, the triad of symptoms – tinnitus, low-frequency hearing loss and vertigo – often occur together, followed by complete remissions lasting for long periods. Tinnitus is typically low frequency and roaring, which corresponds to changes occurring in the low frequency, apical region of the cochlea. Quite profound changes in cochlear micromechanics occur as a result of the increase in endolymphatic pressure producing a deformity of both Reisner's membrane and the basilar membrane. This might result in significant changes in spontaneous activity in the auditory nerve and could produce temporary strong perceptions of tinnitus. Ménière's syndrome, together with *acute acoustic trauma*, are unique in that peripheral pathology may be the principal entity with respect to tinnitus perception. Although the tinnitus may well herald the onset of a Ménière's attack in the early stages, it usually disappears between attacks, even though there may have been some permanent damage to the cochlea. Tinnitus tends to become more continuous in those patients who have frequent vertigo attacks and there is continuous "monitoring" of the ear to identify the early symptoms of the onset of distressing vertigo.

In patients where hearing loss has become permanent, the additional "straining to hear" phenomenon will be responsible for the continued experience of tinnitus, although this symptom is generally not as troublesome as the vertigo. In the early stages of Ménière's syndrome, after treatment with drugs such as diuretics or betahistine, cochlear function may return to near normal. It must be remembered that these treatments, which may be successful in reducing tinnitus in the early stages of Ménière's syndrome, are not effective in the advanced stages. In addition, treatment that might be helpful for vertigo may be ineffective in reducing tinnitus.

The situation is complicated by the fact that any treatment that induces a remission of severe rotational vertigo will greatly reduce stress and may even reverse chronic anxiety states brought about by the complete unpredictability of the episodic vertigo and vomiting. This improvement in chronic anxiety may yield an improvement in tinnitus. It is important not to promote treatments used for Ménière's syndrome, including endolymphatic sac surgery, as a treatment for tinnitus alone.

6.2.8   Auditory nerve compression

Arterial loops in the internal auditory canal have been suggested as being responsible for vertigo, hearing loss and tinnitus in certain patients (Jannetta, 1980). The diagnosis was only made possible with the development of computer tomographic (CT) angiography and may now be more simply made with MRI angiography. The treatment, called microvascular decompression, involves exposing the nerve, moving the arterial loop slightly aside and placing a small piece of teflon sponge to prevent future contact of artery and the nerve. Although this approach was first used to help vertigo, it was later proposed as a treatment for tinnitus (Jannetta 1980, 1987). Initial reports of good results have not been repeatable. There is a risk of interfering with blood flow to the cochlea, and patients have occasionally suffered total loss of hearing and facial paralysis following this procedure. Intra-operative nerve monitoring is strongly recommended by the pioneers of this technique to decrease the possibility of auditory, vestibular or facial nerve damage (Moller et al., 1992a). Vascular loops might be responsible for an extremely small number of patients experiencing clinically significant tinnitus. Just the coexistence of vascular loops and tinnitus does not prove their causal linking, as the prevalence of asymptomatic vascular loops in the internal auditory canals of the general population is probably quite significant.

6.2.9 Somatosounds

Historically, somatosounds were classified as "objective tinnitus." We define them as the perception of sound generated within the body by vibratory rather than neural activity. Even though we consider somatosounds to be a separate entity from tinnitus, many still consider them part of tinnitus. While TRT is effective for somatosounds, it is important to discuss briefly their etiologies and specific treatments.

Several categories of somatosounds have been identified, based on their etiology. The general group of pulsatile somatosounds relate to vascular lesions, congenital arterial alteration, congenital venous anomalies, acquired venous anomalies, some neoplasms, benign intracranial hypertension, great vessel bruits and high cardiac output. The non-pulsatile somatosounds include palatal myoclonus, temporomandibular joint dysfunction (TMD, a common cause of ear pain in adults), tensor tympani muscle spasm and spontaneous otoacoustic emission. Detailed description of their diagnosis and treatment is presented in many papers, e.g. Hazell, 1989; Jastreboff et al., 1998; Perry & Gantz, 2000.

The prevalence of clinically significant somatosounds is low; surgical treatments are only rarely appropriate and frequently carry a high morbidity. This is particularly true with vascular somatosounds involving major arteries or veins. It is important, however, to diagnose properly and treat conditions requiring surgical or medical attention (such as neoplasm), where somatosound is a side effect. As TRT works on the reaction induced by perception of any sound, regardless of whether it is external, internal or phantom, it is highly effective for somatosounds as well. In our experience, very few cases of true somatosound, not indicative of other serious pathology, ended in a surgical procedure, simply because of the sound being perceived.

6.2.10 Summary of surgical approaches

Surgical procedures should be considered only if indicated by conditions other than tinnitus.

At present, there is no evidence that any surgical procedure is effective in treating tinnitus when tinnitus is the only problem. We believe that surgical procedures should be considered only if indicated by conditions other than tinnitus.

6.3 Treatment of medical conditions associated with tinnitus and hyperacusis

Tinnitus, hyperacusis and somatosounds frequently occur in association with other disorders outside the auditory system. These conditions need to be diagnosed and treated independently of tinnitus. In most instances, they are associated with specific symptoms which helps in differential diagnosis. While tinnitus might emerge in association with these conditions, treatment of the condition does not necessarily result in significant improvement of tinnitus.

Impaired articulation of the joint of the jaw (TMD) is a frequent condition, nearly as common as tinnitus itself. As facial pain, earache, tinnitus and other aural symptoms frequently coexist, a causal connection between TMD and tinnitus has been postulated (Costen, 1937; Kempf, Roller & Muhlbradt, 1993; Rubinstein, Axelsson & Carlsson, 1990; Rubinstein & Erlandsson, 1991a, 1991b).

The relationship between TMD and tinnitus is confounded by the fact that TMD occurs commonly in patients with underlying anxiety and stress, which are also common in tinnitus patients. Even though there is no proven direct physiological relation between tinnitus and TMD and the studies published so far have been inadequately controlled (Erlandsson, Rubinstein & Carlsson, 1991), these two phenomena frequently coexist and so treatment of TMD has been recommended for tinnitus itself. The techniques used in TMD clinics relieve pain caused by tension in the powerful muscles attached to the jaw joint, reducing discomfort and also the stress caused by it; this indirectly decreases the impact caused by tinnitus. Conversely, the neurophysiological model would suggest that the extended periods of increased autonomic tone associated with tinnitus distress might result in increased tension in jaw joint and neck musculature, with resultant spasm and pain in these muscle groups.

The auditory pathways receive input from the somatosensory system (Itoh *et al.*, 1987). Many patients after vestibular schwannoma surgery exhibit gaze-related tinnitus, or tinnitus evoked by stimulating a narrow band of skin on the hand (Cacace *et al.*, 1994; Hazell, 1990b). In some patients there is temporary enhancement or suppression of tinnitus during facial manipulation (Levine, 1999) or electrical stimulation of the median nerve (Moller, Moller & Yokota, 1992b). This evidence may help to explain the confusion regarding TMD and tinnitus. Modification of tinnitus by somatosensory stimulation was associated with TMD without assessing if such a link existed. At present, the somatosensory input relating to changes in tinnitus remains of research interest only, and in counseling patients during TRT.

Many tinnitus patients complain about fullness in the ear, and a variety of sensations, including pain, related to the ears. This frequently can be linked to tensor tympani syndrome, which is probably facilitated by increased general and ear-oriented anxiety (Klochoff, 1979). These problems disappear when sufficient improvement, including decrease of anxiety, is observed as a result of the treatment.

It is extremely common to experience increased tinnitus on waking (waking tinnitus) either in the morning or after a "catnap". All the sensory systems, including hearing, are put on alert at the moment of waking, and neuronal activity is greatly increased in the brain. The environment may be quite silent at these times, so it is not surprising that tinnitus is instantly noticed and may be especially intrusive. A very small group of patients has been shown to have increased tinnitus because of low blood sugar on waking (R. Coles personal communication). A simple trial of dextrose (e.g., a proprietary energy drink) can identify if tinnitus is in this category. If blood sugar is low on waking, it is likely that there are other health problems too, and medical advice should be sought. Some diabetics experience fluctuating tinnitus if their diabetes is not well controlled. Low blood sugar seems to increase tinnitus; however, there is no good evidence that diabetes is itself responsible for persistent hearing loss or persistent tinnitus.

Some patients experience tinnitus during migraine attacks. Others, who have in the past suffered from migraine or who experience classical migraine symptoms at other times, may find that proper treatment and prophylaxis will improve their tinnitus.

There is no agreement as to whether hypertension itself is a causative factor in tinnitus emergence or persistence. Increased blood pressure is very common, particularly in older people, who are also more likely to experience tinnitus. Our belief is that these two conditions commonly coexist. Occasionally, tinnitus will improve following control of blood pressure, but in most cases it is unrelated either to the condition or to its treatment. The neurophysiological model of tinnitus indicates that there is frequently a chronic elevation of autonomic activity, which is itself one of the underlying predisposing causes of hypertension.

Thyroid dysfunctions may be associated with hearing loss. Both high and low thyroid functions may result in tinnitus (clinical observation; Elliott, 2000).

Syphilis is a relatively rare condition nowadays, but nevertheless it can produce cochlear damage as well as, in later stages, damage to the central nervous system. Severe cases of tinnitus, usually associated with profound hearing loss, are seen sometimes in congenital syphilis. Appropriate treatment by a specialist in these diseases might improve the situation in the early stages with respect to tinnitus, and this should always be sought.

Occasionally, anemia is responsible for pulsatile somatosounds from increased blood flow. Severe anemia may also result in poor oxygenation of parts of the brain, including the auditory system. Therapies used in anemia, such as iron and vitamin B_{12}, should be administered under appropriate medical care after proper investigation of the problem. Self-administration of supplements is not advised, as it makes subsequent accurate diagnosis of the anemia more difficult.

Much less attention has been paid in the literature to hyperacusis and decreased sound tolerance than to tinnitus. As with tinnitus, hyperacusis occurs alone or as part of an auditory and non-auditory syndromes (Adour & Wingerd, 1974; Fallon *et al.*, 1992; Fukaya & Nomura, 1988; Gopal *et al.*, 2000; Henkin & Daly, 1968; Jastreboff *et al.*, 1999a; Klein *et al.*, 1990; Lader 1994; McCandless & Goering,

1974; Nields *et al.*, 1999; Oen *et al.*, 1997; Vingen *et al.*, 1998; Waddell & Gronwall, 1984; Wayman *et al.*, 1990). In Bell's palsy, which is paralysis of the facial muscles caused by dysfunction of the VII cranial nerve, 29% of patients report hyperacusis. Hyperacusis was described in subjects with Ramsey Hunt syndrome, characterized by facial palsy, herpes zoster and otalgia. Some patients complain of reduced sound tolerance after stapedectomy, perilymphatic fistula and after acute acoustic trauma.

Lyme disease, caused by a tick transmitting a bacterial infection (*Borrelia burgdorferi*), is responsible for a number of neurological problems and has been reported in the USA and in Europe. In one study of Lyme disease, 48% of patients exhibited hyperacusis, and frequently tinnitus (Fallon *et al.*, 1992). These problems often improve with effective antibiotic treatment, but in some cases hyperacusis remains a problem (Nields *et al.*, 1999). These patients typically exhibit worsening of their auditory symptoms for prolonged periods of time as a result of exposure to sounds (Ch. 3, category 4). This is the reason why all category 4 patients should be tested for Lyme disease antibodies. Additionally, some patients with Lyme disease exhibit global hypersensitivity: to light, touch, smell and temperature as well as sound.

Williams syndrome is a rare medical problem. Children affected by this syndrome have characteristic facial appearance, cardiovascular abnormalities, are commonly hyperactive and have a wide variety of medical and developmental problems, which can include mental retardation. Hyperacusis occurs in 95% of children with Williams syndrome (Einfeld *et al.*, 1997; Nigam & Samuel, 1994; Van Borsel Curfs & Fryns, 1997). It is worth noting that hyperacusis was also reported in patients with head injuries, after spinal anesthesia and in children with learning disabilities and autism (Katznell & Segal, 2001; Oen *et al.*, 1997; Waddell & Gronwall, 1984).

6.4 Masking

Tinnitus masking refers to the suppression of tinnitus by external sound, thereby eliminating its perception.

Tinnitus suppression by sound, called tinnitus masking, was proposed by Jones and Knudsen in 1928 and later by Saltzman & Ersner in 1947, using early hearing aids. It was promoted in the late 1970s by Vernon as a highly successful approach to symptomatic tinnitus (Vernon & Schleuning, 1978). The idea was to cover up tinnitus by providing the patient with an external sound, thereby eliminating its perception. Much emphasis was placed on the psychoacoustical properties (the frequency and intensity) of the masking sound to find the most effective spectrum for the masker, with the concept that the masking sound should be "tuned" to the tinnitus pitch. However, when "maskers" generating narrow band noise, tuned specifically to the pitch of tinnitus, were introduced by the 3M Corporation, they were not particularly successful. This is an example of the misleading effect of using the word masking rather than suppression when applied to tinnitus. In reality, as Feldmann demonstrated, tinnitus suppression by external noise is not frequency dependent (Feldmann 1969a,b, 1971). Suppression of tinnitus can be achieved with equal ease by tones far outside the critical band of the perceived tinnitus pitch. It is also easier to achieve suppression with broadband rather than a narrow band of noise (Henry & Meikle, 2000; Kitajima, Kitahara & Kodama, 1987; Shailer, Tyler & Coles, 1981). So tuning the masker to any perceived tinnitus pitch or any particular frequency is irrelevant.

In the past, there were concerns that continuous exposure to high-level masking sounds might result in permanent cochlear damage. This possibility, although unlikely, still cannot be totally excluded. We might expect an accumulation of minor traumas caused by the sometimes quite high levels of masking sound that patients might be exposed to over the years. This problem may be particularly relevant in patients with more marked hearing loss, who would naturally require higher absolute levels of masking sound. Patients treated with the "tinnitus instrument/combination device" consisting of a noise generator and hearing aid combined, could be particularly at risk.

The masking approach reflects the belief that the tinnitus is completely localized in the cochlea. Additionally, it also attempts to relate tinnitus annoyance with the psychoacoustical parameters, such as pitch, loudness, maskability of the tinnitus, disregarding the fact that since 1985 it has been known that there was no such relationship (Hazell *et al.*, 1985b; Henry & Meikle, 2000). One obvious shortcoming of this approach is that maskers cannot be used for the patient on whom it is impossible to mask tinnitus. Unfortunately, a significant proportion of tinnitus patients, at least an estimated 50%, have tinnitus that cannot be masked at all (Mitchell, Vernon & Creedon, 1993; Vernon, Griest & Press, 1990). Furthermore, masking cannot be used by patients with hypersensitivity to sound (associated with tinnitus in about 40%) because the device exceeds loudness discomfort levels (LDLs) and may make symptoms worse.

Frequently, the high level of sound needed to suppress tinnitus interferes with the perception of speech, particularly in noise (Terry & Jones, 1986). Additionally, many patients found that the high levels of sound required to achieve suppression were just as unpleasant as their tinnitus, and they either rejected the treatment or turned the sound down below the level required for suppression (Hazell *et al.*, 1985b).

There are many factors that lead to failure of masking as a treatment for tinnitus. In addition to those already mentioned, there is a problem that once the masker is turned off, most of the patients return to their previous perception of unchanged and annoying tinnitus. Additionally, many subjects who were initially successful in suppressing their tinnitus with the use of maskers found that the external sound had to be continually increased to achieve suppression (Penner & Bilger, 1989). This phenomenon does not seem to reflect an increase of tinnitus loudness but rather habituation to the external suppressing sound. In practical terms, this means that it is difficult to keep tinnitus suppressed, since it will tend to re-emerge, creating an impression that tinnitus is getting louder. This discourages many patients from using masking since they perceive that their tinnitus is getting louder as a result of treatment.

Many patients trying masking simply did not comply with instructions to set the instrument high enough to make their tinnitus inaudible, and used lower sound levels insufficient to suppress the perception of tinnitus. In reality, they set their instruments at comfortable, frequently variable levels. Investigation revealed that in most cases the level of sound was close to the suppression level, and well above the "mixing point" (for explanation see Ch. 3 and Jastreboff *et al.* (1994)). Those patients who reported improvement using this approach have been labeled as using partial masking, a technique that later proved to be partially effective (Hazell *et al.*, 1985b). Note that in TRT the sound levels used are always aimed to be at or below this "mixing point" and always below the level creating annoyance or discomfort.

Partial masking can be partially effective.

It is worthwhile discussing some matters of terminology here. In our opinion the use of the term masking with respect to tinnitus is inappropriate and misleading. The word masking implies total covering of a sound by the other sound, and it has been used for tinnitus with this meaning for many years (Johnson, 1998; Vernon, 1977). The use of the term partial masking has a direct implication that masking, by definition, is total or not at all.

Both concepts were aimed at providing temporary relief. The feeling of control over tinnitus was helpful to some patients. Unfortunately, masking did not provide long-lasting relief and patients who were helped still had to use maskers for the rest of their life to obtain continuous relief. In patients utilizing the partial-masking approach, if the level of sound was low enough, it could facilitate the natural process of habituation and was positively received by some patients (Hazell, Sheldrake & Meerton, 1987).

From the point of view of TRT, masking of tinnitus must be seen as counter-productive, since total suppression of tinnitus by definition prevents habituation of tinnitus. Habituation requires regular exposure to the object to be habituated.

"Residual inhibition" describes a temporary disappearance of tinnitus following brief exposure to sound.

"Residual inhibition," a temporary disappearance of tinnitus following brief exposure to sound (typically 10 dB above minimum suppression level), is a derivative of the masking approach. It refers to the phenomenon of poststimulus inhibition of tinnitus, a better name. Most probably it reflects the neurophysiological rebound phenomenon; temporal change of the level of spontaneous neuronal activity after switching off an external stimulus. Controversial results have been presented regarding the percentage of tinnitus sufferers experiencing residual inhibition (Schleuning, Johnson & Vernon, 1980; Terry *et al.*, 1983). In the past, much hope was generated that it would be possible to prolong the effect of residual inhibition, and in some cases even permanently relieve tinnitus, by proper selection of the physical characteristics of the external sound. Even though the work on residual inhibition started in the late 1970s, these expectations have never been met. It has remained an interesting phenomenon benefiting the occasional patient.

The masking procedure, although still used in some centers, turned out not to be as effective as initially hoped, and the same success rate for maskers and placebo devices has been reported (Erlandsson *et al.*, 1987). Except for the results of the Oregon Center, which reported 64% effectiveness of the treatment, measured as a percentage of patients who purchased hearing aids, tinnitus maskers or tinnitus instruments (combination of hearing aid and masker in one device) (Johnson, 1998), there are no other papers supporting claims of such a high level of success.

6.5 Hearing aids

Many patients with hearing loss report relief from their tinnitus when using hearing aids.

The beneficial effects of early hearing aids in tinnitus patients were first reported by Saltzman and Ersner in 1947. This has been supported by other reports over the years (Brooks & Bulmer, 1981; Kiessling, 1980; Melin *et al.*, 1987; Miller, 1981; Stacey, 1980) and is a very common observation in hearing aid-dispensing practices. While the mechanisms of this effect were unknown, popularization of the masking techniques in the late 1970s led to the suggestion that tinnitus was masked through hearing aids by amplified external sounds. When maskers proved to be much less effective than was originally reported, attention was focused on hearing aids. Again, it was still not clear by what mechanism hearing aids might be conveying this benefit, but they were reported to produce a varying degree of relief from tinnitus in some patients.

The neurophysiological model provides an explanation and rationale for using hearing aids. The model also provides a specific recommendation for the way in which hearing aids should be used in tinnitus patients (see Ch. 3). It is interesting that in some patients tinnitus is suppressed as soon as hearing aids are put on. Although these patients obtain symptomatic relief from their hearing aids, they still complain about tinnitus when the aid is removed, for instance at night. In this group, habituation of tinnitus may be hindered since they are in the same situation as patients who are using masking; the brain cannot retrain and habituate to a stimulus that it cannot detect. It is recommended that hearing aids are deliberately removed for some time every day, enabling tinnitus to be heard while introducing TRT counselling and low, audible, levels of the background sound (sound enrichment).

Certain hearing aids with high internal noise levels have been purposefully recommended to tinnitus patients. Even without proper counseling, or the ability to control the noise level, these patients nevertheless obtained some benefit through these hearing aids, which were acting as both amplifiers and sound generators. Now, it is possible to offer these patients new combination instruments, which contain an independently controlled high-quality hearing aid together with a sound generator.

Recently, programable hearing aids that fully occluded the ear canals and were set with a high level of compression have been promoted as treatment for hyperacusis, even when there was little or no hearing loss. These hearing aids act essentially as ear-plugs, the attenuation being counterbalanced by amplification of lower sound levels. Once sound levels reach a predetermined level, the amplification is automatically decreased, and the aid starts to act as an ear-plug. This approach, by simply offering protection from the sound, does not alleviate the problem. Actually, it would further enhance the hyperacusis and promote development of misophonia. This method reflects a frequent approach to hyperacusis, in which the patient is encouraged to avoid sound by the constant use of ear-plugs and/or ear-muffs. We are against this approach; however, sudden reintroduction of sounds that are creating a strong reaction must be avoided, and a gradual transition from the use of plugs or compression hearing aids must be planned within a program of TRT desensitization.

Modern hearing aids with advanced programs to suppress background environmental noise can also enhance tinnitus, as they will decrease the contribution of low-level background sounds. These sounds are part of sound therapy, and hearing aids with such programs will decrease their impact.

6.6   Psychological treatments

Tinnitus patients reporting severe emotional difficulties, with anxiety, anger, known profound psychological problems or psychosis, as well as those who are significantly distressed, can potentially benefit from specific psychological approaches.

Many psychological treatments can be summarized as coping strategies: teaching patients how to "live with their tinnitus."

There are several centers worldwide promoting cognitive–behavioral therapies for tinnitus patients (Andersson & Lyttkens, 1999; Goebel *et al.*, 1999; Hallam & McKenna, 1999; Hallam, Rachman & Hinchcliffe, 1984; Henry & Wilson, 1999; Sweetow, 2000). These therapies include relaxation training, distraction attention techniques, cognitive reconstruction, imaginary exercises and modification of maladaptive thoughts and behavior. Many of these approaches can be summarized as coping strategies: teaching patients how to "live with their tinnitus."

According to the neurophysiological model, non-specific behavioral training is unlikely to have any permanent effect in inducing tinnitus habituation in the majority of subjects with significant tinnitus.

According to the neurophysiological model, non-specific behavioral training is unlikely to have a permanent effect in inducing tinnitus habituation in the majority of subjects. However, some patients can benefit from these treatments because of improvement in their emotional problems.

Many patients observe a close correlation between their general stress level and tinnitus. Some patients describe an increase in the actual loudness or other physical parameters of tinnitus perception with an increase in stress, while others report just an increase of tinnitus annoyance. Any procedure temporarily or permanently decreasing the degree of stress is helpful for tinnitus patients. At the same time, procedures based entirely on stress alleviation, for example biofeedback and general stress-decreasing counseling, are effective only in a small percentage of patients, the effects are temporary and they are not significantly different from the general placebo effect.

Treatment of tinnitus, aimed at reducing anxiety and tension by using a variety of behavioral techniques, could provide some benefit to patients. Various studies have documented a significant increase of anxiety about disease (somatic anxiety) and depression in tinnitus clinic populations (Halford & Anderson, 1991; Jakes *et al.*, 1985; McKenna, Hallam & Hinchcliffe, 1991; Stephens & Hallam, 1985; Sullivan *et al.*, 1993). Many different techniques have been used, including relaxation training (Jakes *et al.*, 1986), biofeedback (Landis & Landis, 1992; Ogata *et al.*, 1993) and more formal psychotherapy in behavioral training (Kroner-Herwig *et al.*, 1995). In a group of patients who are inherently anxious, a reduction of anxiety will produce a non-specific benefit, with an increased feeling of well-being and a reduction in the number of anxiety and panic attacks. When the threshold for anxiety and panic is reduced by the presence of irritating and intrusive tinnitus, any lowering of activity in the emotional and autonomic centers is likely to result in a transient reduction in symptoms. Patients preoccupied by strong negative beliefs associated with tinnitus and with tendencies to pessimism and somatic anxiety might benefit from engaging in cognitive reconstruction approaches. These techniques identify, explain, interpret, discuss and challenge negative thoughts and beliefs, finally replacing them with more positive thoughts and emotions. Refocusing attention from tinnitus to other stimuli is another technique used in psychology. Some people are helped by learning to switch the focus of attention quickly from one stimulus to another, or by engaging in activities that preoccupy so tinnitus is not the main focus of attention. Distraction techniques may provide symptom relief and be helpful at times of extreme anxiety, but they are not compatible with the habituation approach used in TRT.

Relaxation techniques, aimed at improving general well-being and stress reduction, can be of some help and can be implemented without involving tinnitus at all. Progressive muscle relaxation, breathing exercises, biofeedback, yoga and meditation all reduce tension and improve quality of sleep and life. In addition, they produce physiological changes, such as decreased muscle tension, reduced heart rate, improved respiration, and modify the response to stressful situations. Overall, psychological techniques help in better self-management of distress caused by tinnitus, which, in turn, helps in coping with tinnitus in spite of its presence. Psychological approaches do not have the negative side effects associated with drug therapies and are basically harmless for patients.

## 6.7	Electrical stimulation

Transmission of information within the nervous system requires electrical impulses to travel through neurons and to other neurons. It is possible to activate a neuron as well as interfere, modulate or even block on-going spontaneous and evoked activity using an electrical current. This property of electrical stimulation is the basis of the cochlear implant: electrical stimulation of the auditory nerve for profound deafness.

Electrical stimulation offers the most powerful means of influencing neuronal activity and, in theory, of attenuating tinnitus. Practical results have yet to be achieved.

Electrical stimulation offers the most powerful means of influencing neuronal activity and, in theory, offers a possibility of attenuating tinnitus-related neuronal activity. Practical results, however, lag behind the theoretical potential.

Electrophysiological studies suggest the possibility of blocking nearly any neuronal activity by applying a constant current with proper polarization: "anodal block" (e.g., Vyklicky, Keller & Jastreboff, 1976). Such stimulation cannot be used for long periods, as it would inevitably damage the neurons and tissues through which it passed.

Most attempts at tinnitus attenuation using electrical stimulation have been empirical and not based on any specific theory.

Alternating currents tend to enhance not suppress neuronal activity. Therefore, the majority of work aimed at tinnitus attenuation with electrical stimulation has been with alternating currents, without any specific theory or phenomenology (based on symptoms), and on a trial and error basis. As it is easier to influence neuronal activity when the stimulating electrode is close to it, much work in this field has used cochlear implants. Electrical stimulation through the middle ear, stimulation of the whole head or stimulation of deep brain structure (Martin et al., 1999) yielded mixed results, which were typically worse than with stimulation through cochlear implants.

Electrical stimulation as a treatment for tinnitus is not new (for review of history see Hazell et al. (1993) and Dauman (2000)). Since the discovery of direct current by Volta in 1800, frequent attempts have been made to stimulate the ear with electricity as a proposed cure for either deafness or tinnitus. MacNaughton Jones (1891), who wrote an important treatise on ear disease, also used electrical stimulation for treating tinnitus but commented that the effects of the electricity could not be distinguished from "other therapeutic effects." He was probably the first to note the effect of counseling on the patient with tinnitus, and to identify the difficulty in separating this powerful effect from more specific treatments applied at the same time.

With direct current, anodal suppression of tinnitus was found to be most effective. This finding was reported first by Graham and Hazell (1977) and then by Aran and coworkers (Aran & Cazals, 1981; Portmann et al., 1979). Transtympanic needle electrodes passed through the eardrum, and also round window electrodes, were used to stimulate the ear. Round window stimulation was shown to be more effective than stimulating the bony wall of the promontory over the cochlea in suppressing tinnitus. Aran and coworkers used only direct current and counseled strongly against this treatment because of the likelihood of damage to the cochlea by passing a direct current through it.

The advent of cochlear implants raised the hope that it might be possible to suppress or eliminate tinnitus by electrical stimulation of the cochlea, either in a hearing or a deaf ear. The results of pioneering work from the House Ear Institute in Los Angeles, reported as early as 1976, showed that tinnitus in a profoundly deaf individual could be improved following cochlear implantation (House, 1976). This has been followed by various reports confirming the benefits of cochlear implantation for profoundly deaf tinnitus sufferers. An alternative mode of stimulation, a digitally pulsed current, was applied via an intracochlear, usually multichannel, electrode, thereby delivering a complex speech signal. On a few occasions, cochlear implants have been inserted into the ears of patients with minimal or no hearing loss in an attempt to eliminate tinnitus (Thedinger, House & Edgerton, 1985). Unfortunately, not only was it impossible to suppress the tinnitus, but some patients were actually made worse. However, the majority of deaf people receiving cochlear implants for auditory rehabilitation in a totally deaf ear obtained at least partial relief from tinnitus when the implant was used (Berliner & Cunningham, 1987; Dauman & Tyler, 1993; Dauman, Tyler & Aran, 1993; House & Brackmann, 1981; McKerrow *et al.*, 1991; Tyler & Kelsay, 1990). The question remains as to whether or not this relief was achieved by the provision of an auditory signal that suppressed tinnitus perception by an electrically induced perception of sound (similar to masking) or whether it came from direct interference with tinnitus-related neuronal activity below the level of perception.

In 1995, Hazell, McKinney & Aleksy found that 27% of 800 patients awaiting cochlea implantation had never experienced tinnitus. At the same time, 48% of patients who had troublesome tinnitus reported significant improvement following implantation (Hazell *et al.*, 1995). The benefits in tinnitus suppression correlated weakly with improved communication ability; therefore, part of the mechanism of tinnitus suppression in cochlear implantation may be the removal of the "straining to communicate" phenomenon.

Promising results were reported with the use of an implant delivering sinusoid alternating current to patients with unilateral deafness and severe tinnitus (Fraysse & Lazorthes, 1983; Hazell, Meerton & Conway, 1989; Hazell *et al.*, 1993). It was interesting that a low-frequency alternating current (below 50 Hz) was most effective in suppressing tinnitus, and the mechanism was probably not one of masking (Hazell *et al.*, 1993). Notably, some patients have been monitored for up to five years after surgery and were still obtaining tinnitus suppression from their implant.

Another approach to electrical stimulation for tinnitus is to stimulate the cochlea externally from electrodes placed on the ear canal skin or on the round window. The results to date are not optimistic for people with normal or only partially impaired hearing. However, in patients with a totally deaf ear, and using correct stimulus parameters, it was possible to achieve partial relief from tinnitus on a number of occasions (Hazell *et al.*, 1993). In 1993 the Cochlear Corporation reported the results of a multicenter trial using ear canal sinusoidal stimulation in addition to transtympanic and round window electrodes (S. Staller, 1996, personal communication). Their report agreed with Hazell *et al.* (1993a) that low-frequency sinusoid stimulation was more effective. However, the results were not sufficiently promising to justify development of electrical tinnitus suppressors on a commercial basis.

Various studies have shown that 2–5% of totally deaf subjects with tinnitus experience exacerbation of tinnitus after cochlear implantation. It is possible to improve their tinnitus using TRT so that the implant can eventually be used on an everyday basis. This has been achieved in London on selected patients.

Transcutaneous (across the skin) electrical stimulation has been used effectively in the treatment of pain and in the healing of bone fractures for many years (Candy & Pareson, 1990). There have been a number of reports on the use of electrical stimuli applied to the skin over the mastoid for tinnitus suppression, and it would appear that this approach works in some patients. However, in double-blind control trials using these techniques, there were fewer subjects with positive results in the active than in the placebo group (Dobie *et al.*, 1986; Penner & Bilger, 1989). It is interesting that in the *Scott et al.* (1994) study, there was one subject who consistently obtained tinnitus relief over a three month period whenever the active device was switched on. Thedinger, Karlsen & Schack (1987) found a true benefit in only 7% of patients. Low-intensity square waves or biphasic pulses through an ear or mastoid application have also been tried (Engelberg & Bauer, 1985).

Transcutaneous electrical nerve stimulation for somatosensory stimulation has also been tried for tinnitus relief. This is an established technique for treating musculoskeletal pain, using weak electrical currents passed through electrodes attached to the skin. The electrical current stimulates pain nerve endings and might work in a similar way to acupuncture. Several authorities have tried to use this technique in tinnitus by applying electrodes to the mastoid region. Results were negative or temporary (Giordano *et al.*, 1987; Kaada, Hognestad & Havstad, 1989; Rahko & Kotti, 1997; Scott *et al.*, 1994).

Very recent results utilizing high-frequency (4.8 kHz) stimulation via a modified cochlear implant or an electrode placed on the promontory have indicated attenuation or total blockage of tinnitus for a duration of minutes to hours in about 50% of subjects (Rubinstein *et al.*, 2003). While the success rate was similar to that reported with electrical stimulation performed with other protocols, the interesting observation was that in some patients it was possible to achieve tinnitus suppression without evoking perception of sound induced by this high-frequency stimulation. The question of efficacy and safety of this method remains open.

Electrical tinnitus suppression with implanted electrodes presently has more potential than transdermal stimulation.

Stimulation of deep brain structures has been utilized for treatment of movement disorders, Parkinson disease and chronic pain. It was discovered accidentally that it sometimes also improves tinnitus (Jeanmonod, Magnin & Morel, 1996). The results from seven subjects indicated that three of the patients, receiving deep brain stimulation for reasons other than tinnitus but happening to have tinnitus, achieved temporal attenuation of tinnitus (Martin *et al.*, 1999). While interesting, deep brain stimulation is at the moment at an early experimental stage.

6.8   Alternative therapies

A large number of alternative therapies, outside the field of conventional Western medicine, have been used to treat tinnitus. Most treatments give some patients temporary relief, which may result from the placebo effect or from temporary changes in autonomic activity.

The list of alternative therapies outside the field of conventional Western medicine is very long and reflects the strong desire of tinnitus patients to find relief following the failure of standard treatments (Podoshin *et al.*, 1991). The list includes acupuncture, homeopathy, magnetic stimulation, reflexology, craniosacral therapy and ear-candling. The few available double-blind studies show that none of these approaches is really effective for tinnitus. At the same time, nearly all of them give some patients temporary relief, which may result from the placebo effect or from changes in autonomic activity.

In the USA and Europe, the term alternative medicine refers to treatments that are not part of the "Western medical tradition." This does not infer that they are invalid or ineffective. In Eastern countries, such therapies would be considered conventional. There are, however, particular problems that arise when patients seek help from alternative medicine, which need to be pointed out.

Alternative practitioners are typically general practitioners who are seeing the same wide spectrum of medical disorders that a family physician would see. This does not allow them the opportunity to develop expertise in the management of very specific conditions, even relatively common ones like tinnitus. They may also have minimal training in the underlying basic sciences and are, therefore, unable to apply a mechanism-based approach to therapy. In many areas of alternative medicine, understanding the mechanism may be thought unnecessary, and the approach is purely phenomenological. All these factors contribute to the present situation where very few claims of success can be verified. While the majority of them could be studied by double-blind randomized evaluation, such studies have not been published; where they are available (as in the case of acupuncture) results are negative (Andersson & Lyttkens, 1996; Axelsson, Andersson & Gu, 1996; Dobie, 1999; Park, White & Ernst, 2000).

At the same time, dissatisfaction with Western medical practitioners is one of the reasons why patients turn to alternative therapies. Medical providers seem to have too little time to listen to the many complex problems and complaints tinnitus patients tend to have. The alternative practitioner usually has more time and is often a skilled counselor. The effects of counseling and the use of therapies that may produce relaxation or reduction in anxiety have already been shown to be effective in helping patients to cope with their tinnitus. It is often difficult or impossible to extract the counseling effects of alternative medicine from the effects of more specific therapies that are applied.

6.8.1   Acupuncture

Acupuncture is a part of traditional Chinese medicine that is used extensively around the world. There is no doubt of its effectiveness in treating pain (Longworth & McCarthy, 1997). Acupuncture is capable of producing local anesthesia adequate to perform major surgery in certain patients. A number of studies show varying degrees of success and failure in treating tinnitus (Andersson & Lyttkens, 1996; Gu & Axelsson, 1996; Hansen, 1975; Marks, Emery & Onisiphorou, 1984; Nilsson, Axelsson & Li De, 1992). Occasional successes are overshadowed by the much larger number of patients who have spent much time and money on acupuncture for tinnitus without receiving any long-term benefit (Gu & Axelsson, 1996). Recent double-blind studies have failed to show any benefit of acupuncture for tinnitus (Axelsson *et al.*, 1996; Dobie, 1999; Park *et al.*, 2000; Vilholm, Moller & Jorgensen, 1998).

6.8.2   Transcutaneous "black boxes"

The Therapak, a small black box with flashing lights, has been promoted for the treatment of musculoskeletal aches and pains and suggested in the treatment of tinnitus in the UK. Roland *et al.* (1993) have suggested that this device did give significant help in 45% of patients treated. Unfortunately, we have not detected a single patient obtaining long-term benefit from this treatment. The manufacturer claims that the device produces a variable low-frequency, pulsed, electromagnetic signal, rich in harmonics. Examination of the inside of the box by an electronics engineer suggested that there were no components capable of producing any type of electromagnetic radiation able to penetrate the body.

6.8.3   Homeopathy

Homeopathy is based on the concept of using agents that cause symptoms similar to the disease but in extremely low concentrations. The selection of an appropriate remedy depends on a detailed assessment of a patient's overall physical and emotional state, and it requires extensive contact with the patient. It would be relatively easy to evaluate this therapy by a double-blind trial, but so far this has not been done with tinnitus. Sporadic reports of improvement do not seem to exceed the expectations of temporary improvement as a result of non-specific counseling (Simpson, Donaldson & Davies, 1998).

6.8.4 Ultrasonic stimulation

Following chance observations that tinnitus improved following the use of ultrasound for the diagnosis of sinus disease, a trial of ultrasound applied to the ear was performed. In an initial study (Carrick et al., 1986) of 40 patients, 40% improved with ultrasound and only 7% with a dummy stimulator. A further study (Rendell et al., 1987) failed to confirm these benefits. With 40 subjects in a double-blind controlled trial, there was no difference between ultrasound and placebo and very little change in tinnitus was observed in any subject in either group. Recently, this idea was rekindled by the introduction of two new devices: one producing high-frequency sound (specifically processed music) that still is within hearing range (UltraQuiet[TM]) and the other offering real ultrasound stimulation (HiSonic[®]) in low 20 kHz range together with high-frequency sounds from the hearing range. Presently, there are no clear results regarding their effectiveness.

6.8.5 Magnetic stimulation

In 1987, Takeda reported prolonged reduction of tinnitus a few days after placing powerful magnets near to the tympanic membrane (see Coles, 1998). A subsequent double-blind trial on 50 patients did not reveal any effects (Coles et al., 1991).

6.8.6 Lasers

Several studies of laser treatment in patients and studies on temporal bones to examine the possibility of laser-activated repair mechanisms within the cochlea have shown consistently negative results (Partheniadis-Stumpf, Maurer & Mann, 1993; Shiomi et al., 1997; von Wedel et al., 1995). The controlled human study showed no improvement in tinnitus, and evaluation of the light intensity in the temporal bone study showed that the laser light did not penetrate in the intact ear (Mirz et al., 1999a; Walger et al., 1996).

6.8.7 Hyperbaric oxygen

Hyperbaric oxygen has been used for a long time as an empirical treatment for sudden sensorineural deafness, with the reasoning that increasing cochlear blood flow and concentration of oxygen in the perilymph might induce and facilitate recovery of damaged hair cells (Fattori et al., 1996; Vavrina & Muller, 1995). In Germany, it is also being used extensively for "acute sensorineural tinnitus," with similar justification. While uncontrolled trials have suggested improvement in about 60% of patients, other studies have shown it is much less effective, if at all, and there are no long-term studies. There is no evidence that the emergence of troublesome tinnitus relates to changes in cochlear blood flow, which hyperbaric oxygen therapy is supposed to improve. An attempt to evaluate effectiveness of this method to treat Ménière's syndrome showed no difference between patients receiving hyperbaric oxygen and a control group (Fattori et al., 1996).

6.8.8 Various herbal therapies

For years, a variety of herbal mixtures with attractive names implying their effectiveness for tinnitus have been introduced on the market. The recent explosion of web-based trade has made it easier to reach desperate tinnitus patients. Lack of studies supporting the claims of high effectiveness did not discourage people from buying. The problem is that these products are actually making tinnitus worse, as patients receive another confirmation that "nothing works for tinnitus" once the temporary placebo effect disappears. Furthermore, as these products are not the subject of normal governmental control, their composition is frequently unknown and it often does not match description of contents. Consequently, it is impossible to predict what potential negative interaction there might be with medications that patients may be taking for other conditions, or the effect it might have on tinnitus or decreased sound tolerance.

6.8.9 Music therapies

Music-based therapies have a long tradition in psychology and medicine (Cabrera & Lee, 2000; Good, 1996; Lipe, 2002; Watkins, 1997) and recently elements were proposed for tinnitus treatment. As with any treatment decreasing general stress levels and inducing relaxation, this therapy could be used as an adjunct to TRT but, on their own, would be predicted to have only a temporary effect by altering autonomic activity. Systematic studies are needed, however, to determine if the introduction of music may have any additional beneficial effect.

6.8.10 Reflexology, hypnosis, aromatherapy, craniosacral therapy

Reflexology, hypnosis, aromatherapy and craniosacral therapy are non-specific treatments (in terms of conventional medicine) that are widely used for the reduction of stress and stress-related conditions such as a headache, anxiety, digestive problems, etc. Having the scalp muscles or the soles of the feet massaged, or pleasant-smelling oil applied over the body, may produce significant feelings of relaxation and well-being. The treatments are typically applied by therapists without any specialist knowledge of audiology, or the neurophysiology of tinnitus, making diagnosis of these conditions a haphazard process. Tinnitus patients have sometime reported improvement, particularly in feelings of anxiety, following these therapies.

6.8.11 Alternative treatments for hyperacusis: ear protection, pink noise, auditory integration

Compared with tinnitus, the number of treatments that have been proposed for hyperacusis is limited. The most common approach is to encourage ear protection, typically by ear-plugs. In some cases, tightly fitted hearing aids set for minimal gain and with high compression are recommended. These hearing aids are acting as earplugs with sound intensity-dependent attenuation. So called "pink-noise therapy," in which patients are exposed to relatively high levels of sound but with certain frequencies removed, is also recommended. Note that the term "pink noise" is not related to acoustical pink noise, which is a noise with energy decreasing inversely with frequency. Auditory integration, which with varying degrees of success is used for autistic children (Mudford *et al.*, 2000), is used as well. So far there are no clear data supportive of any of these approaches. As presented elsewhere in the book, TRT provides a high level of success for hyperacusis, including a cure for some patients.

6.9   Conclusions

Tinnitus is a common and troublesome condition. Therefore, it is not surprising that many attempts have been made to find a cure, or at least a treatment that could reduce the symptoms. The studies presented in the literature, and outlined here, show that the proportion of patients reported to improve is close to the placebo effect, which makes claims of their effectiveness doubtful.

There are rare causes of tinnitus where medical or surgical treatment of underlying pathology can benefit the patient. However, it is always necessary to consider that many of these treatments may have significant side effects and to select an optimal approach adjusted for the individual patient.

7

General conclusions and future directions

In this book, the main points of the neurophysiological model and TRT are reviewed, stressing the importance of extra-auditory connections in the brain responsible for the clinically significant tinnitus and decreased sound tolerance. TRT has to date proved the most effective treatment for tinnitus and decreased sound tolerance; moreover it can be applied to all patients regardless of the etiology of tinnitus.

The authors are optimistic about future developments, which should increase the speed of treatment and make it more effective, particularly for some classes of patient, such as those with profound deafness. Recent advances in neuroscience, brain imaging techniques, pharmacology, genetics and cell biology hold promise for a better life for tinnitus sufferers in the future.

In this book, we have presented a neurophysiological approach to tinnitus, aimed at habituation of the tinnitus-induced reaction and its perception. The model described stresses that tinnitus perception results from compensatory activity within the auditory pathways to otherwise small and irrelevant disturbances. These originate in most cases in the periphery but undergo enhancement and create feedback mechanisms involving the limbic and autonomic nervous systems that form a vicious circle resulting in strong annoyance and distress for the patient. The level of annoyance is not related to physical characteristics of perceived tinnitus sounds – their loudness, pitch or ability to be suppressed by external sounds – but reflects negative associations related to perception of tinnitus. The approach does not aim to eliminate or attenuate the tinnitus source, but to prevent the signal from reaching the limbic and autonomic nervous systems and from activating high cortical areas involved in tinnitus awareness. Therefore, properties of the tinnitus signal, and its perception, are irrelevant in achieving habituation.

The clear implication of the neurophysiological model of tinnitus is that the initial reason for emergence of the tinnitus signal is irrelevant. Tinnitus perception might result from noise-induced cochlear damage, viral infection, drugs, ageing, etc. We are not trying to attenuate the source, which at this moment we do not believe is possible, but attempting to block this signal above the source to prevent it from activating the limbic and autonomic nervous systems, giving rise to anxiety, annoyance and so on (habituation of reactions) and also higher levels of the auditory system (habituation of perception). As the method for blocking this signal is not dependent on its specifics or characteristics, TRT is effective regardless of the source, trigger or underlying cause of emergence of the tinnitus signal.

As habituation is achievable to any kind of tinnitus or external sound, it is irrelevant if it can be "masked" (suppressed by sound) or not, or if it is loud, soft or of any particular pitch. This feature alone separates TRT from other treatments, which tend to target specific subtypes or clinical diagnoses of tinnitus and thus cannot be used on a general population of tinnitus patients. TRT does not require selection of patients. Data coming from our centers, and others around the world, show over 80% of patients have significant improvement following TRT, without any preselection of those to treat.

Another positive aspect of TRT is that treatment does not have to be continued indefinitely. Usually 12 to 18 months are sufficient for inducing, and sustaining, habituation and to achieve permanent plastic changes within the nervous system for tinnitus habituation. As a result, the patient does not require any additional treatments or procedures except for following general instructions about avoiding very loud sounds and total silence. This is in contrast to other treatments, which require continuous use to provide relief (e.g., masking). Furthermore, TRT utilizes the normal processes and features of the brain to achieve habituation and does not have side effects.

It is worth noting that TRT works at two levels: habituation of reaction to tinnitus and habituation of tinnitus perception. The time course and the extent of habituation of reaction and perception vary from patient to patient. In most cases, as a first step, we will achieve reduction of reaction to tinnitus before achieving habituation of tinnitus perception. Our data indicate the possibility of removal of tinnitus perception for periods of time, in some cases, to the extent that patients are unable to perceive their tinnitus even if they are trying to focus their attention on it. We would like to stress that this is not the aim of TRT, and that this requires a longer time. Nevertheless, this finding indicates that further improvement in TRT can be achieved beyond the stated goal of habituation of tinnitus reaction.

One of the postulates of the neurophysiological model is that enhanced gain within the auditory pathways contributes to tinnitus, predicting that a large percentage of people with tinnitus will be affected by decreased sound tolerance as well. Therefore, part of TRT is directed toward decreasing this hypersensitivity.

What is the weakness of TRT? The main problem is that time is needed to achieve sustained habituation and it, therefore, requires substantial effort by both therapist and patient. As TRT is not taught in graduate schools and it requires specific knowledge and expertise, a dedicated commitment by physician and audiologist is needed in learning new skills. There also needs to be wider availability of TRT courses.

We are the first to realize that this approach, even if it seems to be highly effective, can be further improved. We still have a small percentage of patients whom we cannot help; furthermore TRT at present may take up to 12–18 months. We believe this time can be shorten significantly, perhaps to just a few months, if, simultaneously with TRT, it was possible to attenuate even partially the tinnitus source or tinnitus-related neuronal activity in the brain.

This opens a new avenue for drug therapy and other therapies, to decrease the tinnitus signal or stress, or generally improve patients' well-being. Previously, for a drug to be of clinical interest, it would be necessary to attenuate tinnitus by at least 50% or more. If, however, we combine a drug that offers partial attenuation of tinnitus, even by 10–20%, with TRT, then treatment should be shortened significantly. Such a drug must not, of course, interfere with the habituation process itself and, particularly, should not hinder plasticity of the brain. Other methods (e.g., electrical stimulation) partially able to suppress the tinnitus signal would be equally helpful.

It is crucial to understand what are the specific characteristics differentiating TRT from all other methods. There is substantial confusion in this respect and many believe that it is essential to have special instruments or use a particular sound level (mixing point) for TRT.

We hope that in this book we have conveyed the following key points.

- The fundamental feature of TRT is specific (retraining) counseling, based on, and following the principles of the neurophysiological model of tinnitus. The model includes information and direction about the need for avoiding silence and for enrichment of the auditory background (sound therapy)
- While new skills need to be learned in the fitting of sound generators and hearing aids in patients with tinnitus and decreased sound tolerance, instruments are not always necessary, and indeed TRT may be performed without them, albeit with suboptimal results in certain cases. The specific method of sound delivery is of secondary importance.
- There is no need to set the sound at any specific level (e.g., the mixing point); a range of sound levels can be used providing that all the listed criteria are fulfilled. Similarly there are a number of rules regarding sound use that patients are taught.
- Sound used for enriching the auditory background must never evoke annoyance or discomfort of any type.
- Sound levels close to the threshold of hearing should be extended as they might induce stochastic resonance and consequently enhance the tinnitus signal.

- The sound level is set by increasing it from the threshold of hearing until one of the following conditions is met:
  - the sound induces annoyance if used for a prolonged period of time
  - the sound has reached the mixing point.

The sound is then set slightly below the level determined by these conditions.

Note that the restriction of setting the sound to below the mixing point automatically excludes the possibility of tinnitus suppression (masking) as the mixing point denotes the beginning of partial masking and is always below the level required for masking.

Another important point is the issue of a cure for tinnitus. If we are aiming to totally remove tinnitus perception, then presently there is no cure. However, as we have argued in this book, the problem for clinically significant tinnitus is not its perception, which is very common and natural, but the reactions induced by the tinnitus signal. TRT can decrease or even remove these reactions; when this happens, then there is a cure for clinically significant tinnitus. From the patients' point of view, the final effect of fully successful TRT treatment is that tinnitus disappears completely as an issue, rather than an entity or experience. In practice, it is the same as if tinnitus was gone: a cure of tinnitus.

The future for hearing restoration looks much more very exciting now. There are expectations about the possibility of regeneration of hair cells in the cochlea, and through this improvement of hearing and potentially of tinnitus. Both regeneration and the transplantation of hair cells are still very much in the early stages of research. However, findings published in June 2003 showing regeneration of hair cells and axon of neurons traveling toward these new cells in living animals (Kawamoto *et al.*, 2003) are extremely encouraging. There is the possibility that within the next decade or so a restoration of damaged hair cells might be achieved.

It appears, however, that while this might help hearing, it might actually induce tinnitus, or enhance already existing tinnitus. As argued in previous chapters, tinnitus perception might result from the compensation occurring from heterogeneous activation of outer and inner hair cells (IHC) systems; therefore, it is reasonable to expect that even when regeneration is achieved, innervation will not be restored to a perfect state and more heterogeneity will be induced. This would result in inducing new tinnitus sources or enhancing pre-existing tinnitus.

Patients with very profound deafness create a significant challenge. Although TRT counseling is very effective in this group, sound therapy is difficult or impossible to apply. Direct stimulation of the auditory pathways by electrical stimulation is needed to enhance the level of background neuronal activity normally achieved by sound therapy. As a ramification of work on electrical stimulation, it is possible to expect that some form of electrical stimulation might be applicable in patients with milder hearing loss, or even with normal hearing.

People with severe hyperacusis offer another challenge. A number of them experience prolonged increase of their tinnitus and hyperacusis as a result of exposure to any sound (category 4), and they are particularly difficult to treat. More work is needed to understand the mechanisms of hyperacusis, particularly in this subgroup, and through this to achieve better results. The same reasoning applies to tinnitus. By better understanding the mechanisms of tinnitus generation and through this devising mechanism-specific ways of attenuating the tinnitus source and the tinnitus-related neuronal activity, we should be able to achieve significant improvement in treatment. The enhancement of brain plasticity should result in facilitating habituation as well. Work using an animal model of tinnitus offers great hope in achieving this goal.

The issue of how tinnitus-related neuronal activity is processed within the nervous system is basically still open. There are only a few papers on this issue, and work has just started to find out which neurotransmitters and neuronal systems are involved (Andersson *et al.*, 2000; Chen & Jastreboff, 1995; Jastreboff & Sasaki, 1986; Marriage & Barnes, 1995; Melcher *et al.*, 2000; Milbrandt *et al.*, 2000; Mirz *et al.*, 1999a, 2000a, b; Muhlnickel *et al.*, 1998; Sahley & Nodar, 2001; Simpson & Davies, 2000). Preliminary results indicate that there are as many surprises as in the field of psychoacoustics. For example, centers in the auditory pathways that are receiving multisensory information, particularly from the somatosensory system (touch), are involved in processing the tinnitus signal (Levine, 1999). By finding out which neuronal centers, receptors and transmitters are involved, it should be possible to design and utilize new methods and drugs that would attenuate the tinnitus signal and decrease abnormal gain in the auditory pathways. Again, improvement should be achieved faster if this approach is combined with TRT.

This book is not the last word on tinnitus theory and treatment. However, it outlines TRT, which is seen as a significant step in removing tinnitus as a problem and eliminating the suffering caused by it.

Appendix 1: interview forms

The following forms are used in the interviews of a tinnitus patient, before commencing treatment and at follow-up.

TINNITUS / HYPERACUSIS
INITIAL INTERVIEW FORM

Clinic # :
Name :
DOB :
SSN :
Insurance :
Date :

T&HC#:

tel:
e-mail:

T I N N I T U S

RE / LE / Both / Head = >   Intermittent / Constant
                             Fluctuations in volume Y / N
Description of T sound(s)

Onset: Gradual / Sudden   When
"Bad days" Y / N   Frequency

Activities prevented or affected:
○ Concentration ○ Sleep ○ QRA ○ Work
○ Restaurants ○ Sports ○ Social ○ Other

Effect of sound: None / Louder / Softer
        How long: min / hours / days

Ear overprotection Y / N   % of time
            in quiet Y / N

% of time when: Aware   Annoyed
Severity: 0 1 2 3 4 5 6 7 8 9 10
Annoyance: 0 1 2 3 4 5 6 7 8 9 10
Effect on Life: 0 1 2 3 4 5 6 7 8 9 10

Any other T specific treatments

Why is T a problem

Comments:

S O U N D   T O L E R A N C E

Oversensitivity: Y / N   Physical discomfort? Y / N
Description of troublesome sounds

"Bad days" Y / N   Frequency

Activities prevented or affected:
○ Concerts ○ Shopping ○ Movies ○ Work
○ Restaurants ○ Driving ○ Sports ○ Church
○ Housekeeping ○ Childcare ○ Social ○ Other

Effect of sound: None / Stronger / Weaker
        How long: min / hours / days

Ear overprotection Y / N   % of time
            in quiet Y / N

Severity: 0 1 2 3 4 5 6 7 8 9 10
Annoyance: 0 1 2 3 4 5 6 7 8 9 10
Effect on Life: 0 1 2 3 4 5 6 7 8 9 10

Any other ST specific treatments

Why is ST a problem

Comments:

H L

Hearing problem   Y / N
Hearing Aid(s)   Y / N type:
Ever recommended Y / N

Category:
Recommendation:

Ranking problems: Tinnitus: 0 1 2 3 4 5 6 7 8 9 10
        Sound tolerance: 0 1 2 3 4 5 6 7 8 9 10
                Hearing: 0 1 2 3 4 5 6 7 8 9 10

Ptn decision:
Next visit:

T - tinnitus   ST - sound tolerance (hyperacusis + phonophobia)
Is you T preventing or affecting any activities in your life.
QRA - quiet recreational activities: Is your T interfering with QRA such as reading or meditating.
% of time when: Aware - What % of time were you aware of your T over last month?
                Annoyed - What % of the time over last months T bothered you?
Severity - How strong or loud was your T on average over last month? 0 - no T, 10 - as strong as you can imagine.
Annoyance - How much was T annoying you on average over last month 0 - not at all; 10 - as much as you can imagine.
Effect on life - How much was T affecting your life on average over last month. 0 - no effect; 10 - as much as you can imagine.
Any other T specific treatments - Are you using any other treatments for your T.
Sound tolerance - Is your tolerance to louder sounds the same as people around you?
Hearing - Do you think you have a hearing problem?
Ranking - rank importance of your problems with 0 - no problem, 10 - as large as you can imagine   MM & PJ Jastreboff, 1999

Appendix 1. Fig. A

FU

TINNITUS / HYPERACUSIS
FOLLOW-UP INTERVIEW FORM

CATEGORY:
Date of init. couns.
T&HC#:   Date of instr. fitt.
SG:
tel: HA:
FUQ #:
Month #:
Type of visit:

Clinic #   :
Name   :
DOB   :
SSN   :
Insurance :
Date   :

T I N N I T U S

Activities prevented or affected: Changes: Y / N
◯◯Concentration ◯◯Sleep   ◯◯QRA   ◯◯Work
◯◯Restaurants ◯◯Sports   ◯◯Social ◯◯Other

% of time when: Aware   (1st   ) Annoyed   (1st   )
Has it changed
Severity: 0 1 2 3 4 5 6 7 8 9 10
Annoyance: 0 1 2 3 4 5 6 7 8 9 10
Effect on Life: 0 1 2 3 4 5 6 7 8 9 10

Comments:

"Bad days" Y / N   Frequency
Are they: as frequent Y /N   as bad Y / N

Effect of sound: None / Louder / Softer
How long: min / hours / days

Ear overprotection Y / N   % of time
in quiet Y / N
Any other T specific treatments

S O U N D   T O L E R A N C E

Description of troublesome sounds

Activities prevented or affected: Changes: Y / N
◯◯Concerts   ◯◯Shopping   ◯◯Movies ◯◯Work
◯◯Restaurants   ◯◯Driving   ◯◯Sports ◯◯Church
◯◯Housekeeping ◯◯Childcare   ◯◯Social ◯◯Other

Severity: 0 1 2 3 4 5 6 7 8 9 10
Annoyance: 0 1 2 3 4 5 6 7 8 9 10
Effect on Life: 0 1 2 3 4 5 6 7 8 9 10

Comments:

"Bad days" Y / N   Frequency
Are they: as frequent Y /N   as bad Y / N

Effect of sound: None / Stronger/ Weaker
How long: min / hours / days

Ear overprotection Y / N   % of time
in quiet Y / N
Any other ST specific treatments

H L

Hearing problem

Recommendation:

The problem in general: Same / Better / Worse
Ranking problems: Tinnitus: 0 1 2 3 4 5 6 7 8 9 10
Sound tolerance: 0 1 2 3 4 5 6 7 8 9 10
Hearing: 0 1 2 3 4 5 6 7 8 9 10

Next visit:

How would you feel if you had to give back your instruments
Are you glad you started this program? Y / N / NS
Main problems discussed:

T - tinnitus   ST - sound tolerance (hyperacusis + phonophobia)
Is you T preventing or affecting any activities in your life.
QRA - quiet recreational activities: Is your T interfering with QRA such as reading or meditating.
% of time when: Aware - What % of time were you aware of your T over last month?
Annoyed - What % of the time over last months T bothered you?
Severity - How strong or loud was your T on average over last month. 0 - no T, 10 - as strong as you can imagine.
Annoyance - How much was T annoying you on average over last month; 0 - not at all; 10 - as much as you can imagine.
Effect on life - How much was T affecting your life on average over last month. 0 - no effect; 10 - as much as you can imagine.
Any other T specific treatments - Are you using any other treatments for your T.
Sound tolerance - Is your tolerance to louder sounds the same as people around you?
Hearing - Do you think you have a hearing problem?
Ranking - rank importance of your problems with 0 - no problem, 10 - as large as you can imagine

Type of visit: - phone, fax, e-mail, office visit
●◯ - an activity affected at first visit
◯● - an activity affected as for today

MM & PJ Jastreboff, 1999

Appendix 1. Fig. B

Appendix 2: representative examples used in counseling

New neighbor

Imagine a new neighbor has moved next door. You exhibit mild interest to start with, but your anxiety increases very soon when you observe small packages being delivered to the front door on a regular basis by different individuals who quickly depart. You guess that your neighbor is perhaps a drugs dealer, and the prospect of spending many years next door to such criminal activity fills you with great alarm. You are constantly looking through the window monitoring the activities next door and experience much anxiety and depression by constantly thinking of the inevitable and desperate outcome for yourself and your young family of living next door to such a person. Some time later you learn, quite by chance, that your neighbor is involved in collecting food parcels for the homeless. The realization that you have wrongly assessed the situation results in a sudden change of attitude. You lose your dislike for your neighbor and stop monitoring his activities. You even feel foolish at your inappropriate initial assessment, realizing that you are all too likely to think the worst of people.

Because of the common traditional beliefs about tinnitus being an untreatable disease, which can destroy life quality, it is very understandable that those perceiving it often become anxious and depressed and find it impossible not to monitor every tiny variation of its behavior. Once the truth about tinnitus, its natural, benign and fundamentally normal origin, is known and understood, all the unpleasant reactions gradually disappear.

Inability to shift attention from a stimulus indicating danger

Let us imagine that in the interview room, in place of a chair we have, in the corner of the room, a live tiger. Even if I tell you that this tiger is very gentle and has not eaten any patients since last week, and I am instructing you to focus your attention exclusively on this important explanation of the neurophysiological model of tinnitus, so important for your treatment, you would not be able to avoid monitoring the behavior of this tiger even if you have a reasonable trust in my opinion. In this case, a stimulus is placed high on the priority list demanding our attention, and we are subconsciously forced to monitor its status, even against our will. Similarly, tinnitus, once it has acquired negative associations indicating danger, is periodically forcing our attention on it, against our will, distracting us from other worthwhile tasks.

Hanging by your hands

Hanging by your hands in the air from the edge of the roof may be acceptable for a short period of time, but it will produce feelings of extreme exhaustion, over a longer period. Stimulation of the autonomic nervous system results in the preparation of the body for fight or flight. It involves the increased secretion of certain hormones, increased heart rate and respiration, increasing muscle tension, etc. At the same time, activities associated with pleasure (positive reinforcement) are suppressed; we lose our appetite when we are frightened or in a potentially dangerous situation. Similarly, tinnitus producing even mildly elevated levels of activity in the autonomic nervous system can produce high levels of exhaustion if present for prolonged periods of time.

Catching a plane in the early morning

Let us imagine that you have to fly to a meeting in the morning, which necessitates leaving the house at about 5:00 am. Several alarm clocks are set to ensure that you wake; your spouse is primed to wake you, and your colleague will telephone you at the same time. Despite all these precautions, typically your sleep will be very shallow and fitful during the night, and you will eventually become wide awake sometime before the alarm clock goes off. This reflects an elevated level of activity in the autonomic nervous system, preparing you to wake up on time and be ready for immediate action in order to avoid missing the plane. Imagine having to repeat this scenario on a daily basis, moving from one city to another, catching early morning planes. Going to bed early will not improve the quality of your sleep, which will still be fitful and disturbed. Similarly, tinnitus inducing even mild activation of the autonomic nervous system is promoting a prolonged "catch the morning plane" situation and might profoundly affect your sleep patterns.

Glossary

Addison's disease Adrenocortical insufficiency usually caused by idiopathic atrophy or destruction of both adrenal glands by tuberculosis, an autoimmune process or other diseases characterized by fatigue, decreased blood pressure, weight loss, increased melanin pigmentation of the skin and mucous membranes, anorexia and nausea or vomiting; without appropriate replacement therapy, it can progress to acute adrenocortical insufficiency. Syn: addisonian syndrome, hyposupradrenalism, morbus Addisonii (*Stedman's Concise Medical Dictionary* 1997).

agonist A drug capable of combining with receptors to initiate drug actions; it possesses affinity and intrinsic activity (*Stedman's Concise Medical Dictionary* 1997).

angiography Radiography of vessels after the injection of a radioopaque contrast material. It usually requires percutaneous insertion of a radioopaque catheter and positioning under fluoroscopic control (*Stedman's Concise Medical Dictionary* 1997).

antagonist Something opposing or resisting the action of another; certain structures, agents, diseases or physiologic processes that tend to neutralize or impede the action or effect of others (*Stedman's Concise Medical Dictionary* 1997).

asymptomatic Without symptoms, or producing no symptoms (*Stedman's Concise Medical Dictionary* 1997).

audiogram The graphic record drawn from the results of hearing tests with the audiometer. It charts the threshold of hearing at various frequencies against sound intensity in decibels (*Stedman's Concise Medical Dictionary* 1997).

auditory imagery The phantom perception of musical tunes, or of voices without any understandable speech.

auditory (cochlear) nerve The nerve connecting the cochlea with the cochlear nuclei in the brainstem. It consists of two types of neural fibers: type I innervating inner hair cells and type II innervating outer hair cells.

auditory periphery This includes the external and middle ear, the cochlea and the auditory nerve.

auditory pathways Neural paths and connections within the central nervous system, beginning at the organ of Corti's hair cells, continuing along the eighth (auditory) nerve and terminating at the auditory cortex (*Stedman's Concise Medical Dictionary* 1997).

autonomic nervous system   The part of the nervous system that represents the motor inner-vation of smooth muscle, cardiac muscle and gland cells. It consists of two physio-logically and anatomically distinct components, which are mutually antagonistic: the sympathetic and parasympathetic systems. In both, the pathway of innervation consists of a synaptic sequence of two motor neurons, one of which lies in the spinal cord or brainstem as the preganglionic neuron. This has a thin but myelin-ated axon (preganglionic or B fiber), which emerges with an outgoing spinal or cranial nerve and synapses with one or more of the postganglionic (or, more strictly, ganglionic) neurons composing the autonomic ganglia. The unmyelinated postganglionic fibers, in turn, innervate the smooth muscle, cardiac muscle or gland cells. The preganglionic neurons of the sympathetic system lie in the inter-mediolateral cell column of the thoracic and upper two lumbar segments of the spinal gray matter; those of the parasympathetic system compose the visceral motor (visceral efferent) nuclei of the brainstem as well as the lateral column of the sec-ond to fourth sacral segments of the spinal cord. The ganglia of the sympathetic section are the paravertebral ganglia of the sympathetic trunk and the prevertebral or collateral ganglia; those of the parasympathetic section lie either near the organ to be innervated or as intramural ganglia within the organ itself except in the head, where there are four discrete parasympathetic ganglia (ciliary, otic, pterygopalatine and submandibular). Impulse transmission from preganglionic to postganglionic neuron is mediated by acetylcholine in both the sympathetic and parasympathetic sections; transmission from the postganglionic fiber to the visceral effector tis-sues is classically said to be by acetylcholine in the parasympathetic part and by norepinephrine in the sympathetic part. Recent evidence suggests the existence of further non-cholinergic, non-adrenergic classes of postganglionic fiber. Syn: pars autonomica, systema nervosum autonomicum, autonomic part, involuntary ner-vous system, vegetative nervous system, visceral nervous system (*Stedman's Concise Medical Dictionary* 1997).

axon   The single process of a nerve cell that under normal conditions conducts nervous impulses away from the cell body and its remaining processes (dendrites). It is a relatively even filamentous process varying in thickness from 0.25 approximately to more than 10 μm. In contrast to dendrites, which rarely exceed 1.5 mm in length, axons can extend great distances from the parent cell body (some axons of the pyramidal tract are 40 to 50 cm long). Axons 0.5 μm thick or over are generally enveloped by a segmented myelin sheath provided by oligodendroglia cells (in brain and spinal cord) or Schwann cells (in peripheral nerves). Like dendrites and nerve cell bodies, axons contain a large number of neurofibrils. With some exceptions, nerve cells synaptically transmit impulses to other nerve cells or to effector cells (muscle cells, gland cells) exclusively by way of the synaptic terminals of their axon (*Stedman's Concise Medical Dictionary* 1997).

basilar membrane   The membrane extending from the bony spiral membrane to the basilar crest of the cochlea. It forms the greater part of the floor of the cochlear duct, separating the latter from the scala tympani, and it supports the organ of Corti (*Stedman's Concise Medical Dictionary* 1997).

Bell's palsy   Paresis or paralysis, usually unilateral, of the facial muscles caused by dysfunction of the VII cranial nerve. It is probably caused by a viral infection, usually demyelinating in type. Syn: peripheral facial paralysis (*Stedman's Concise Medical Dictionary* 1997).

BICROS   A hearing aid system providing bilateral contralateral routing and amplification of sound.

bruits   An abnormal sound made by internal organs, such as the heart and blood vessels. They can be detected by stethoscope or other amplifying device.

categories in tinnitus retraining therapy   Classification of treatments based on the neurophysiological model of tinnitus for implementation of TRT. There are five main categories; the specifics are different for each category but there is a common element of counseling and use of sound.

cerebral cortex   The gray cellular mantle (1 to 4 mm thick) covering the entire surface of the cerebral hemisphere of mammals. It is characterized by a laminar organization of cellular and fibrous components such that its nerve cells are stacked in defined layers (*Stedman's Concise Medical Dictionary* 1997).

cochlea   A cone-shaped cavity in the petrous portion of the temporal bone, forming one of the divisions of the labyrinth or internal ear. It consists of a spiral canal making two and a half turns around a central core of spongy bone, the modiolus; this spiral canal of the cochlea contains the membranous cochlea, or cochlear duct, in which is the spiral organ (Corti) (*Stedman's Concise Medical Dictionary* 1997).

cochlear implant   An electronic device implanted under the skin that has electrodes in the middle ear on the promontory or cochlear window or in the inner ear in the cochlea. It is intended to create sound sensation in total sensory deafness. Syn: cochlear prosthesis (*Stedman's Concise Medical Dictionary* 1997).

computed tomography (CT)   An imaging method providing anatomical information for a cross-sectional plane of the body. Each image is generated by a computed synthesis of X-ray transmission data obtained in many different directions in a given plane. Syn: computed axial tomography. CT was developed in 1967 by the British electronics engineer Godfrey Hounsfield and it has revolutionized diagnostic medicine. Hounsfield linked X-ray sensors to a computer and worked out a mathematical technique called algebraic reconstruction for assembling images from transmission data. In 1973, the Mayo Clinic began operating the first machine in the USA. Early machines yielded digital images with at least 100 times the clarity of normal radiographs. Subsequently, the speed and accuracy of machines has improved many times over. CT scans reveal both bone and soft tissues, including organs, muscles and tumors. Image tones can be adjusted to highlight tissues of similar density, and, through graphics software, the data from multiple cross-sections can be assembled into three-dimensional images. CT aids diagnosis, surgery and other treatments such as radiation therapy, in which effective dosage is highly dependent on the precise density, size and location of a tumor (*Stedman's Concise Medical Dictionary* 1997).

conditioned reflex   A learnt reflex in which a stimulus initially incapable of evoking a reaction acquires the ability to do so by repeated pairing with another stimulus that does elicit the response. The second stimulus produces reinforcement (reward or punishment). Subsequent presentation of the first sensory stimulus will then elicit the reaction alone. Creating a conditioned reflex is associated with new functional connections being formed within the brain; once established it is stable and cannot be modified by conscious effort. Note that emotional reactions such as fear can be conditioned as well, e.g. by the presentation of a sound. If the sound was previously associated with a threatening situation, fear will be induced by this specific sound presentation.

contralateral   Opposite side.

critical band   A narrow band of frequencies surrounding the tone contributing to the masking of the tone.

CROS   An aid providing contralateral routing of sound.

dB (decibel)   A unit used to express relative difference in power or intensity, usually between two acoustic or electric signals, equal to ten times the common logarithm of the ratio of the two levels (*American Heritage Dictionary* 1994).

decreased sound tolerance   A reduced ability to tolerate external sound. Can result from hyperacusis, misophonia or phonophobia, or any combinations of these phenomena. Decreased sound tolerance is not related to hearing threshold and can exist with normal hearing or with profound hearing loss.

demystification   Teaching the mechanisms of hearing, tinnitus and decreased sound tolerance using the neurophysiological model. Allaying fears by providing knowledge and understanding; an important facet of TRT.

disinhibition   A decrease of inhibition.

distortion product otoacoustic emission (DPOAE)   A method for measuring the function of outer hair cells.

double-blind study   A study in which neither the experimenter/assessor nor the participants know which group is subject to which procedure, thus helping to assure that the biases or expectations of either will not influence the results (*Stedman's Concise Medical Dictionary* 1997).

endolymph   Fluid in the central channel in the inner ear.

eustachian tube   A tube leading from the tympanic cavity to the nasopharynx; it enables equalization of pressure within the tympanic cavity with ambient air pressure, referred to commonly as "popping of the ears" (*Stedman's Concise Medical Dictionary* 1997).

frequency   The number of vibrations, cycles or other recurrences in unit time. For a sinusoidal signal such as sound, it is the number of periods occurring in one second and is expressed in hertz (Hz) or cycles per second.

habituation   The decline of a conditioned response following repeated exposure to the conditioned stimulus (*American Heritage Dictionary* 1994).

habituation of perception   The disappearance of perception of a stimulus resulting from repeated presentation of a non-significant stimulus without reinforcement.

habituation of reaction   The disappearance of reaction resulting from repeated presentation of a non-significant stimulus without reinforcement.

hallucination   The apparent, often strong, subjective perception of an object or event when no such stimulus or situation is present. It may be visual, auditory, olfactory, gustatory or tactile (*American Heritage Dictionary* 1994).

hearing level   A standardized scale for measuring human hearing represented as a deviation from the average hearing of a normal-hearing population.

hearing threshold   Weakest sound perceived for a given frequency, typically described in decibels as a deviation from a standard value for a normal-hearing human population (*see* hearing level).

Hertz (Hz)   A unit of frequency equivalent to 1 cycle per second.

hydrops   Increased pressure in the inner ear endolymph.

hyperacusis   Abnormally strong reaction to sound occurring within the auditory pathways. At the behavioral level, it is manifested by a patient experiencing physical discomfort as a result of exposure to sound (quiet, medium or loud). The same sound would not evoke a similar reaction in an average listener. The strength of the reaction is controlled by the physical characteristics of the sound (e.g., its spectrum and intensity). It can result from both peripheral and central auditory dysfunction.

hyperbaric oxygen therapy   Treatment in which oxygen is provided in a sealed chamber at an ambient pressure greater than 1 atmosphere (*Stedman's Concise Medical Dictionary* 1997).

inner hair cells (IHC)   Receptor cells in the cochlea that tranduce mechanical vibrations of sound into electrical impulses within the auditory nerve. These are subsequently perceived as a sound.

intensity   "Intensity is the sound power transmitted through a given area in a sound field" (Moore 1995). The term is used in general meaning to indicate the amount of sound.

ipsilateral   The same side.

kindling   A word used in epilepsy to describe the process whereby a weak electrical stimulus, as a result of repetitive presentation, induces a full epileptic attack. In the case of tinnitus, the term is used to describe the prolonged worsening of tinnitus and/or hyperacusis as a result of exposure to a relatively short period of moderate or loud sound.

labyrinthectomy   An operation for destroying all the hearing and balance function in the inner ear.

limbic system   Collective term denoting a heterogeneous array of brain structures at or near the edge (limbus) of the medial wall of the cerebral hemisphere, in particular the hippocampus, amygdala and fornicate gyrus. The term is often used to include also the interconnections of these structures and their connections with the septal area, the hypothalamus and the medial zone of the mesencephalic tegmentum. By way of these connections, the limbic system exerts an important influence upon the endocrine and autonomic motor system; its functions also appear to affect motivational and mood states. Syn: visceral brain (*Stedman's Concise Medical Dictionary* 1997).

loudness discomfort levels (LDL)   Audiological measurements determining sound levels that are uncomfortable to a subject because of their loudness.

Lyme disease   A chronic infection transmitted by the animal tick *Borrelia burgdorferi*, which affects the nervous system among other effects. Hyperacusis is frequently one of the symptoms. Lyme disease is treatable with large doses of antibiotics.

magnetic resonance imaging (MRI)   A diagnostic radiological modality using the magnetic nuclei (especially protons) of a patient. These are aligned in a strong, uniform magnetic field, absorb energy from the tuned radiofrequency pulses and emit radiofrequency signals as their excitation decays. These signals, which vary in intensity according to nuclear abundance and molecular chemical environment, are converted into sets of tomographic images by using field gradients in the magnetic field, which permits three-dimensional localization of the point sources of the signals. (Syn: nuclear magnetic resonance imaging, NMR imaging, nuclear magnetic resonance tomography.) The basic idea of MRI was conceived in 1948 but could not be implemented until the advent of computers and the mathematical technique known as algebraic reconstruction. Unlike conventional radiography or CT, MRI does not expose patients to ionizing radiation. In addition, it provides superior images of the body's interior, delineating muscle, bone, blood vessel, nerve, organ and tumor tissue (*Stedman's Concise Medical Dictionary* 1997).

masking   The amount by which the threshold of audibility for one sound is raised by the presence of another (masking) sound. Commonly masking is understood as total disappearance of perception of a sound as a result of the presence of a masking sound.

Ménière syndrome   This is characterized clinically by vertigo, nausea, vomiting, tinnitus and progressive deafness owing to swelling of the endolymphatic system. Syn: auditory vertigo, endolymphatic hydrops, labyrinthine vertigo, Ménière's disease.

minimal masking level   Now known as minimal suppression level (q.v.).

minimal suppression level (MSL)   Minimal level of white noise necessary to suppress the perception of tinnitus.

misophonia   Abnormally strong reactions of the autonomic and limbic systems resulting from enhanced connections between the auditory and limbic systems. Importantly, misophonia and phonophobia do not involve a significant activation of the auditory system.

monotonic   Sequences where the successive members consistently either increase or decrease but do not oscillate in relative value. Each member of a monotone increasing sequence is greater than or equal to the preceding member; each member of a monotone decreasing sequence is less than or equal to the preceding member (*American Heritage Dictionary* 1994).

myringoplasty   Operative repair of a damaged tympanic membrane.

neuron   The morphological and functional unit of the nervous system. A neuron comprises a nerve cell body, short radiating processes called dendrites and one long process called the axon. The axon plus its covering or sheath is the nerve fiber. Syn: nerve cell.

neurophysiology   Branch of science involving the physiological mechanism of nervous system function.

neurotransmitter   A group of substances released by a presynaptic cell, upon excitation. The neurotransmitter crosses the synapse to stimulate or inhibit the postsynaptic cell. More than one may be released at any given synapse. Examples are acetylcholine, norepinephrine and glutamate.

otosclerosis   A new formation of spongy bone about the stapes and fenestra vestibuli (oval window), resulting in progressively increasing deafness without signs of disease in the eustachian tube or tympanic membrane (*Stedman's Concise Medical Dictionary* 1997).

otosclerosis surgery   Surgery aimed at removing the effects of stapes fixation to improve hearing.

ototoxic   Damaging to the inner ear.

outer hair cells (OHC)   Receptor cells in the cochlea that act as a biomechanical amplifier for weak sounds up to about 50dB. They are not necessary for sound transduction and their gain is variable. Their dysfunction may trigger compensatory action in the auditory system, resulting in tinnitus.

palatal myoclonus   Rhythmic contractions of the soft palate, sometimes including pharyngeal muscles, causing clicking sound in the ears.

pattern recognition   Detection of a specific sequence of neuronal activity at a behavioral level; detection and classification of a design.

perilymph   The fluid contained within the osseus labyrinth, surrounding and protecting the membranous labyrinth. Perilymph resembles extracellular fluid in composition (sodium salts are the predominate positive electrolyte) and, via the perilymphatic duct, is in continuity with cerebrospinal fluid (*Stedman's Concise Medical Dictionary* 1997).

perilymphatic fistula   Leak of perilymph caused by damage to the cochlea.

phantom perception   Perception without a corresponding physical stimulus, for example the sensation that an amputated limb is still present, often associated with painful paresthesia (phantom 1 imb).

phenomenological   The systematic description and classification of phenomena without attempt at explanation or interpretation; based only on observation and not on any theory.

phobia   Any objectively unfounded morbid dread or fear that arouses a state of panic. The word is used as a combining form in many terms expressing the object that inspires the fear (e.g., a morbid fear of spiders, arachnophobia).

phonophobia   A specific form of misophonia when fear of sound is the dominant emotion.

pitch of a sound   "Attribute of auditory sensation in terms of which sound may be ordered on a musical scale" (Moore, 1995).

placebo effect   The placebo effect is the report of a change while the patient is only receiving a regimen containing no active ingredient: a placebo. A placebo needs to be as identical in appearance as possible to the active ingredients. The appropriate method for controlling the placebo effect is a double-blind study (q.v.) where the specific effects of the treatment can be distinguished from the non-specific effects of believing that treatment is occurring.

presbyacusis   Loss of ability to perceive or discriminate sounds as a part of the ageing process; the pattern and age of onset may vary. Syn: presbyacousia, presbycusis (*Stedman's Concise Medical Dictionary* 1997).

promontory of tympanic cavity   A rounded eminence on the labyrinthine wall of the middle ear, caused by the first coil of the cochlea. Syn: promontorium cavi tympani, tuber cochleae, tympanic promontory (*Stedman's Concise Medical Dictionary* 1997).

psychoacoustical evaluation of tinnitus   Determination of tinnitus pitch, loudness and minimal suppression levels using psychoacoustical methodology.

psychoacoustics   A discipline combining experimental psychology and physics; it deals with the physical features of sound as related to audition, as well as with the physiology and psychology of sound reception processes (*Stedman's Concise Medical Dictionary* 1997).

pure-tone audiometry   Audiometry utilizing tones of various frequencies and intensities as auditory stimuli to measure hearing, including comparisons of results from testing air conduction and bone conduction (*Stedman's Concise Medical Dictionary* 1997).

Ramsay Hunt syndrome   A set of symptoms caused by herpes zoster infection of the vii cranial nerve and geniculate ganglion, including facial paralysis, deafness and otalgia.

recruitment   A term used in the testing of hearing: the unequal reaction of the ear to equal steps of increasing intensity, measured in decibels, when such inequality of response results in a greater than normal increment of loudness (*Stedman's Concise Medical Dictionary* 1997). Recruitment is typically referred to in audiology as an abnormally high slope of loudness growth; it may coexist with decreased sound tolerance, but these phenomena are not causally linked. It is a necessary outcome of sensorineural hearing loss and is usually the result of a reduction in the outer hair cell population.

residual inhibition   Disappearance or decreased loudness of tinnitus perception for some time after exposure to loud sound; typically sound with an intensity 10 dB higher than minimal suppression level is used.

sensation level   A hearing level for a given frequency in reference to the hearing threshold of a given subject.

somatosensory   Sensation received in the skin and deep tissues.

somatosound   A perceived natural body sound, for example palatal myoclonus, vascular sounds, audible otoacoustic emissions.

sound pressure level (SPL)   A measure of sound energy relative to 0.0002 dynes/cm^2, expressed in decibels (*Stedman's Concise Medical Dictionary* 1997).

spontaneous otoacoustic emissions (SOAE)   Emission of sound from the cochlea resulting from mechanical vibration of the outer hair cells.

stapedectomy   Operation to remove the stapes footplate in whole or part and to replace its superstructure (crura) with a metal or plastic prosthesis. It is used for otosclerosis with stapes fixation to overcome a conductive hearing loss.

stapedotomy   The surgical creation of a small opening in the footplate of the stapes. This is a recent improvement in surgery for otosclerosis where the integrity of the cochlea is maintained by extreme precision in opening the footplate, with the opening carefully sealed by vein graft under a specially designed piston.

subcortical   Below the level of the brain cortex.

syndromic tinnitus   Tinnitus associated with a specific medical condition, e.g. Ménière's syndrome, otosclerosis.

tinnitus matching   Determining the psychoacoustical parameters of tinnitus by matching with external sounds.

tinnitus-related neuronal activity   The neuronal activity, perception of which results in tinnitus.

tonal tinnitus   Tinnitus perceived as close to a pure tone.

tonotopic   A spatial arrangement of structures such that certain tone frequencies are transmitted along a particular portion of the structure, as in the cochlea in the auditory pathway.

Williams syndrome   A congenital disorder characterized by mental retardation, mild growth deficiency, elfin facies, supravalvular aortic stenosis and, occasionally, elevated blood calcium; it may be associated with hypersensitivity to vitamin D or excess ingestion of the vitamin during pregnancy (*Stedman's Concise Medical Dictionary* 1997). Hyperacusis is a common symptom.

winding-up effect   Worsening of a symptom as the result of exposure to an initial non-obtrusive stimulus. This is well recognized in pain; in tinnitus and hyperacusis it describes the significant worsening to even very low levels of sound. The same sound presented for shorter periods of time has no effect.

Abbreviations

CT	computed/computerised tomography
dB	decibel
DPOAE	distortion product otoacoustic emission
Hz	hertz
IHC	inner hair cells
LDL	loudness discomfort levels
MML	minimal masking level (now known as minimal suppression level (MSL))
MRI	magnetic resonance imaging
OHC	outer hair cells
SOAE	spontaneous otoacoustic emissions
SPL	sound pressure level
THI	Tinnitus Handicap Inventory
TMD	temporomandibular joint dysfunction

References

Adour, K. K. & Wingerd, J. (1974) Idiopathic facial paralysis (Bell's palsy): factors affecting severity and outcome in 446 patients. *Neurology*, **24**, 1112–1116.

Alberts, D. S. & Noel, J. K. (1995) Cisplatin-associated neurotoxicity: can it be prevented? *Anticancer Drugs*, **6**, 369–383.

Alster, J., Shemesh, Z., Ornan, M. & Attias, J. (1993) Sleep disturbance associated with chronic tinnitus. *Biol. Psychiatry*, **34**, 84–90.

American Heritage Dictionary, 3rd edn (1994) SoftKey International.

American National Standards Institute (1969) *Specifications for Audiometers.* pp. S3.6 New York: ANSI.

Anari, M., Axelsson, A., Elies, W. & Magnusson, L. (1999) Hypersensitivity to sound: questionnaire data, audiometry and classification. *Scand. Audiol.*, **28**, 219–230.

Anderson, H., Wagstaff, J., Crowther, D., *et al.* (1988) Comparative toxicity of cisplatin, carboplatin (CBDCA) and iproplatin (CHIP) in combination with cyclophosphamide in patients with advanced epithelial ovarian cancer. *Eur. J. Cancer Clin. Oncol.*, **24**, 1471–1479.

Andersson, G. & Lyttkens, L. (1996) Acupuncture for tinnitus: time to stop? *Scand. Audiol.*, **25**, 273–275.

Andersson, G. & Lyttkens, L. (1999) Effects of psychological treatment for tinnitus: a meta-analytic review. In *Proceedings of the Sixth International Tinnitus Seminar*, ed. Hazell, J. W. P., pp. 125–127. London: Tinnitus & Hyperacusis Centre.

Andersson, G., Kinnefors, A., Ekvall, L. & Rask-Andersen, H. (1997) Tinnitus and translabyrinthine acoustic neuroma surgery. *Audiol. Neurootol.*, **2**, 403–409.

Andersson, G., Lyttkens, L., Hirvela, C., Furmark, T., Tillfors, M. & Fredrikson, M. (2000) Regional cerebral blood flow during tinnitus: a PET case study with lidocaine and auditory stimulation. *Acta Otolaryngol.*, **120**, 967–972.

anon. (1981a) Definition and classification of tinnitus. *Tinnitus. CIBA Foundation Symposium* **85**, ed. Evered, D. & Lawrenson, G., pp. 300–302. London: Pitman.

anon. (1981b) Doctors' discussion. *Am. J. Otol.*, **2**, 291–293.

Aran, J. M. & Cazals, Y. (1981) Electrical suppression of tinnitus. *CIBA Found. Symp.*, **85**, 217–231.

Axelsson, A., Andersson, S. & Gu, L. D. (1996) Acupuncture in the management of tinnitus: a placebo-controlled study. In *Proceedings of the Fifth International Tinnitus Seminar*, ed. Vernon, J. A. & Reich, G., pp. 71–73. Portland, OR: American Tinnitus Association.

Baguley, D. M. & Andersson, G. (2003) Factor analysis of the Tinnitus Handicap Inventory. *Am. J. Audiol.*, **12**, 31–34.

Baguley, D. M., Moffat, D. A. & Hardy, D. G. (1992) What is the effect of translabyrinthine acoustic schwannoma removal upon tinnitus? *J. Laryngol. Otol.*, **106**, 329–331.

Baguley, D. M., Beynon, G. J., Grey, P. L., Hardy, D. G. & Moffat, D. A. (1997) Audio-vestibular findings in meningioma of the cerebello–pontine angle: a retrospective review. *J. Laryngol. Otol.*, **111**, 1022–1026.

Barkats, M., Venault, P., Christen, Y. & Cohen-Salmon, C. (1994) Effect of long-term treatment with EGb 761 on age-dependent structural changes in the hippocampi of three inbred mouse strains. *Life Sci.*, **56**, 213–222.

Bartnik, G., Fabijanska, A. & Rogowski, M. (1999) Our experience in treatment of patients with tinnitus and/or hyperacusis using the habituation method. In *Proceedings of the Sixth International Tinnitus Seminar*, ed. Hazell, J. W. P., pp. 415–417. London: Tinnitus & Hyperacusis Centre.

Bartoshuk, L. M., Kveton, J. F., Yanagisawa, K. & Catalanotto, F. C. (1994) Taste loss and taste phantoms: a role of inhibition in the taste system. In *Olfaction and Taste XI, Proceedings of the 11th International Symposium on Olfaction and Taste, 1993*, ed. Kurihara, K., Suzuki, N. & Ogawa, H., pp. 557–560. Tokyo: Springer-Verlag.

Basheer, R., Magner, M., McCarley, R. W. & Shiromani, P. J. (1998) REM sleep deprivation increases the levels of tyrosine hydroxylase and norepinephrine transporter mRNA in the locus coeruleus. *Brain Res. Mol. Brain Res.*, **57**, 235–240.

Bast, T., Zhang, W. N. & Feldon, J. (2001) The ventral hippocampus and fear conditioning in rats. Different anterograde amnesias of fear after tetrodotoxin inactivation and infusion of the GABA(A) agonist muscimol. *Exp. Brain Res.*, **139**, 39–52.

Beasley, N. J. & Jones, N. S. (1996) Ménière's disease: evolution of a definition. *J. Laryngol. Otol.*, **110**, 1107–1113.

Beckers, T., Wagemans, J., Boucart, M. & Giersch, A. (2001a) Different effects of lorazepam and diazepam on perceptual integration. *Vision Res.*, **41**, 2297–2303.

(2001b) Different effects of lorazepam and diazepam on perceptual integration. *Vision Res.*, **41**, 2297–2303.

Berliner, K. I. & Cunningham, J. K. (1987) Tinnitus suppression in cochlear implantation. In *Tinnitus*, ed. Hazell, J. W. P., London: Churchill Livingstone.

Berliner, K. I., Shelton, C., Hitselberger, W. E. & Luxford, W. M. (1992) Acoustic tumors: effect of surgical removal on tinnitus. *Am. J. Otol.*, **13**, 13–17.

Berrios, G. E. (1991) Musical hallucinations: a statistical analysis of 46 cases. *Psychopathology*, **24**, 356–360.

Berrios, G. E. & Rose, G. S. (1992) Psychiatry of subjective tinnitus: conceptual, historical and clinical aspects. *Neurol. Psychol. Brain Res.*, **1**, 76–82.

Berry, J. A., Gold, S. L., Frederick, E. A., Gray, W. C. & Staecker, H. (2002) Patient-based outcomes in patients with primary tinnitus undergoing tinnitus retraining therapy. *Arch. Otolaryngol. Head Neck Surg.*, **128**, 1153–1157.

Bertran, J. M. & Alvarez, D.C. (1999) [Results of surgery of the endolymphatic sac.] *Acta Otorrinolaringol. Esp.*, **50**, 179–183.

Bian, L. & Chertoff, M. E. (2001) Distinguishing cochlear pathophysiology in 4-aminopyridine and furosemide treated ears using a nonlinear systems identification technique. *J. Acoust. Soc. Am.*, **109**, 671–685.

Black, F. O. & Homer, L. (1996) Platform posturography. *Arch. Otolaryngol. Head Neck Surg.*, **112**, 1273–1274.

Bobbin, R. P., Jastreboff, P. J., Fallon, M. & Littman, T. (1990) Nimodipine, an L-channel Ca^{2+} antagonist, abolishes the negative summating potential recorded from the guinea pig cochlea. *Hearing Res.*, **46**, 277–288.

Boettcher, F. A. & Salvi, R. J. (1993) Functional changes in the ventral cochlear nucleus following acute acoustic overstimulation. *J. Acoust. Soc. Am.*, **94**, 2123–2134.

Bohne, B. A. & Clark, W. W. (1982) Growth of hearing loss and cochlear lesion with increasing duration of noise exposure. In *New Perspectives on Noise-induced Hearing Loss*, ed. Hamernik, R. P., Henderson, D. & Salvi, R., pp. 283–302. New York: Raven Press.

Bolanos-Jimenez, F., Manhaes de Castro, R., Sarhan, H., Prudhomme, N., Drieu, K. & Fillion, G. (1995) Stress-induced 5-HT_{1A} receptor desensitization: protective effects of *Ginkgo biloba* extract (EGb 761). *Fundam. Clin. Pharmacol.*, **9**, 169–174.

Brennan, J. F. & Jastreboff, P. J. (1991) Generalization of conditioned suppression during salicylate-induced phantom auditory perception in rats. *Acta Neurobiol. Exp.*, **51**, 15–27.

Brooks, C. M. (1987) Autonomic nervous systems, nature and functional role. In *Encyclopedia of Neuroscience*, ed. Adelman, G., pp. 96–98. Boston, MA: Birkhauser.

Brooks, D. N. & Bulmer, D. (1981) Survey of binaural hearing aid users. *Ear Hear.*, **2**, 220–224.

Brummett, R. E. (1995) A mechanism for tinnitus? In *Mechanisms of Tinnitus*, ed. Vernon, J. A. & Moller, A. R., pp. 7–10. Boston, MA: Allyn and Bacon.

Buchel, C. & Dolan, R. J. (2000) Classical fear conditioning in functional neuroimaging. *Curr. Opin. Neurobiol.*, **10**, 219–223.

Budd, R. J. & Pugh, R. (1996) Tinnitus coping style and its relationship to tinnitus severity and emotional distress. *J. Psychosom. Res.*, **41**, 327–335.

Busto, U. E. (1999) Benzodiazepines: the science and the myths. *Can. J. Clin. Pharmacol.*, **6**, 185–186.

Busto, U. E., Sellers, E. M., Naranjo, C. A., Cappell, H., Sanchez-Craig, M. & Sykora, K. (1986) Withdrawal reaction after long-term therapeutic use of benzodiazepines. *N. Engl. J. Med.*, **315**, 854–859.

Butefisch, C. M., Davis, B. C., Wise, S. P., *et al.* (2000) Mechanisms of use-dependent plasticity in the human motor cortex. *Proc. Natl. Acad. Sci.* **97**, 3661–3665.

Cabrera, I. N. & Lee, M. H. (2000) Reducing noise pollution in the hospital setting by establishing a department of sound: a survey of recent research on the effects of noise and music in health care. *Prev. Med.*, **30**, 339–345.

Cacace, A. T., Lovely, T. J., Winter, D. F., Parnes, S. M. & McFarland, D. J. (1994) Auditory perceptual and visual-spatial characteristics of gaze-evoked tinnitus. *Audiology*, **33**, 291–303.

Cacace, A. T., Cousins, J. P., Parnes, S. M., *et al.* (1999a) Cutaneous-evoked tinnitus II. Review of neuroanatomical, physiological and functional imaging studies. *Audiol.* **4**, 258–268.

(1999b) Cutaneous-evoked tinnitus I. Phenomenology, psychophysics and functional imaging. *Audiol. Neuro-Otology*, **4**, 247–257.

Candy, P. J. & Pareson, D. C. (1990) A 10 year review of union and non-union with an implanted bone growth stimulator. *Clin. Orthop.*, **259**, 216–222.

Cardinaal, R. M., De Groot, J. C., Huizing, E. H., Veldman, J. E. & Smoorenburg, G. F. (2000) Cisplatin-induced ototoxicity: morphological evidence of spontaneous outer hair cell recovery in albino guinea pigs? *Hear. Res.*, **144**, 147–156.

Carrick, D. G., Davies, W. M., Fielder, C. P. & Bihari, J. (1986) Low-powered ultrasound in the treatment of tinnitus: a pilot study. *Br. J. Audiol.*, **20**, 153–155.

Catalano, P. J. & Post, K. D. (1996) Elimination of tinnitus following hearing preservation surgery for acoustic neuromas. *Am. J. Otol.*, **17**, 443–445.

Causse, J. B., Causse, J. R., Bel, J., *et al.* (1985) [Prognosis for tinnitus after surgery for otospongiosis.] *Ann. Otolaryngol. Chir. Cervicofac.*, **102**, 407–413.

Champlin, C. A., Muller, S. P. & Mitchell, S. A. (1990) Acoustic measurements of objective tinnitus. *J. Speech Hear. Res.*, **33**, 816–821.

Chen, G. D. & Fechter, L. D. (2003) The relationship between noise-induced hearing loss and hair cell loss in rats. *Hear. Res.*, **177**, 81–90.

Chen, G. D. & Jastreboff, P. J. (1995) Salicylate-induced abnormal activity in the inferior colliculus of rats. *Hear. Res.*, **82**, 158–178.

Cirelli, C. & Tononi, G. (1999) Differences in brain gene expression between sleep and waking as revealed by mRNA differential display and cDNA microarray technology. *J. Sleep Res.*, **8** (Suppl. 1), 44–52.

Clemis, J. D. & McBrien, M. M. (1996) The therapeutic use of histamine in cochleovestibular disorders and tinnitus. In *Proceedings of the Fifth International Tinnitus Seminar*, ed. Vernon, J. A. & Reich, G., pp. 203–209. Portland, OR: American Tinnitus Association.

Cloninger, C. R., Martin, R. L., Guze, S. B. & Clayton, P. J. (1985) Diagnosis and prognosis in schizophrenia. *Arch. Gen. Psychiatry*, **42**, 15–25.

Coles, R. (1988) Trial of an extract of *Ginkgo biloba* (EGB) for tinnitus and hearing loss. *Clin. Otolaryngol.*, **13**, 501–502.

Coles, R., Bradley, P., Donaldson, I. & Dingle, A. (1991) A trial of tinnitus therapy with ear-canal magnets. *Clin. Otolaryngol.*, **16**, 371–372.

Coles, R. R., Thompson, A. C. & O'Donoghue, G. M. (1992) Intra-tympanic injections in the treatment of tinnitus. *Clin. Otolaryngol.*, **17**, 240–242.

Coles, R. R. A. (1984) Epidemiology of tinnitus: (1) prevalence. *J. Laryngol. Otol. Suppl.* **9**: 7–15.

(1987) Epidemiology of tinnitus. In *Tinnitus*, ed. Hazell, J. W. P., pp. 46–70. Edinburgh: Churchill Livingstone.

(1996) Epidemiology, aetiology and classification, In *Proceedings of the Fifth International Tinnitus Seminar*, ed. Vernon, J. A. & Reich, G., pp. 25–30. Portland, OR: American Tinnitus Association.

(1998) Therapeutic blind alleys. In *Tinnitus Treatment and Relief* ed. Vernon, J. A. pp. 8–19. New York: Allyn & Bacon.

Costen, J. B. (1937) Summary of neuralgias and ear symptoms associated with the mandibular joint. *Mississippi Doctor*, **15**, 33.

Coull, J. T., Frith, C. D. & Dolan, R. J. (1999) Dissociating neuromodulatory effects of diazepam on episodic memory encoding and executive function. *Psychopharmacology* (Berl.), **145**, 213–222.

Culebras, A. (1992) Update on disorders of sleep and the sleep–wake cycle. *Psychiatr. Clin. North Am.*, **15**, 467–489.

Dauman, R. (2000) Electrical stimulation for tinnitus suppression. In *Tinnitus Handbook*, ed. Tyler, R., pp. 377–398. San Diego, CA: Singular, Thomson Learning.

Dauman, R. & Tyler, R. S. (1993) Tinnitus suppression in cochlear implant users. *Adv. Otorhinolaryngol.*, **48**, 168–173.

Dauman, R., Tyler, R. S. & Aran, J. M. (1993) Intracochlear electrical tinnitus reduction. *Acta Otolaryngol.* (Stockh.), **113**, 291–295.

Davies, E., Knox, E. & Donaldson, I. (1994) The usefulness of nimodipine, an L-calcium channel antagonist, in the treatment of tinnitus. *Br. J. Audiol.*, **28**, 125–129.

Davis, A. (1996) The aetiology of tinnitus: risk factors for tinnitus in the UK population – a possible role for conductive pathologies? In *Proceedings of the Fifth International Tinnitus Seminar*, ed. Vernon, J. A. & Reich, G., pp. 38–45. Portland, OR: American Tinnitus Association.

Davis, A. & El Refaie, A. (2000) Epidemiology of tinnitus. In *Tinnitus Handbook*, ed. Tyler, R., pp. 1–23. San Diego, CA: Singular, Thomson Learning.

Davis, M. & Whalen, P. J. (2001) The amygdala: vigilance and emotion. *Mol. Psychiatry*, **6**, 13–34.

Deberdt, W. (1994) Interaction between psychological and pharmacological treatment in cognitive impairment. *Life Sci.*, **55**, 2057–2066.

de Las, C. C., Sanz, E. J., de la Fuente, J. A., Padilla, J. & Berenguer, J. C. (2000) The Severity of Dependence Scale (SDS) as screening test for benzodiazepine dependence: SDS validation study. *Addiction*, **95**, 245–250.

den Hartigh, J., Hilders, C. G., Schoemaker, R. C., Hulshof, J. H., Cohen, A. F. & Vermeij, P. (1993) Tinnitus suppression by intravenous lidocaine in relation to its plasma concentration. *Clin. Pharmacol. Ther.*, **54**, 415–420.

Denk, D. M., Heinzl, H., Franz, P. & Ehrenberger, K. (1997) Caroverine in tinnitus treatment. A placebo-controlled blind study. *Acta Otolaryngol.*, **117**, 825–830.

Dobie, R. A. (1999) A review of randomized clinical trials in tinnitus. *Laryngoscope*, **109**, 1202–1211.

Dobie, R. A., Hoberg, K. E. & Rees, T. S. (1986) Electrical tinnitus suppression: a double-blind crossover study. *Otolaryngol. Head Neck Surg.*, **95**, 319–323.

Dobie, R. A., Sakai, C. S., Sullivan, M. D., Katon, W. J. & Russo, J. (1993) Antidepressant treatment of tinnitus patients: report of a randomized clinical trial and clinical prediction of benefit. *Am. J. Otol.*, **14**, 18–23.

Donaldson, I. (1978) Tinnitus: a theoretical view and a therapeutic study using amylobarbitone. *J. Laryngol. Otol.*, **92**, 123–130.

(1981) Tegretol: a double blind trial in tinnitus. *J. Laryngol. Otol.*, **95**, 947–951.

Drew, S. & Davies, E. (2001) Effectiveness of *Ginkgo biloba* in treating tinnitus: double blind, placebo controlled trial. *Br. Med. J.*, **322**, 73.

Duckert, L. G. & Rees, T. S. (1983) Treatment of tinnitus with intravenous lidocaine: a double-blind randomized trial. *Otolaryngol. Head Neck Surg.*, **91**, 550–555.

(1984) Placebo effect in tinnitus management. *Otolaryngol. Head Neck Surg.*, **92**, 697–699.

Duverger, D., De Feudis, F. V. & Drieu, K. (1995) Effects of repeated treatment with an extract of *Ginkgo biloba* (EGb 761) on cerebral glucose utilization in the rat: an autoradiographic study. *Gen. Pharmacol.*, **26**, 1375–1383.

Eggermont, J. J. (1990) On the pathophysiology of tinnitus; a review and a peripheral model. *Hear. Res.*, **48**, 111–123.

Ehrenberger, K. & Brix, R. (1983) Glutamic acid and glutamic acid diethylester in tinnitus treatment. *Acta Otolaryngol.* (Stockh.), **95**, 599–605.

Einfeld, S. L., Tonge, B. J., Florio, T., Van Borsel, J., Curfs, L. M. & Fryns, J. P. (1997) Behavioral and emotional disturbance in individuals with Williams syndrome hyperacusis in Williams syndrome: a sample survey study. *Am. J. Ment. Retard.*, **8**, 121–126.

Elliott, B. (2000) Diagnosing and treating hypothyroidism. *Nurse Pract.*, **25**, 92–105.

Emmerich, E., Richter, F., Reinhold, U., Linss, V. & Linss, W. (2000) Effects of industrial noise exposure on distortion product otoacoustic emissions (DPOAEs) and hair cell loss of the cochlea: long term experiments in awake guinea pigs. *Hear. Res.*, **148**, 9–17.

Emmett, J. R. & Shea, J. J. (1980) Treatment of tinnitus with tocainide hydrochloride. *Otolaryngol. Head Neck Surg.*, **88**, 442–446.

Engelberg, M. & Bauer, W. (1985) Transcutaneous electrical stimulation for tinnitus. *Laryngoscope*, **95**, 1167–1173.

Erlandsson, S., Ringdahl, A., Hutchins, T. & Carlsson, S. G. (1987) Treatment of tinnitus: a controlled comparison of masking and placebo. *Br. J. Audiol.*, **21**, 37–44.

Erlandsson, S. I., Rubinstein, B. & Carlsson, S. G. (1991) Tinnitus: evaluation of biofeedback and stomatognathic treatment. *Br. J. Audiol.*, **25**, 151–161.

Estes, W. K. & Skinner, B. F. (1941) Some quantitative properties of anxiety. *J. Exp. Psychol.*, **29**, 390–400.

Fallon, B. A., Nields, J. A., Burrascano, J. J., Liegner, K., DelBene, D. & Liebowitz, M. R. (1992) The neuropsychiatric manifestation of Lyme borreliosis. *Psychiatr. Q.*, **63**, 95–117.

Fattori, B., De Iaco, G., Vannucci, G., Casani, A. & Ghilardi, P. L. (1996) Alternobaric and hyperbaric oxygen therapy in the immediate and long-term treatment of Ménière's disease. *Audiology*, **35**, 322–334.

Feldmann, H. (1969a) [Studies on the masking of subjective tinnitus: a contribution to the pathophysiology of tinnitus.] *Z. Laryngol. Rhinol. Otol.*, **48**, 528–545.

(1969b) [Homolateral and contralateral masking of subjective tinnitus by broad spectrum noise, narrow spectrum noise and pure tones.] *Arch. Klin. Exp. Ohren. Nasen. Kehlkopfheilkd.*, **194**, 460–465.

(1971) Homolateral and contralateral masking of tinnitus by noise-bands and by pure tones. *Audiology*, **10**, 138–144.

(1992) Mechanisms of tinnitus. Medical and audiometric investigation. In *Audiology in Europe, an Academic Conference*, Cambridge, 1992, abstract 18.

Fisch, U. (1970) Transtemporal surgery of the internal auditory canal. Report of 92 cases, technique, indications and results. *Adv. Otorhinolaryngol.*, **17**, 203–240.

Fleishaker, J. C., Garzone, P. D., Chambers, J. H., Sirocco, K. & Weingartner, H. (1995) Comparison of the spectrum of cognitive effects of alprazolam and adinazolam after single doses in healthy subjects. *Psychopharmacology* (Berl.), **120**, 169–176.

Freeman, S., Plotnik, M., Elidan, J. & Sohmer, H. (1999) Differential effect of the loop diuretic furosemide on short latency auditory and vestibular-evoked potentials. *Am. J. Otol.*, **20**, 41–45.

Fucci, M. J., Sataloff, R. T. & Myers, D. L. (1994) Vestibular nerve section. *Am. J. Otolaryngol.*, **15**, 180–189.

Fukaya, T. & Nomura, Y. (1988) Audiological aspects of idiopathic perilymphatic fistula. *Acta Otolaryngol. Suppl.* (Stockh.), **456**, 68–73.

Gananca, M. M., Mangabeira Albernaz, P. L., Caovilla, H. H. & Ito, Y. I. (1988) Controlled clinical trial of pentoxifylline versus cinnarizine in the treatment of labyrinthine disorders. *Pharmatherapeutica*, **5**, 170–176.

George, R. N. & Kemp, S. (1991) A survey of New Zealanders with tinnitus. *Br. J. Audiol.*, **25**, 331–336.

Gerak, L. R., Woolverton, W. L., Nader, M. A., *et al.* (2001) Behavioral effects of flunitrazepam: reinforcing and discriminative stimulus effects in rhesus monkeys and prevention of withdrawal signs in pentobarbital-dependent rats. *Drug Alcohol Depend.*, **63**, 39–49.

Gerken, G. M. (1979) Central denervation hypersensitivity in the auditory system of the cat. *J. Acoust. Soc. Am.*, **66**, 721–727.

   (1992) Central auditory temporal processing: alterations produced by factors involving the cochlea. In *Effect of Noise on the Auditory System*, ed. Dancer, A., Henderson, D., Salvi, R. & Hamernik, R., pp. 146–155. Philadelphia, PA: Mosby.

   (1993) Alteration of central auditory processing of brief stimuli: a review and a neural model. *J. Acoust. Soc. Am.*, **93**, 2038–2049.

   (1996) Central tinnitus and lateral inhibition: an auditory brainstem model. *Hear. Res.*, **97**, 75–83.

Gerken, G. M., Saunders, S. S. & Paul, R. E. (1984) Hypersensitivity to electrical stimulation of auditory nuclei follows hearing loss in cats. *Hear. Res.*, **13**, 249–259.

Gerken, G. M., Saunders, S. S., Simhadri-Sumithra, R. & Bhat, K. H. V. (1985) Behavioral thresholds for electrical stimulation applied to auditory brainstem nuclei in cat are altered by injurious and noninjurious sound. *Hear. Res.*, **20**, 221–231.

Gerken, G. M., Simhadri-Sumithra, R. & Bhat, K. H. V. (1986) Increase in central auditory responsiveness during continuous tone stimulation or following hearing loss. In *Basic and Applied Aspects of Noise-induced Hearing Loss*, ed. Salvi, R. J., Henderson, D., Hamernik, R. P. & Colletti, V., pp. 195–211. New York: Plenum.

Gersdorff, M., Robillard, T., Stein, F., Declaye, X. & van der Bemden, S. (1987a) [The zinc sulfate overload test in patients suffering from tinnitus associated with low serum zinc. Preliminary report.] *Acta Otorhinolaryngol.* (Belg.), **41**, 498–505.

   (1987b) A clinical correlation between hypozincemia and tinnitus. *Arch. Otorhinolaryngol.*, **244**, 190–193.

Giordano, C., Bona Galvagno, M., Brosio, R., Schieroni, M. P. & Revello, M. P. (1987) [Treatment of tinnitus with the TENS stimulator in cervico-arthrosis patients. Preliminary results.] *Minerva Med.*, **78**, 861–864.

Goebel, G., Rubler, D., Stepputat, F., Hiller, W., Heuser, J. & Ficher, M. M. (1999) Controlled prospective study of tinnitus retraining therapy compared to tinnitus coping therapy and broad-band noise generator therapy. In *Proceedings of the Sixth International Tinnitus Seminar*, ed. Hazell, J. W. P., pp. 302–306. London: Tinnitus & Hyperacusis Centre.

Good, M. (1996) Effects of relaxation and music on postoperative pain: a review. *J. Adv. Nurs.*, **24**, 905–914.

Goodwin, P. E. (1980) Tinnitus and auditory imagery. *Am. J. Otol.*, **2**, 5–9.

Goosens, K. A. & Maren, S. (2001) Contextual and auditory fear conditioning are mediated by the lateral, basal, and central amygdaloid nuclei in rats. *Learn. Mem.*, **8**, 148–155.

Gopal, K. V., Daly, D. M., Daniloff, R. G. & Pennartz, L. (2000) Effects of selective serotonin reuptake inhibitors on auditory processing: case study. *J. Am. Acad. Audiol.*, **11**, 454–463.

Graham, J. M. & Hazell, J. W. (1977) Electrical stimulation of the human cochlea using a transtympanic electrode. *Br. J. Audiol.*, **11**, 59–62.

Gu, L. & Axelsson, A. (1996) Acupuncture for tinnitus: a review from 5 years of clinical investigations. In *Proceedings of the Fifth International Tinnitus Seminar*, ed. Vernon, J. A. & Reich, G., pp. 84–89. Portland, OR: American Tinnitus Association.

Gukovich, V. A., Avramenko, L. V. & Moroz, B. S. (1974) [Characteristics and dynamics of tinnitis in otosclerosis.] *Zh. Ushn. Nos. Gorl. Bolezn.*, 41–47.

Guth, P., Risey, J., Amedee, R. G. & Norris, C. H. (1992) A pharmacological approach to the treatment of tinnitus. In *Tinnitus 91. Proceedings of the Fourth International Tinnitus Seminar, 1991*, ed. Aran, J.-M. & Dauman, R., pp. 115–118. Amsterdam: Kugler & Ghedini.

Gutschmidt, K. U., Stenkamp, K., Buchheim, K., Heinemann, U. & Meierkord, H. (1999) Anticonvulsant actions of furosemide in vitro. *Neuroscience*, **91**, 1471–1481.

Halford, J. B. & Anderson, S. D. (1991) Anxiety and depression in tinnitus sufferers. *J. Psychosom. Res.*, **35**, 383–390.

Hallam, R. & McKenna, L. (1999) A neuropsychological study of concentration problems in tinnitus patients. In *Proceedings of the Sixth International Tinnitus Seminar*, ed. Hazell, J. W. P., pp. 108–113. London: Tinnitus & Hyperacusis Centre.

Hallam, R. S., Rachman, S. & Hinchcliffe, R. (1984) Psychological aspects of tinnitus. In *Contributions to Medical Psychology*, 3rd edn, ed. Rachman, R., pp. 31–34. Oxford: Pergamon Press.

Hammeke, T. A., McQuillen, M. P. & Cohen, B. A. (1983) Musical hallucinations associated with acquired deafness. *J. Neurol. Neurosurg. Psychiatry*, **46**, 570–572.

Hansen, J. E. (1975) Acupuncture in otolaryngology. *Am. J. Chin. Med.*, **3**, 281–284.

Harcourt, J., Thomsen, J. & Tos, M. (1997) Translabyrinthine vestibular schwannoma surgery: postoperative tinnitus and cochlear nerve integrity. *Auris Nasus Larynx*, **24**, 21–26.

Harris, S., Brismar, J. & Cronqvist, S. (1979) Pulsatile tinnitus and therapeutic embolization. *Acta Otolaryngol.* (Stockh.), **88**, 220–226.

Haynes, B. F., Pikus, A., Kaiser-Kupfer, M. & Fauci, A. S. (1981) Successful treatment of sudden hearing loss in Cogan's syndrome with corticosteroids. *Arthritis Rheum.*, **24**, 501–503.

Hazell, J. W. P. (1981) A tinnitus synthesizer physiological considerations. *J. Laryngol. Otol. Suppl.*, **10**, 187–195.

(1989) Tinnitus II: surgical management of conditions associated with tinnitus and somatosounds. *Can. J. Otolaryngol. Head Neck Surg.*, **103**, 739–742.

(1990a) Tinnitus. II: surgical management of conditions associated with tinnitus and somatosounds. *J. Otolaryngol.*, **19**, 6–10.

(1990b) Tinnitus and disability with ageing: adaptation and management. *Acta Otolaryngol. Suppl.* (Stockh.), 1–7.

Hazell, J. W. P. & McKinney, C. J. (1996) Support for a neurophysiological model of tinnitus: research data and clinical experience. In *Proceedings of the Fifth International Tinnitus Seminar*, ed. Vernon, J. A. & Reich, G., pp. 51–57. Portland, OR: American Tinnitus Association.

Hazell, J. W. P. & Sheldrake, J. B. (1992) Hyperacusis and tinnitus. In *Tinnitus 91. Proceedings of the Fourth International Tinnitus Seminar*, ed. Aran, J.-M. & Dauman, R., pp. 245–248. Amsterdam: Kugler & Ghedini.

Hazell, J. W. P., Wood, S. M., Cooper, H. R., *et al.* (1985a) A clinical study of tinnitus maskers. *Br. J. Audiol.*, **19**, 65–146.

(1985b) A clinical study of tinnitus maskers. *Br. J. Audiol.*, **19**, 65–146.

Hazell, J. W. P., Sheldrake, J. B. & Meerton, L. J. (1987) Tinnitus masking: is it better than counseling alone? In *Proceedings of the Third International Tinnitus Seminar*, ed. Feldmann, H., pp. 239–250. Karlsruhe: Harsch Verlag.

Hazell, J. W. P., Meerton, L. J. & Conway, M. J. (1989) Electrical tinnitus suppression (ETS) with a single channel cochlear implant. *J. Laryngol. Otol. Suppl.*, **18**, 39–44.

Hazell, J. W. P., von Schoenberg, M., Meerton, L. J. & Sheldrake, J. B. (1992a) Tinnitus and the unilateral dead ear. In *Tinnitus 91. Proceedings of the Fourth International Tinnitus Seminar*, ed. Aran, J.-M. & Dauman, R., pp. 261–264. Amsterdam: Kugler & Ghedini.

Hazell, J. W. P., Fraser, J. G. & Robinson, P. J. (1992b) Positional audiometry in the diagnosis of perilymph fistula. *Am. J. Otol.*, **13**, 263–269.

Hazell, J. W. P., Jastreboff, P. J., Meerton, L. E. & Conway, M. J. (1993) Electrical tinnitus suppression: frequency dependence of effects. *Audiol.*, **32**, 68–77.

Hazell, J. W. P., McKinney, C. J. & Aleksy, W. (1995) Mechanisms of tinnitus in profound deafness. *Ann. Otol. Rhinol. Laryngol. Suppl.*, **166**, 418–420.

Heilbrun, A. B., Jr, Diller, R., Fleming, R. & Slade, L. (1986) Strategies of disattention and auditory hallucinations in schizophrenics. *J. Nerv. Ment. Dis.*, **174**, 265–273.

Heitzmann, T., Rubio, L., Cardenas, M. R. & Zofio, E. (1999) The importance of continuity in TRT patients: results at 18 months. In *Proceedings of the Sixth International Tinnitus Seminar*, ed. Hazell, J. W. P., pp. 509–511. London: Tinnitus & Hyperacusis Centre.

Heller, M. F. & Bergman, M. (1953) Tinnitus in normally hearing persons. *Ann. Otol.*, **62**, 73–93.

Henkin, R. I. & Daly, R. L. (1968) Auditory detection and perception in normal man and in patients with adrenal cortical insufficiency: effect of adrenal cortical steroids. *J. Clin. Invest.*, **47**, 1269–1280.

Henry, J. A. & Meikle, M. B. (2000) Psychoacoustic measures of tinnitus. *J. Am. Acad. Audiol.*, **11**, 138–155.

Henry, J. A., Jastreboff, M. M., Jastreboff, P. J., Schechter, M. A. & Fausti, S. A. (2003) Guide to conducting Tinnitus Retraining Therapy (TRT) initial and follow-up interviews. *J. Rehab. Res. Dev.*, **40**, 157–178.

Henry, J. L. & Wilson, P. H. (1999) Cognitive–behavioural therapy for tinnitus-related distress: an experimental evaluation of initial treatment and relapse prevention. In *Proceedings of the*

Sixth International Tinnitus Seminar, ed. Hazell, J. W. P., pp. 118–124. London: Tinnitus & Hyperacusis Centre.

Hentzer, E. (1968) Objective tinnitus of the vascular type. A follow-up study. *Acta Otolaryngol.* (Stockh.), **66**, 273–281.

Herraiz, C., Hernandez, F. J., Machado, A., De Lucas, P. & Tapia, M. C. (1999) Tinnitus retraining therapy: our experience. In *Proceedings of the Sixth International Tinnitus Seminar*, ed. Hazell, J. W. P., pp. 483–484. London: Tinnitus & Hyperacusis Centre.

Higson, J. M., Haggard, M. P. & Field, D. L. (1994) Validation of parameters for assessing obscure auditory dysfunction: robustness of OAD status across samples and test methods. *Br. J. Audiol.*, **28**, 27–39.

Hochman, D. W., Baraban, S. C., Owens, J. W. & Schwartzkroin, P. A. (1995) Dissociation of synchronization and excitability in furosemide blockade of epileptiform activity. *Science*, **270**, 99–102.

Hoffmann, F., Beck, C., Schutz, A. & Offermann, P. (1994) [Ginkgo extract EGb 761 (tenobin)/HAES versus naftidrofuryl (Dusodril)/HAES. A randomized study of therapy of sudden deafness.] *Laryngorhinootologie*, **73**, 149–152.

Holgers, K. M., Axelsson, A. & Pringle, I. (1994) *Ginkgo biloba* extract for the treatment of tinnitus. *Audiology*, **33**, 85–92.

Holgers, K. M., Zöger, S., Svedlund, J. & Erlandsson, S. I. (1999) Psychiatric profile of tinnitus patients referred to an audiological clinic. In *Proceedings of the Sixth International Tinnitus Seminar, 1999*, ed. Hazell, J. W. P., pp. 283–285. London: Tinnitus & Hyperacusis Centre.

House, J. W. & Brackmann, D. E. (1981) Tinnitus: surgical treatment. *Ciba. Found. Symp.*, **85**, 204–216.

House, W. F. (1976) Cochlear implants. *Ann. Otol. Rhinol. Laryngol.*, **85**, 1–93.

Huguet, F., Drieu, K. & Piriou, A. (1994) Decreased cerebral 5-HT$_{1A}$ receptors during ageing: reversal by *Ginkgo biloba* extract (EGb 761). *J. Pharm. Pharmacol.*, **46**, 316–318.

Hulshof, J. H. & Vermeij, P. (1984) The effect of intra-venous lidocaine and several different doses of oral tocainide HCl on tinnitus. A dose-finding study. *Acta Otolaryngol.* (Stockh.), **98**, 231–238.

(1985) The value of tocainide in the treatment of tinnitus. A double-blind controlled study. *Arch. Otorhinolaryngol.*, **241**, 279–283.

(1986) The value of flunarizine in the treatment of tinnitus. *ORL J. Otorhinolaryngol. Relat. Spec.*, **48**, 33–36.

(1987) The effect of nicotinamide on tinnitus: a double-blind controlled study. *Clin. Otolaryngol.*, **12**, 211–214.

Hultcrantz, E. (1988) Clinical treatment of vascular inner ear diseases. *Am. J. Otolaryngol.*, **9**, 317–322.

Huynh, L. & Fields, S. (1995) Alprazolam for tinnitus. *Ann. Pharmacother.*, **29**, 311–312.

Israel, J. M., Connelly, J. S., McTigue, S. T., Brummett, R. E. & Brown, J. (1982) Lidocaine in the treatment of tinnitus aurium. A double-blind study. *Arch. Otolaryngol.*, **108**, 471–473.

Itoh, K., Kamiya, H., Mitani, A., Yasui, Y., Takada, M. & Mizuno, N. (1987) Direct projections from the dorsal column nuclei and the spinal trigeminal nuclei to the cochlear nuclei in the cat. *Brain Res.*, **400**, 145–150.

Jakes, S. C., Hallam, R. S., Chambers, C. & Hinchcliffe, R. (1985) A factor analytical study of tinnitus complaint behaviour. *Audiology*, **24**, 195–206.

Jakes, S. C., Hallam, R. S., Rachman, S. & Hinchcliffe, R. (1986) The effects of reassurance, relaxation training and distraction on chronic tinnitus sufferers. *Behav. Res. Ther.*, **24**, 497–507.

Jannetta, P. J. (1980) Neurovascular compression in cranial nerve and systemic disease. *Ann. Surg.*, **192**, 518–525.

(1987) Microvascular decompression of the cochlear nerve as treatment of tinnitus. In *Proceedings of the Third International Tinnitus Seminar*, ed. Feldmann, H., pp. 348–352. Karlsruhe: Harsch Verlag.

Jastreboff, M. M. & Jastreboff, P. J. (2001a) Component of decreased sound tolerance: hyperacusis, misophonia, phonophobia. *ITHS News Lett.*, **2**, 5–7.

(2001b) Hyperacusis. *Audiology On-line*, www.audiologyonline.com (accessed 18 June 2001).

(2002) Decreased sound tolerance and Tinnitus Retraining Therapy (TRT). *Aust. N. Z. J. Audiol.*, **21**, 74–81.

Jastreboff, P. J. (1990) Phantom auditory perception (tinnitus): mechanisms of generation and perception. *Neurosci. Res.*, **8**, 221–254.

(1992) Mechanisms of tinnitus. Experimental animal models, In *Audiology in Europe, an Academic Conference, Cambridge*, 1992, abstract 19.

(1995) Tinnitus as a phantom perception: theories and clinical implications, In *Mechanisms of Tinnitus*, ed. Vernon, J. & Moller, A. R., pp. 73–94. Boston, MA: Allyn & Bacon.

(1996a) Clinical implications of the neurophysiological model of tinnitus. In *Proceedings of the Fifth International Tinnitus Seminar*, ed. Vernon, J. A. & Reich, G., pp. 500–507. Portland, OR: American Tinnitus Association.

(1996b) Processing of the tinnitus signal within the brain. In *Proceedings of the Fifth International Tinnitus Seminar*, ed. Vernon, J. A. & Reich, G. pp. 58–68. Portland, OR: American Tinnitus Association.

(1998) Tinnitus. In *Current Therapy in Otolaryngology: Head and Neck Surgery*, 6th edn, ed. Gates, G. A., pp. 90–95. St Louis, MO: Mosby.

(1999a) Categories of the patients and the treatment outcome. In *Proceedings of the Sixth International Tinnitus Seminar*, ed. Hazell, J. W. P., pp. 394–398. London: Tinnitus & Hyperacusis Centre.

(1999b) How TRT derives from the neurophysiological model. In *Proceedings of the Sixth International Tinnitus Seminar*, ed. Hazell, J. W. P., pp. 87–91. London: Tinnitus & Hyperacusis Centre.

(1999c) Optimal sound use in TRT: theory and practice. In *Proceedings of the Sixth International Tinnitus Seminar*, ed. Hazell, J. W. P., pp. 491–494. London: Tinnitus & Hyperacusis Centre.

(1999d) The neurophysiological model of tinnitus and hyperacusis. In *Proceedings of the Sixth International Tinnitus Seminar*, ed. Hazell, J. W. P., pp. 32–38. London: Tinnitus & Hyperacusis Centre.

(2000) Tinnitus habituation therapy (THT) and tinnitus retraining therapy (TRT). In *Tinnitus Handbook*, ed. Tyler, R., pp. 357–376. San Diego, CA: Singular, Thomson Learning.

Jastreboff, P. J. & Brennan, J. F. (1988) Specific effects of nimodipine on the auditory system. *Ann. N. Y. Acad. Sci.*, **522**, 716–718.

(1996) Mechanisms of L-type calcium channel antagonist action on tinnitus. In *Proceedings of the Fifth International Tinnitus Seminar*, ed. Vernon, J. A. & Reich, G., pp. 234–236. Portland, OR: American Tinnitus Association.

Jastreboff, P. J. & Jastreboff, M. M. (2000a) Tinnitus Retraining Therapy (TRT) as a method for treatment of tinnitus and hyperacusis patients. *J. Am. Acad. Audiol.*, **11**, 156–161.

(2000b) Potential impact of stochastic resonance on tinnitus and its treatment. In *The 23rd Annual Midwinter Meeting of the Association for Research in Otolaryngology*, p. 5542.

(2001c) The neurophysiological model of tinnitus and its practical implementation: Current status. In *Advances in Otolaryngology-Head and Neck Surgery, vol 15*, ed. Myers, E. N., Bluestone, C. D., Brackman, D. E., Krause, C. J. & Tutchko, M. J., St. Louis: Mosby.

(2003a) Tinnitus and hyperacusis. In *Ballenger's Otorhinolaryngology Head and Neck Surgery*, 16th edn. ed. Snow, J. B., Jr. & Ballenger, J. J., pp. 456–475. Hamilton, Ontario, Canada: BC Decker.

(2003b) Tinnitus Retraining Therapy for patients with tinnitus and decreased sound tolerance. *Otolaryngologic Clinics of North America*, **36**, 321.

Jastreboff, P. J. & Sasaki, C. T. (1986) Salicylate-induced changes in spontaneous activity of single units in the inferior colliculus of the guinea pig. *J. Acoust. Soc. Am.*, **80**, 1384–1391.

(1994) An animal model of tinnitus: a decade of development. *Am. J. Otol.*, **15**, 19–27.

Jastreboff, P. J., Brennan, J. F., Coleman, J. K. & Sasaki, C. T. (1988) Phantom auditory sensation in rats: an animal model for tinnitus. *Behav. Neurosci.*, **102**, 811–822.

Jastreboff, P. J., Brennan, J. F. & Sasaki, C. T. (1991) Quinine-induced tinnitus in rats. *Arch. Otolaryngol. Head Neck Surg.*, **117**, 1162–1166.

Jastreboff, P. J., Hazell, J. W. P. & Graham, R. L. (1994) Neurophysiological model of tinnitus: dependence of the minimal masking level on treatment outcome. *Hear. Res.*, **80**, 216–232.

Jastreboff, P. J., Gray, W. C. & Gold, S. L. (1996) Neurophysiological approach to tinnitus patients. *Am. J. Otol.*, **17**, 236–240.

Jastreboff, P. J., Zhou, S., Jastreboff, M. M., Kwapisz, U. & Gryczynska, U. (1997) Attenuation of salicylate-induced tinnitus by *Ginkgo biloba* extract in rats. *Audiol Neurootol.*, **2**, 197–212.

Jastreboff, P. J., Gray, W. C. & Mattox, D. E. (1998) Tinnitus and Hyperacusis, *In Otolaryngology Head and Neck Surgery*, 3rd edn, ed. Cummings, C. W., Fredrickson, J. M., Harker, L. A., Krause, C. J., Richardson, M. A. & Schuller, D. E., pp. 3198–3222. St Louis, MO: Mosby.

Jastreboff, P. J., Jastreboff, M. M. & Sheldrake, J. B. (1999a) Audiometrical characterization of hyperacusis patients before and during TRT. In *Proceedings of the Sixth International Tinnitus Seminar*, ed. Hazell, J. W. P., pp. 495–498. London: Tinnitus & Hyperacusis Centre.

Jastreboff, P. J., Jastreboff, M. M., Kwon, O., Shi, J. & Hu, S. (1999) An animal model of noise induced tinnitus. In *Proceedings of the Sixth International Tinnitus Seminar, 1999, Cambridge, UK*, ed. Hazell, J. W. P., pp. 198–202. London: Tinnitus & Hyperacusis Centre.

Jastreboff, P. J., Jastreboff, M. M. & Mattox, D. E. (2001) *Statistical analysis of the progress of tinnitus treatment during Tinnitus Retraining Therapy (TRT)*. In *The 24th Annual Midwinter Meeting of the Association for Research in Otolaryngology, abstract 21630*.

Jeanmonod, D., Magnin, M. & Morel, A. (1996) Low-threshold calcium spike bursts in the human thalamus. Common physiology for sensory, motor and limbic positive systems. *Brain*, 119, 363–375.

Johnson, J. & Lalwani, A. K. (2003) Ménière's disease, vestibular neuronitis, paroxysmal positional vertigo, and cerebellopontine angle tumors. In *Ballenger's Otorhinolaryngology Head and Neck Surgery*, 16th edn, ed. Snow, J. B., Jr & Ballenger, J. J., pp. 408–442. Hamilton, Ontario: BC Decker.

Johnson, R. M. (1998) The masking of tinnitus. In *Tinnitus Treatment and Relief*, ed. Vernon, J. A., pp. 164–186. Boston, MA: Allyn and Bacon.

Johnson, R. M., Brummett, R. & Schleuning, A. (1993) Use of alprazolam for relief of tinnitus. A double-blind study. *Arch. Otolaryngol. Head Neck Surg.*, 119, 842–845.

Jones, I. H. & Knudsen, V. O. (1928) Certain aspects of tinnitus particularly treatment. *Laryngoscope*, 38, 597–611.

Juergens, S. (1991) Alprazolam and diazepam: addiction potential. *J. Subst. Abuse Treat.*, 8, 43–51.

Kaada, B., Hognestad, S. & Havstad, J. (1989) Transcutaneous nerve stimulation (TNS) in tinnitus. *Scand. Audiol.*, 18, 211–217.

Kaltenbach, J. A. (2000) Neurophysiologic mechanisms of tinnitus. *J. Am. Acad. Audiol.*, 11, 125–137.

Kaltenbach, J. A. & Afman, C. E. (2000) Hyperactivity in the dorsal cochlear nucleus after intense sound exposure and its resemblance to tone-evoked activity: a physiological model for tinnitus. *Hear. Res.*, 140, 165–172.

Kaltenbach, J. A., Zhang, J. & Afman, C. E. (2000) Plasticity of spontaneous neural activity in the dorsal cochlear nucleus after intense sound exposure. *Hear. Res.*, 147, 282–292.

Kaltenbach, J. A., Rachel, J., Mathog, T. A. & Zhang, J. (2001) Cisplatin induced hyperactivity in the DCN: *relation to outer hair cell loss*. In *The 24th Annual Midwinter Meeting of the Association for Research in Otolaryngology*, p. 20653.

Katznell, U. & Segal, S. (2001) Hyperacusis: review and clinical guidelines. *Otol. Neurotol.*, 22, 321–326.

Kau, R. J., Sendtner-Gress, K., Ganzer, U. & Arnold, W. (1997) Effectiveness of hyperbaric oxygen therapy in patients with acute and chronic cochlear disorders. *ORL J. Otorhinolaryngol. Relat. Spec.*, 59, 79–83.

Kawamoto, K., Ishimoto, S., Minoda, R., Brough, D. E. & Raphael, Y. (2003) *Math1* gene transfer generates new cochlear hair cells in mature guinea pigs in vivo. *J. Neurosci.*, 23, 4395–4400.

Kay, N. J. (1981) Oral chemotherapy in tinnitus. *Br. J. Audiol.*, 15, 123–124.

Kempf, H. G., Roller, R. & Muhlbradt, L. (1993) [Correlation between inner ear disorders and temporomandibular joint diseases.] *HNO*, 41, 7–10.

Keppel, G. (1991) *Design and Analysis: A Researcher's Handbook*, 3rd edn. Englewood Cliffs, NJ: Prentice-Hall.

Kiessling, J. (1980) [Masking of tinnitus aurium by maskers and hearing aids.] *HNO*, 28, 383–388.

Kilic, C., Curran, H. V., Noshirvani, H., Marks, I. M. & Basoglu, M. (1999) Long-term effects of alprazolam on memory: a 3.5 year follow-up of agoraphobia/panic patients. *Psychol. Med.*, 29, 225–231.

Kimberg, D. Y., Aguirre, G. K. & D'Esposito, M. (2000) Modulation of task-related neural activity in task-switching: an fMRI study. *Brain Res. Cogn. Brain Res.*, **10**, 189–196.

Kitajima, K., Kitahara, M. & Kodama, A. (1987) Can tinnitus be masked by band erased filtered masker? Masking tinnitus with sounds not covering the tinnitus frequency. *Am. J. Otol.*, **8**, 203–206.

Kitano, H., Kitahara, M., Uchida, K. & Kitajima, K. (1987) Treatment of tinnitus with muscle relaxant. In *Proceedings of the Third International Tinnitus Seminar*, ed. Feldmann, H., pp. 327–330. Karlsruhe: Harsch Verlag.

Klein, A. J., Armstrong, B. L., Greer, M. K. & Brown, F. R. (1990) Hyperacusis and otitis media in individuals with Williams syndrome. *J. Speech Hear. Disord.*, **55**, 339–344.

Klochoff, I. (1979) *Impedance Fluctuation and a "Tensor Tympani Syndrome"*, pp. 69–76. Lisbon: Universidad Nova de Lisboa Ed Penha & Pizarro.

Klostermann, W., Vieregge, P. & Kömpf, D. (1992) Musical pseudo-hallucination in acquired hearing loss. *Fortschr. Neurol. Psychiatr.*, **60**, 262–273.

Knox, G. W. & McPherson, A. (1997) Ménière's disease: differential diagnosis and treatment. *Am. Fam. Physician*, **55**, 1185–1190, 1193–1194.

Konorski, J. (1948) *Conditioned Reflexes and Neuronal Organization*. Cambridge: Cambridge University Press.

Kopelman, J., Budnick, A. S., Sessions, R. B., Kramer, M. B. & Wong, G. Y. (1988) Ototoxicity of high-dose cisplatin by bolus administration in patients with advanced cancers and normal hearing. *Laryngoscope*, **98**, 858–864.

Kroner-Herwig, B., Hebing, G., van Rijn-Kalkmann, U., Frenzel, A., Schilkowsky, G. & Esser, G. (1995) The management of chronic tinnitus: comparison of a cognitive–behavioural group training with yoga. *J. Psychosom. Res.*, **39**, 153–165.

Kveton, J. F. & Bartoshuk, L. M. (1994) The effect of unilateral chorda tympani damage on taste. *Laryngoscope*, **104**, 25–29.

Kwon, O., Jastreboff, M. M., Hu, S., Shi, J. & Jastreboff, P. J. (1999) Modification of single-unit activity related to noise-induced tinnitus in rats. In *Proceedings of the Sixth International Tinnitus Seminar*, ed. Hazell, J. W. P., pp. 459–462. London: Tinnitus & Hyperacusis Centre.

Lader, M. (1994) Anxiolytic drugs: dependence, addiction and abuse. *Eur. Neuropsychopharmacology*, **4**, 85–91.

    (1999) Limitations on the use of benzodiazepines in anxiety and insomnia: are they justified? *Eur. Neuropsychopharmacol.*, **9** (Suppl. 6), S399–S405.

Laffrëe, J. B., Vermeij, P. & Hulshof, J. H. (1989) The effect of iontophoresis of lignocaine in the treatment of tinnitus. *Clin. Otolaryngol.*, **14**, 401–404.

Lamour, Y., Holloway, H. W., Rapoport, S. I. & Soncrant, T. T. (1992) *Ginkgo biloba* extract decreases local glucose utilization in the adult rat brain. In *Effects of* Ginkgo biloba *Extract (EGb 761) on the Central Nervous System*, ed. Christen, Y., Costentin, J. & Lacour, M., pp. 19–25. Paris: Elsevier.

Landis, B. & Landis, E. (1992) Is biofeedback effective for chronic tinnitus? An intensive study with seven subjects. *Am. J. Otolaryngol.*, **13**, 349–356.

Lenarz, T. (1986) Treatment of tinnitus with lidocaine and tocainide. *Scand. Audiol. Suppl.*, **26**, 49–51.

Lenarz, T., Schreiner, C., Snyder, R. L. & Ernst, A. (1993) Neural mechanisms of tinnitus. *Eur. Arch. Otorhinolaryngol.*, **249**, 441–446.

Leone, C. A., Edgerton, B., Berliner, K. & House, J. W. (1984) [House cochlear implant for the control of tinnitus: preliminary results.] *Acta Otorhinolaryngol. Ital.*, **4**, 163–170.

Levi, H. & Chisin, R. (1987) Can tinnitus mask hearing? A comparison between subjective audiometric and objective electrophysiological thresholds in patients with tinnitus. *Audiology*, **26**, 153–157.

Levine, R. A. (1999) Somatic (craniocervical) tinnitus and the dorsal cochlear nucleus hypothesis. *Am. J. Otolaryngol.*, **20**, 351–362.

Levo, H., Blomstedt, G. & Pyykko, I. (2000) Tinnitus and vestibular schwannoma surgery. *Acta Otolaryngol. Suppl.* (Stockh.), **543**, 28–29.

Liberman, M. C. & Kiang, N. Y. S. (1978) Acoustic trauma in cats. *Acta Otolaryngol. Suppl.* (Stockh.), **358**, 1–63.

Lipe, A. W. (2002) Beyond therapy: music, spirituality, and health in human experience: a review of literature. *J Music Ther.*, **39**, 209–240.

Longo, L. P. & Johnson, B. (2000) Addiction: Part I. Benzodiazepines: side effects, abuse risk and alternatives. *Am. Fam. Physician*, **61**, 2121–2128.

Longridge, N. S. (1979) A tinnitus clinic. *J. Otolaryngol.*, **8**, 390–395.

Longworth, W. & McCarthy, P. W. (1997) A review of research on acupuncture for the treatment of lumbar disk protrusions and associated neurological symptomatology. *J. Altern. Complement. Med.*, **3**, 55–76.

Lux-Wellenhof, G. (1999) Treatment history of incoming patients to the Tinnitus & Hyperacusis Centre in Frankfurt/Main. In *Proceedings of the Sixth International Tinnitus Seminar*, ed. Hazell, J. W. P., pp. 502–506. London: Tinnitus & Hyperacusis Centre.

Lux-Wellenhof, G. & Hellweg, F. C. (2002) Longterm follow up study of TRT in Frankfurt. In *Proceedings of the Seventh International Tinnitus Seminar*, ed. Patuzzi, R., pp. 277–279. Perth, Australia: University of Western Australia.

MacNaughton Jones, H. (1891) *Subjective Noises in the Head and Ears: Their Etiology, Diagnosis and Treatment*. London: Baillière, Tindall and Cox.

Man-Son-Hing, M., Wells, G. & Lau, A. (1998) Quinine for nocturnal leg cramps: a meta-analysis including unpublished data. *J. Gen. Intern. Med.*, **13**, 600–606.

Mansbach, A. L. & Freyens, P. (1983) [Tinnitus: current data and treatment with sodium valproate.] *Acta Otorhinolaryngol. Belg.*, **37**, 697–705.

Marchbanks, R. (1997) Why monitor perilymphatic pressure in Ménière's disease? *Acta Otolaryngol. Suppl.* (Stockh.), **526**, 27–29.

Marks, N. J., Emery, P. & Onisiphorou, C. (1984) A controlled trial of acupuncture in tinnitus. *J. Laryngol. Otol.*, **98**, 1103–1109.

Marriage, J. & Barnes, N. M. (1995) Is central hyperacusis a symptom of 5-hydroxytryptamine (5-HT) dysfunction? *J. Laryngol. Otol.*, **109**, 915–921.

Martin, W. H., Shi, Y.-B., Burchiel, K. J. & Anderson, V. C. (1999) Deep brain stimulation effects on hearing function and tinnitus. In *Proceedings of the Sixth International Tinnitus Seminar*, ed. Hazell, J. W. P., pp. 68–72. London: Tinnitus & Hyperacusis Centre.

Matthies, C. & Samii, M. (1997) Management of 1000 vestibular schwannomas (acoustic neuromas): clinical presentation. *Neurosurgery*, **40**, 1–9.

McCandless, G. A. & Goering, D. M. (1974) Changes in loudness after stapedectomy. *Arch. Otolaryng.*, **100**, 344–350.

McFadden, D. (Chairman of Working Group 89 of CHABA)(1982) *Tinnitus: Facts, Theories, and Treatments*. Washington, DC: National Academy Press. http://books.nap.edu/books/0309033284/html/R1.html

McIlwain, J. C. (1987) Glutamic acid in the treatment of tinnitus. *J. Laryngol. Otol.*, **101**, 552–554.

McKenna, L. (2000) Tinnitus and insomnia. In *Tinnitus Handbook*, ed. Tyler, R., pp. 59–84. San Diego, CA: Singular, Thomson Learning.

McKenna, L., Hallam, R. S. & Hinchcliffe, R. (1991) The prevalence of psychological disturbance in neurotology outpatients. *Clin. Otolaryngol.*, **16**, 452–456.

McKerrow, W. S., Schreiner, C. E., Snyder, R. L., Merzenich, M. M. & Toner, J. G. (1991) Tinnitus suppression by cochlear implants. *Ann. Otol. Rhinol. Laryngol.*, **100**, 552–558.

McKinney, C. J., Hazel, J. W. P. & Graham, R. L. (1999) An evaluation of the TRT method. In *Proceedings of the Sixth International Tinnitus Seminar*, ed. Hazell, J. W. P., pp. 99–105. London: Tinnitus & Hyperacusis Centre.

Melcher, J. R., Sigalovsky, I. S., Guinan, J. J., Jr & Levine, R. A. (2000) Lateralized tinnitus studied with functional magnetic resonance imaging: abnormal inferior colliculus activation. *J. Neurophysiol.*, **83**, 1058–1072.

Melin, L., Scott, B., Lindberg, P. & Lyttkens, L. (1987) Hearing aids and tinnitus: an experimental group study. *Br. J. Audiol.*, **21**, 91–97.

Melzack, R. (1989) Phantom limbs, the self and the brain (The D. O. Hebb memorial lecture). *Can. Psychol.*, **30**, 1–16.

(1990) Phantom limbs and the concept of a neuromatrix. *Trends Neurosci.*, **13**, 88–92.

(1992) Phantom limbs. *Sci. Am.*, **266**, 120–126.

Merchant, S. N., Rauch, S. D. & Nadol, J. B., Jr (1995) Ménière's disease. *Eur. Arch. Otorhinolaryngol.*, **252**, 63–75.

Meyer, B. (1986) [Multicenter randomized double-blind drug vs. placebo study of the treatment of tinnitus with *Ginkgo biloba* extract.] *Presse Med.*, **15**, 1562–1564.

Mihail, R. C., Crowley, J. M., Walden, B. E., Fishburne, J., Reinwall, J. E. & Zajtchuk, J. T. (1988) The tricyclic trimipramine in the treatment of subjective tinnitus. *Ann. Otol. Rhinol. Laryngol.*, **97**, 120–123.

Milbrandt, J. C., Holder, T. M., Wilson, M. C., Salvi, R. J. & Caspary, D. M. (2000) GAD levels and muscimol binding in rat inferior colliculus following acoustic trauma. *Hear. Res.*, **147**, 251–260.

Miller, M. H. (1981) Tinnitus amplification: the high frequency hearing aid. *J. Laryngol. Otol. Suppl.*, **10**, 71–75.

Mirz, F., Zachariae, R., Andersen, S. E., *et al.* (1999a) The low-power laser in the treatment of tinnitus. *Clin. Otolaryngol.*, **24**, 346–354.

Mirz, F., Pedersen, B., Ishizu, K., *et al.* (1999b) Positron emission tomography of cortical centers of tinnitus. *Hear. Res.*, **134**, 133–144.

Mirz, F., Gjedde, A., Ishizu, K. & Pedersen, C. B. (2000a) Cortical networks subserving the perception of tinnitus: a PET study. *Acta Otolaryngol. Suppl*, **543**, 241–243.

Mirz, F., Gjedde, A., Sodkilde-Jrgensen, H. & Pedersen, C. B. (2000b) Functional brain imaging of tinnitus-like perception induced by aversive auditory stimuli. *NeuroReport*, **11**, 633–637.

Mitchell, C. R. & Creedon, T. A. (1995) Psychophysical tuning curves in subjects with tinnitus suggest outer hair cell lesions. *Otolaryngol. Head Neck Surg.*, **113**, 223–233.

Mitchell, C. R., Vernon, J. A. & Creedon, T. A. (1993) Measuring tinnitus parameters: loudness, pitch, and maskability. *J. Am. Acad. Audiol.*, **4**, 139–151.

Moffat, D. A. (1997) Endolymphatic mastoid shunt surgery in unilateral Ménière's disease. *Ear Nose Throat J.*, **76**, 642–8, 650.

Moffat, D. A., Baguley, D. M., Beynon, G. J. & Da Cruz, M. (1998) Clinical acumen and vestibular schwannoma. *Am. J. Otol.*, **19**, 82–87.

Moller, A. R. (1984) Pathophysiology of tinnitus. *Ann. Otol. Rhinol. Laryngol.*, **93**, 39–44.

(1992) Central neurophysiological processes in tinnitus. In *Tinnitus 91. Proceedings of the Fourth International Tinnitus Seminar*, ed. Aran, J.-M. & Dauman, R., pp. 165–179. Amsterdam: Kugler & Ghedini.

(1995) Pathophysiology of tinnitus. In *Mechanisms of tinnitus*, ed. Vernon, J. A. & Moller, A. R., pp. 207–217. Needham Heights, MA: Allyn & Backon.

(1997) Similarities between chronic pain and tinnitus. *Am. J. Otol.*, **18**, 577–585.

Moller, A. R., Moller, M. B., Jannetta, P. J. & Jho, H. D. (1992a) Compound action potentials recorded from the exposed eight nerve in patients with intractable tinnitus. *Laryngoscope*, **102**, 187–197.

Moller, A. R., Moller, M. B. & Yokota, M. (1992b) Some forms of tinnitus may involve the extralemniscal auditory pathway. *Laryngoscope*, **102**, 1165–1171.

Mongan, E., Kelly, P., Nies, K., Porter, W. W. & Paulus, H. E. (1973) Tinnitus as an indication of therapeutic serum salicylate levels. *J. Am. Med. Assoc.*, **226**, 141–145.

Moore, B. C. J. (1995) *An Introduction to the Psychology of Hearing*, 3rd edn.

Moroso, M. J. & Blair, R. L. (1983) A review of cis-platinum ototoxicity. *J. Otolaryngol.*, **12**, 365–369.

MRC-IHR (Medical Research Council's Institute of Hearing Research) (1981) Epidemiology of tinnitus. *CIBA Found. Symp.*, **85**, 16–34.

Mudford, O. C., Cross, B. A., Breen, S., *et al.* (2000) Auditory integration training for children with autism: no behavioral benefits detected. *Am. J. Ment. Retard.*, **105**, 118–129.

Muhlnickel, W., Elbert, T., Taub, E. & Flor, H. (1998) Reorganization of auditory cortex in tinnitus. *Proc. Natl. Acad. Sci. USA*, **95**, 10340–10343.

Munte, T. F., Gehde, E., Johannes, S., Seewald, M. & Heinze, H. J. (1996) Effects of alprazolam and bromazepam on visual search and verbal recognition memory in humans: a study with event-related brain potentials. *Neuropsychobiology*, **34**, 49–56.

Murai, K., Tyler, R. S., Harker, L. A. & Stouffer, J. L. (1992) Review of pharmacologic treatment of tinnitus. *Am. J. Otol.*, **13**, 454–464.

Narayan, S. S., Temchin, A. N., Recio, A. & Ruggero, M. A. (1998) Frequency tuning of basilar membrane and auditory nerve fibers in the same cochleae. *Science*, **282**, 1882–1884.

Newman, C. W., Jacobson, G. P. & Spitzer, J. B. (1996) Development of the Tinnitus Handicap Inventory. *Arch. Otolaryngol. Head Neck Surg.*, **122**, 143–148.

Nields, J. A., Fallon, B. A. & Jastreboff, P. J. (1999) Carbamazepine in the treatment of Lyme disease-induced hyperacusi. *J. Neuropsychiatry Clin. Neurosci.*, **11**, 97–99.

Nigam, A. & Samuel, P. R. (1994) Hyperacusis and Williams syndrome. *J. Laryngol. Otol.*, **108**, 494–496.

Nilsson, S., Axelsson, A. & Li De, G. (1992) Acupuncture for tinnitus management. *Scand. Audiol.*, **21**, 245–251.

Norton, S. J., Schmidt, A. R. & Stover, L. J. (1990) Tinnitus and otoacoustic emissions: is there a link? *Ear Hear.*, **11**, 159–166.

Ochi, K. & Eggermont, J. J. (1997) Effects of quinine on neural activity in cat primary auditory cortex. *Hear. Res.*, **105**, 105–118.

Oen, J. M., Begeer, J. H., Staal-Schreinemachers, A. & Tijmstra, T. (1997) Hyperacusis in children with spina bifida: a pilot-study. *Eur. J. Pediatr. Surg., Suppl.* **1**, 46.

Oestreicher, E., Arnold, W., Ehrenberger, K. & Felix, D. (1999) New approaches for inner ear therapy with glutamate antagonists. *Acta Otolaryngol.*, **119**, 174–178.

Ogata, Y., Sekitani, T., Moriya, K. & Watanabe, K. (1993) Biofeedback therapy in the treatment of tinnitus. *Auris. Nasus. Larynx*, **20**, 95–101.

Olsen, S. O. (1999) The relationship between the uncomfortable loudness level and the acoustic reflex threshold for pure tones in normally-hearing and impaired listeners: a meta-analysis. *Audiology*, **38**, 61–68.

Olsen, S. O., Rasmussen, A. N., Nielsen, L. H. & Borgkvist, B. V. (1999) The acoustic reflex threshold: not predictive for loudness perception in normally-hearing listeners. *Audiology*, **38**, 303–307.

Oosterveld, W. J. (1984) Betahistine dihydrochloride in the treatment of vertigo of peripheral vestibular origin. A double-blind placebo-controlled study. *J. Laryngol. Otol.*, **98**, 37–41.

Overstreet, E. H., Temchin, A. N. & Ruggero, M. A. (2002) Basilar membrane vibrations near the round window of the gerbil cochlea. *Jaro*, **3**, 351–361.

Paaske, P. B., Pedersen, C. B., Kjems, G. & Sam, I. L. (1991) Zinc in the management of tinnitus. Placebo-controlled trial. *Ann. Otol. Rhinol. Laryngol.*, **100**, 647–649.

Park, J., White, A. R. & Ernst, E. (2000) Efficacy of acupuncture as a treatment for tinnitus: a systematic review. *Arch. Otolaryngol. Head Neck Surg.*, **126**, 489–492.

Partheniadis-Stumpf, M., Maurer, J. & Mann, W. (1993) [Soft laser therapy in combination with tebonin i.v. in tinnitus.] *Laryngorhinootologie*, **72**, 28–31.

Penner, M. J. (1992) Linking spontaneous otoacoustic emissions and tinnitus. *Br. J. Audiol.*, **26**, 115–123.

(1993) Synthesizing tinnitus from sine waves. *J. Speech Hear. Res.*, **36**, 1300–1305.

Penner, M. J. & Bilger, R. C. (1989) Adaptation and the masking of tinnitus. *J. Speech Hear. Res.*, **32**, 339–346.

Penner, M. J. & Burns, E. M. (1987) The dissociation of SOAEs and tinnitus. *J. Speech Hear. Res.*, **30**, 396–403.

Penner, M. J. & Coles, R. R. (1992) Indications for aspirin as a palliative for tinnitus caused by SOAEs: a case study. *Br. J. Audiol.*, **26**, 91–96.

Perry, B. P. & Gantz, B. J. (2000) Medical and surgical evaluation and management of tinnitus. In *Tinnitus Handbook*, ed. Tyler, R., pp. 221–241. San Diego, CA: Singular, Thomson Learning.

Pilgramm, M., Lamm, H. & Schumann, K. (1985) [Hyperbaric oxygen therapy in sudden deafness.] *Laryngol. Rhinol. Otol.* (Stuttg.), **64**, 351–354.

Plath, P. & Olivier, J. (1995) Results of combined low-power laser therapy and extracts of *Ginkgo biloba* in cases of sensorineural hearing loss and tinnitus. *Adv. Otorhinolaryngol.*, **49**, 101–104.

Podoshin, L., Ben David, Y., Fradis, M., Gerstel, R. & Felner, H. (1991) Idiopathic subjective tinnitus treated by biofeedback, acupuncture and drug therapy. *Ear Nose Throat J.*, **70**, 284–289.

Podoshin, L., Fradis, M. & David, Y. B. (1992) Treatment of tinnitus by intratympanic instillation of lignocaine (lidocaine) 2 per cent through ventilation tubes. *J. Laryngol. Otol.*, **106**, 603–606.

Portmann, M., Cazals, Y., Negrevergne, M. & Aran, J. M. (1979) Temporary tinnitus suppression in man through electrical stimulation of the cochlea. *Acta Otolaryngol.* (Stockh.), **87**, 294–299.

Pugh, R., Budd, R. J. & Stephens, S. D. (1995) Patients' reports of the effect of alcohol on tinnitus. *Br. J. Audiol.*, **29**, 279–283.

Pujol, R. (1992) Neuropharmacology of the cochlea and tinnitus. In *Tinnitus 91. Proceedings of the Fourth International Tinnitus Seminar*, ed. Aran, J.-M. & Dauman, R., pp. 103–107. Amsterdam: Kugler & Ghedini.

Pujol, R., Puel, J. L., Gervais, A. & Eybalin, M. (1993) Pathophysiology of the glutamatergic synapses in the cochlea. *Acta Otolaryngol.* (Stockh.), **113**, 330–334.

Pulec, J. L. (1995) Cochlear nerve section for intractable tinnitus. *Ear Nose J.*, **74**, 468, 470–476.

Rahko, T. & Hakkinen, V. (1979) Carbamazepine in the treatment of objective myoclonus tinnitus. *J. Laryngol. Otol.*, **93**, 123–127.

Rahko, T. & Kotti, V. (1997) Tinnitus treatment by transcutaneous nerve stimulation (TNS). *Acta Otolaryngol. Suppl.* (Stockh.), **529**, 88–89.

Rapin, J. R., Lamproglou, I., Drieu, K. & DeFeudis, F. V. (1994) Demonstration of the anti-stress activity of an extract of *Ginkgo biloba* (EGb 761) using a discrimination learning task. *Gen. Pharmac.*, **25**, 1009–1016.

Rendell, R. J., Carrick, D. G., Fielder, C. P., Callaghan, D. E. & Thomas, K. J. (1987) Low-powered ultrasound in the inhibition of tinnitus. *Br. J. Audiol.*, **21**, 289–293.

Rice, C. G. (1994) Annoyance due to low frequency hums. *Br. Med. J.*, **308**, 355–356.

Rickels, K., Lucki, I., Schweizer, E., Garcia-Espana, F. & Case, W. G. (1999) Psychomotor performance of long-term benzodiazepine users before, during, and after benzodiazepine discontinuation. *J. Clin. Psychopharmacol.*, **19**, 107–113.

Ridgman, W. J. (1975) *Experimentation in Biology.* Glasgow: Blackie.

Rigby, P. L., Shah, S. B., Jackler, R. K., Chung, J. H. & Cooke, D. D. (1997) Acoustic neuroma surgery: outcome analysis of patient-perceived disability. *Am. J. Otol.*, **18**, 427–435.

Risey, J., Guth, P. S. & Amedee, R. G. (1996) Furosamide distinguishes between central and peripheral tinnitus. In *Proceedings of the Fifth International Tinnitus Seminar*, ed. Vernon, J. A. & Reich, G., pp. 237–242. Portland, OR: American Tinnitus Association.

Robles, L. & Ruggero, M. A. (2001) Mechanics of the mammalian cochlea. *Physiol. Rev.*, **81**, 1305–1352.

Roche, R. J., Silamut, K., Pukrittayakamee, S., *et al.* (1990) Quinine induces reversible high-tone hearing loss. *Br. J. Clin. Pharmacol.*, **29**, 780–782.

Rodriguez de Turco, E. B., Droy-Lefaix, M. T. & Bazan, N. G. (1993) EGb 761 inhibits stress-induced polydipsia in rats. *Physiol. Behav.*, **53**, 1001–1002.

Roland, N. J., Hughes, J. B., Daley, M. B., Cook, J. A., Jones, A. S. & McCormick, M. S. (1993) Electromagnetic stimulation as a treatment of tinnitus: a pilot study. *Clin. Otolaryngol.*, **18**, 278–281.

Rosenfeld, R. M. (2001) Evidence, outcomes, and common sense. *Otolaryngol. Head Neck Surg.*, **124**, 123–124.

Rubinstein, B. & Erlandsson, S. I. (1991a) A stomatognathic analysis of patients with disabling tinnitus and craniomandibular disorders (CMD). *Br. J. Audiol.*, **25**, 77–83.

 (1991b) Tinnitus and craniomandibular disorders: is there a link? A stomatognathic analysis of patients with disabling tinnitus and craniomandibular disorders (CMD). *Swed. Dent. J. Suppl.*, **25**, 77–83.

Rubinstein, B., Axelsson, A. & Carlsson, G. E. (1990) Prevalence of signs and symptoms of craniomandibular disorders in tinnitus patients. *J. Craniomandib. Disord.*, **4**, 186–192.

Rubinstein, J. T., Tyler, R. S., Johnson, A. & Brown, C. J. (2003) Electrical suppression of tinnitus with high-rate pulse trains. *Otol. Neurootol.*, **24**, 478–485.

Ruggero, M. A., Narayan, S. S., Temchin, A. N. & Recio, A. (2000) Mechanical bases of frequency tuning and neural excitation at the base of the cochlea: comparison of basilar-membrane vibrations and auditory-nerve-fiber responses in chinchilla. *Proc. Natl. Acad. Sci. USA*, **97**, 11744–11750.

Rush, C. C., Higgins, S. S., Bickel, W. W. & Hughes, J. J. (1994) Acute behavioral effects of lorazepam and caffeine, alone and in combination, in humans. *Behav. Pharmacol.*, **5**, 245–254.

Ryan, R. M. & Hazell, J. W. P. (1995) Ménières disease: are investigations of any value? A retrospective study. *J. Audiol. Med.*, **3**, 160–170.

Sahley, T. L. & Nodar, R. H. (2001) A biochemical model of peripheral tinnitus. *Hear. Res.*, **152**, 43–54.

Sallanon-Moulin, M., Touret, M., Didier-Bazes, M., *et al.* (1994) Glutamine synthetase modulation in the brain of rats subjected to deprivation of paradoxical sleep. *Brain Res. Mol. Brain Res.*, **22**, 113–120.

Saltzman, M. & Ersner, M. S. (1947) A hearing aid for the relief of tinnitus aurium. *Laryngoscope*, **57**, 358–366.

Salvi, R. J., Powers, N. L., Saunders, S. S., Boettcher, F. A. & Clock, A. E. (1992) Enhancement of evoked response amplitude and single unit activity after noise exposure. In *Noise-Induced Hearing Loss*, ed. Dancer, A. L., Henderson, D., Salvi, R. J. & Hamernik, R., pp. 156–171. St Louis, MO: Mosby.

Salvi, R. J., Wang, J. & Powers, N. (1996) Rapid functional reorganization in the inferior colliculus and cochlear nucleus after acute cochlear damage. In *Auditory System Plasticity and Regeneration*, ed. Salvi, R. J., Henderson, D., Fiorino, F. & Colletti, V., pp. 275–296. New York: Thieme.

Sanchez, T. G., Guerra, G. C. Y., Lorenzi, M. C., Brandao, A. L. & Bento, R. F. (2002) The influence of voluntary muscle contractions upon the onset and modulation of tinnitus. *Audiol. Neuro-Otology*, 7, 370–375.

Schleuning, A. J., Johnson, R. M. & Vernon, J. A. (1980) Evaluation of a tinnitus masking program: a follow-up study of 598 patients. *Ear Hear.*, 1, 71–74.

Schuknecht, H. (1981) The pathophysiology of Ménière's Disease. In *Ménière's Disease*, ed. Vosteen, K. H., Schuknecht, H., Pfaltz, C. R., *et al.*, pp. 10–15. Stuttgart: Thieme.

Schultz, G. & Melzack, R. (1991) The Charles Bonnet syndrome: "phantom visual images." *Perception*, 20, 809–825.

Scott, B., Larsen, H. C., Lyttkens, L. & Melin, L. (1994) An experimental evaluation of the effects of transcutaneous nerve stimulation (TNS) and applied relaxation (AR) on hearing ability, tinnitus and dizziness in patients with Ménière's disease. *Br. J. Audiol.*, 28, 131–140.

Seligmann, H., Podoshin, L., Ben-David, J., Fradis, M. & Goldsher, M. (1996) Drug-induced tinnitus and other hearing disorders. *Drug Saf.*, 14, 198–212.

Shailer, M. J., Tyler, R. S. & Coles, R. R. (1981) Critical masking bands for sensorineural tinnitus. *Scand. Audiol.*, 10, 157–162.

Shambaugh, G. E., Jr (1986) Zinc for tinnitus, imbalance, and hearing loss in the elderly. *Am. J. Otol.*, 7, 476–477.

(1989) Zinc: the neglected nutrient. *Am. J. Otol.*, 10, 156–160.

Shea, J. J. (1981) Otosclerosis and tinnitus. *J. Laryngol. Otol. Suppl.*, 10, 149–150.

Shea, J. J., Jr & Ge, X. (1996) Dexamethasone perfusion of the labyrinth plus intravenous dexamethasone for Ménière's disease. *Otolaryngol. Clin. North Am.*, 29, 353–358.

Shea, J. J. & Xianxi, G. (2000) IV Lidocaine for tinnitus. In *Proceedings of the American Otological Society Annual Spring Meeting*.

Shea, J. J., Emmett, J. R., Orchik, D. J., Mays, K. & Webb, W. (1981) Medical treatment of tinnitus. *Ann. Otol.*, 90, 601–609.

Sheldrake, J. B., Jastreboff, P. J. & Hazell, J. W. P. (1996) Perspectives for the total elimination of tinnitus perception. In *Proceedings of the Fifth International Tinnitus Seminar*, ed. Vernon, J. A. & Reich, G., pp. 531–536. Portland, OR: American Tinnitus Association.

Sheldrake, J. B., Hazell, J. W. P. & Graham, R. L. (1999) Results of tinnitus retraining therapy. In *Proceedings of the Sixth International Tinnitus Seminar*, ed. Hazell, J. W. P., pp. 292–296. London: Tinnitus & Hyperacusis Centre.

Shengtai, Z., Kwapisz, U., Jastreboff, M. M., Gryczynska, U. & Jastreboff, P. J. (1996) Evaluation of the effectiveness of EGB 761 in an animal model of tinnitus. In *Proceedings of the Fifth International Tinnitus Seminar*, ed. Vernon, J. A. & Reich, G., pp. 245–248. Portland, OR: American Tinnitus Association.

Shiomi, Y., Takahashi, H., Honjo, I., Kojima, H., Naito, Y. & Fujiki, N. (1997) Efficacy of transmeatal low power laser irradiation on tinnitus: a preliminary report. *Auris. Nasus. Larynx*, 24, 39–42.

Shulman, A. (1985) External electrical stimulation in tinnitus control. *Am. J. Otol.*, **6**, 110–115.
 (1988) Diagnosis of tinnitus. In *Tinnitus: Pathophysiology and Management*, ed. Kitahara, M.,
 pp. 53–63. Tokyo: Igaku-Shoin.

Silverstein, H., Haberkamp, T. & Smouha, E. (1986) The state of tinnitus after inner ear surgery.
 Otolaryngol. Head Neck Surg., **95**, 438–441.

Silverstein, H., Choo, D., Rosenberg, S. I., Kuhn, J., Seidman, M. & Stein, I. (1996) Intratympanic
 steroid treatment of inner ear disease and tinnitus (preliminary report). *Ear Nose Throat J.*,
 75, 468–474.

Simpson, J. J. & Davies, W. E. (2000) A review of evidence in support of a role for 5-HT in the
 perception of tinnitus. *Hear. Res.*, **145**, 1–7.

Simpson, J. J., Donaldson, I. & Davies, W. E. (1998) Use of homeopathy in the treatment of
 tinnitus. *Br. J. Audiol.*, **32**, 227–233.

Simpson, J. J., Gilbert, A. M., Weiner, G. M. & Davies, W. E. (1999) The assessment of lamotrigine,
 an antiepileptic drug, in the treatment of tinnitus. *Am. J. Otol.*, **20**, 627–631.

Snow, J. B., Doty, R. L., Bartoshuk, L. M. & Getchell, T. V. (1991) Categorization of chemosensory
 disorders. In *Smell and Taste in Health and Disease*, ed. Getchell, T. V., Doty, R. L., Snow,
 J. B. & Bartoshuk, L. M., pp. 445–447. New York: Raven.

Soderman, A. C., Bergenius, J., Bagger-Sjoback, D., Tjell, C. & Langius, A. (2001) Patients' subjective evaluations of quality of life related to disease- specific symptoms, sense of coherence,
 and treatment in Ménière's disease. *Otol. Neurootol.*, **22**, 526–533.

Sprengelmeyer, R., Young, A. W., Schroeder, U., *et al.* (1999) Knowing no fear. *Proc. R. Soc. Lond.
 B, Biol. Sci.*, **266**, 2451–2456.

Stacey, J. S. (1980) Apparent total control of severe bilateral tinnitus by masking, using hearing
 aids. *Br. J. Audiol.*, **14**, 59–60.

Stanford, S. C. (1996) Prozac: panacea or puzzle. *Trends Pharmacol. Sci.*, **17**, 150–154.

Stedman's Concise Medical Dictionary. (1997) New York: Williams & Wilkins.

Stephens, D., Pugh, R. & Jones, G. (1996) Alcohol and tinnitus: beneficial effects. In *Proceedings of
 the Fifth International Tinnitus Seminar*, ed. Vernon, J. A. & Reich, G., pp. 243–244. Portland,
 OR: American Tinnitus Association.

Stephens, S. D. (1984) The treatment of tinnitus: a historical perspective. *J. Laryngol. Otol.*, **98**,
 963–972.

Stephens, S. D. & Hallam, R. S. (1985) The Crown–Crisp experiential index in patients complaining of tinnitus. *Br. J. Audiol.*, **19**, 151–158.

Stephens, S. D., Hallam, R. S. & Jakes, S. C. (1986) Tinnitus: a management model. *Clin. Otolaryngol.*, **11**, 227–238.

Stopp, P. E. (1983) Effects on guinea pig cochlea from exposure to moderately intense broad-band
 noise. *Hear. Res.*, **11**, 55–72.

Sullivan, M., Katon, W., Russo, J., Dobie, R. & Sakai, C. (1993) A randomized trial of nortriptyline
 for severe chronic tinnitus. Effects on depression, disability, and tinnitus symptoms. *Arch.
 Intern. Med.*, **153**, 2251–2259.

 (1994) Coping and marital support as correlates of tinnitus disability. *Gen. Hosp. Psychiatry*,
 16, 259–266.

Swanson, L. W. (1987) Limbic system. In *Encyclopedia of Neuroscience*, ed. Adelman, G.,
 pp. 589–591. Boston, MA: Birkhauser.

Sweetow, R. (2000) Cognitive behavioral modification. In *Tinnitus Handbook*, ed. Tyler, R., pp. 297–312. San Diego, CA: Singular, Thomson Learning.

Szczepaniak, W. S. & Moller, A. R. (1996) Effects of (−)-baclofen, clonazepam, and diazepam on tone exposure-induced hyperexcitability of the inferior colliculus in the rat: possible therapeutic implications for pharmacological management of tinnitus and hyperacusis. *Hear. Res.*, **97**, 46–53.

Tandon, R., Grunhaus, L. & Greden, J. F. (1987) Imipramine and tinnitus. *J. Clin. Psychiatry*, **48**, 109–111.

Terry, A. M. & Jones, D. M. (1986) Preference for potential tinnitus maskers: results from annoyance ratings. *Br. J. Audiol.*, **20**, 277–297.

Terry, A. M., Jones, D. M., Davis, B. R. & Slater, R. (1983) Parametric studies of tinnitus masking and residual inhibition. *Br. J. Audiol.*, **17**, 245–256.

Tewary, A. K., Riley, N. & Kerr, A. G. (1998) Long-term results of vestibular nerve section. *J. Laryngol. Otol.*, **112**, 1150–1153.

Thedinger, B., House, W. F. & Edgerton, B. J. (1985) Cochlear implant for tinnitus. Case reports. *Ann. Otol. Rhinol. Laryngol.*, **94**, 10–13.

Thedinger, B. S., Karlsen, E. & Schack, S. H. (1987) Treatment of tinnitus with electrical stimulation: an evaluation of the Audimax Theraband. *Laryngoscope*, **97**, 33–37.

Thiel, C. M., Henson, R. N., Morris, J. S., Friston, K. J. & Dolan, R. J. (2001) Pharmacological modulation of behavioral and neuronal correlates of repetition priming. *J. Neurosci.*, **21**, 6846–6852.

Thompson, R. F. (1987) Learning and memory, neural mechanisms. In *Encyclopedia of Neuroscience*, ed. Adelman, G., pp. 574–576. Boston, MA: Birkhauser.

Thomsen, J., Bonding, P., Becker, B., Stage, J. & Tos, M. (1998) The non-specific effect of endolymphatic sac surgery in treatment of Ménière's disease: a prospective, randomized controlled study comparing "classic" endolymphatic sac surgery with the insertion of a ventilating tube in the tympanic membrane. *Acta Otolaryngol.*, **118**, 769–773.

Thormodsen, M., Hjortdahl, P., Farbrot, T., *et al.* (1999) [From valium to the happy pill?] *Tidsskr. Nor. Laegeforen.*, **119**, 2157–2160.

Tonndorf, J. (1980) Acute cochlear disorders: the combination of hearing loss, recruitment, poor speech discrimination, and tinnitus. *Ann. Otol. Rhinol. Laryngol.*, **89**, 353–358.

   (1987) The analogy between tinnitus and pain: a suggestion for a physiological basis of chronic tinnitus. *Hear. Res.*, **28**, 271–275.

Tyler, R. (2000) Psychoacoustical measurements. In *Tinnitus Handbook*, ed. Tyler, R., pp. 149–180. San Diego, CA: Singular, Thomson Learning.

Tyler, R. S. & Baker, L. J. (1983) Difficulties experienced by tinnitus sufferers. *J. Speech Hear. Disord.*, **48**, 150–154.

Tyler, R. S. & Kelsay, D. (1990) Advantages and disadvantages reported by some of the better cochlear-implant patients. *Am. J. Otol.*, **11**, 282–289.

van Benthem, P. P. G., Klis, S. F. L., Albers, F. W. J., *et al.* (1994) The effect of nimodipine on cochlear potentials and Na^+ / K^+ - ATPase activity in normal and hydropic cochleas of the albino guinea pig. *Hear. Res.*, **77**, 9–18.

Van Borsel, J., Curfs, L. M. & Fryns, J. P. (1997) Hyperacusis in Williams syndrome: a sample survey study. *Genet. Couns.*, **8**, 121–126.

van Leeuwen, J. P., Braspenning, J. C., Meijer, H. & Cremers, C. W. (1996) Quality of life after acoustic neuroma surgery. *Ann. Otol. Rhinol. Laryngol.*, **105**, 423–430.

Vavrina, J. & Muller, W. (1995) Therapeutic effect of hyperbaric oxygenation in acute acoustic trauma. *Rev. Laryngol. Otol. Rhinol.* (Bord)., **116**, 377–380.

Vermeij, P. & Hulshof, J. H. (1986) Dose finding of tocainide in the treatment of tinnitus. *Int. J. Clin. Pharmacol. Ther. Toxicol.*, **24**, 207–212.

Vernon, J. (1977) Attemps to relieve tinnitus. *J. Am. Audiol. Soc.*, **2**, 124–131.

(1987) Pathophysiology of tinnitus: a special case – hyperacusis and a proposed treatment. *Am. J. Otol.*, **8**, 201–202.

Vernon, J. & Schleuning, A. (1978) Tinnitus: a new management. *Laryngoscope*, **88**, 413–419.

Vernon, J., Griest, S. & Press, L. (1990) Attributes of tinnitus and the acceptance of masking. *Am. J. Otolaryngol.*, **11**, 44–50.

Verwey, B., Eling, P., Wientjes, H. & Zitman, F. G. (2000) Memory impairment in those who attempted suicide by benzodiazepine overdose. *J. Clin. Psychiatry*, **61**, 456–459.

Vidailhet, P., Danion, J. M., Chemin, C. & Kazes, M. (1999) Lorazepam impairs both visual and auditory perceptual priming. *Psychopharmacology* (Berl.), **147**, 266–273.

Vilholm, O. J., Moller, K. & Jorgensen, K. (1998) Effect of traditional Chinese acupuncture on severe tinnitus: a double-blind, placebo-controlled, clinical investigation with open therapeutic control. *Br. J. Audiol.*, **32**, 197–204.

Vingen, J. V., Pareja, J. A., Storen, O., White, R. L. & Stovner, L. J. (1998) Phonophobia in migraine. *Cephalgia*, **18**, 243–249.

von Wedel, H., Calero, L., Walger, M., Hoenen, S. & Rutwalt, D. (1995) Soft-laser/Ginkgo therapy in chronic tinnitus. A placebo-controlled study. *Adv. Otorhinolaryngol.*, **49**, 105–108.

Vyklicky, L., Keller, O. & Jastreboff, P. J. (1976) Anodal blocking of A delta tooth pulp afferents. *Adv. Pain. Res. Ther.*, **1**, 411–414.

Waddell, P. A. & Gronwall, D. M. A. (1984) Sensitivity to light and sound following minor head injury. *Acta Neurol. Scand.*, **69**, 270–276.

Walger, M., von Wedel, H., Hoenen, S. & Calero, L. (1996) Transmission of low powered laser rays to the human cochlea. In *Proceedings of the Fifth International Tinnitus Seminar*, ed. Vernon, J. A. & Reich, G., pp. 99–100. Portland, OR: American Tinnitus Association.

Wang, Z.-X., Ryan, A. F. & Woolf, N. K. (1987) Pentobarbital and ketamine alter the pattern of 2-deoxyglucose uptake in the central auditory system of the gerbil. *Hear. Res.*, **27**, 145–155.

Watanabe, I., Imai, S., Ikeda, M. & Ishida, A. (1997) Time series analysis of the course of Ménière's disease. *Acta Otolaryngol. Suppl.* (Stockh.), **528**, 97–102.

Watkins, G. R. (1997) Music therapy: proposed physiological mechanisms and clinical implications. *Clin. Nurse Spec.*, **11**, 43–50.

Wayman, D. M., Pham, H. N., Byl, F. M. & Adour, K. K. (1990) Audiological manifestations of Ramsay Hunt syndrome. *J. Laryngol. Otol.*, **104**, 104–108.

Welkoborsky, H. J. & Bumb, P. (1988) [Results of tinnitus therapy using lidocaine iontophoresis.] *Laryngol. Rhinol. Otol.* (Stuttg.), **67**, 289–293.

Westerberg, B. D., Roberson, J. B., Jr & Stach, B. A. (1996) A double-blind placebo-controlled trial of baclofen in the treatment of tinnitus. *Am. J. Otol.*, **17**, 896–903.

Wiegand, D. A., Ojemann, R. G. & Fickel, V. (1996) Surgical treatment of acoustic neuroma (vestibular schwannoma) in the United States: report from the Acoustic Neuroma Registry. *Laryngoscope*, **106**, 58–66.

Willatt, D., O'Sullivan, G., Stoney, P. J., Jackson, S. R., Pritchard, J. & McCormick, M. S. (1987) A sequential double blind crossover trial of iontophoresis. In *Proceedings of the Third International Tinnitus Seminar*, ed. Feldmann, H., pp. 316–319. Karlsruhe: Harsch Verlag.

Wyant, G. M. (1979) Chronic pain syndromes and their treatment. II. Trigger points. *Can. Anaesth. Soc. J.*, **26**, 216–219.

Zenner, H. P. & Ernst, A. (1993) Cochlear-motor, transduction and signal-transfer tinnitus: models for three types of cochlear tinnitus. *Eur. Arch. Otorhinolaryngol.*, **249**, 447–454.

Ziemann, U., Hallett, M. & Cohen, L. G. (1998) Mechanisms of deafferentation-induced plasticity in human motor cortex. *J. Neurosci.*, **18**, 7000–7007.

Ziemann, U., Muellbacher, W., Hallett, M. & Cohen, L. G. (2001) Modulation of practice-dependent plasticity in human motor cortex. *Brain*, **124**, 1171–1181.

Zwicker, E. & Schorn, K. (1978) Psychoacoustical tuning curves in audiology. *Audiology*, **17**, 120–140.

Index

Numbers in italics refer to *tables* and *figures*; f indicates footnote.